HEALTHY HEART MIRACLE DIET

HEALTHY HEART MIRACLE DIET

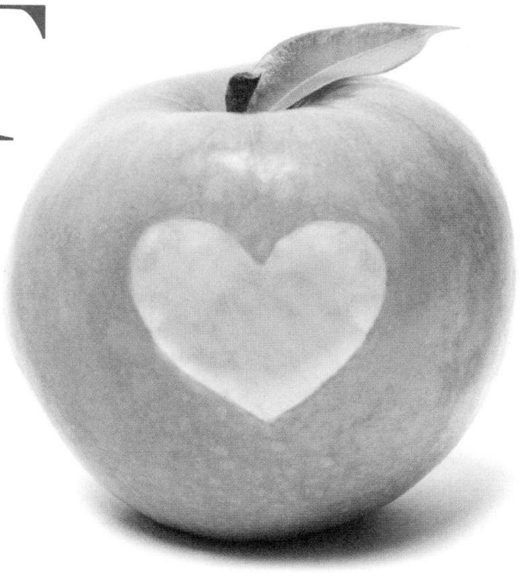

Lose Weight
Look Fabulous
Live Longer

JOHN HASTINGS, coauthor of *ChangeOne*
Dr. Lori Mosca, medical advisor

Reader's Digest
The Reader's Digest Association, Inc.
New York, NY / Montreal

First printing in paperback 2012.

Library of Congress Cataloging in Publication Data is available upon request.

ISBN 978-1-60652-412-1 (paperback)
ISBN 978-1-60652-968-3 (hardcover)

We are committed to both the quality of our products and the service we provide to our customers. We value your comments, so please feel free to contact us.

The Reader's Digest Association, Inc.
Adult Trade Publishing
44 S. Broadway
White Plains, NY 10601

For more Reader's Digest products and information, visit our website:
www.rd.com (in the United States)
www.readersdigest.ca (in Canada)

Printed in China
1 3 5 7 9 10 8 6 4 2 (paperback)
1 3 5 7 9 10 8 6 4 2 (hardcover)

Note to Readers
The information in this book should not be substituted for, or used to alter, medical therapy without your doctor's advice. For a specific health problem, consult your physician for guidance. The mention of any products, retail businesses, or Web sites in this book does not imply or constitute an endorsement by the authors or by The Reader's Digest Association, Inc.

Primary Contributors

John Hastings is a writer and editor with 20 years of experience covering health, fitness, nutrition and medicine. He has served as the Health Editor for *O The Oprah Magazine*; Deputy Editor of *Prevention* magazine; Senior Staff Editor at Reader's Digest; and Senior Editor at *Health* magazine. He is the co-author of *ChangeOne, The Diet and Fitness Plan*, the official weight-loss program of Reader's Digest and a worldwide bestseller. He lives with his family in the suburbs of New York City.

Lori Mosca, MD, MPH, PhD, is Professor of Medicine at Columbia University Medical Center and Director of Preventive Cardiology at New York-Presbyterian Hospital. Her research focuses on lifestyle and family-centered interventions to prevent heart disease. She is Principal Investigator of three National Institutes of Health (NIH) funded studies. Her research contributions were recognized by the American Medical Women's Association with the 2007 Women in Science Award. Dr. Mosca received her medical degree from SUNY Upstate Medical University in Syracuse, and her Masters in Public Health and PhD in Epidemiology from Columbia University. She is author of *Heart to Heart: A Personal Plan for Creating a Heart-Healthy Family.* She is also a competitive triathlete and Hawaii Ironman finisher.

Marie Simmons is a cookbook author, cooking teacher, and food writer based in the San Francisco Bay Area. She has written or co-written 20 cookbooks, several of which have won the food industry's top honors, including Julia Child IACP book awards and James Beard Awards. Marie began her career in the test kitchens of *Woman's Day* Magazine and then moved on to become the food editor for *Cuisine* magazine. Her monthly column, "Cooking for Health," appeared in *Bon Appetit* magazine for 18 years.

Marianne Wait has conceived and developed more than 20 health and wellness books for The Reader's Digest Association, Inc., many of them which have gone on to become global bestsellers. In addition, she is the founding editor of *Walk It Off* and *Reverse Diabetes* magazines.

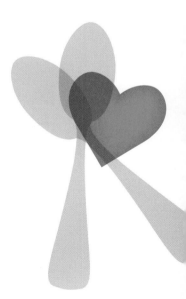

Contents

Introduction: The Future of Healthy Eating **8**

PART ONE

The New View: Heart Disease and Your Diet, 13

1 Are You Eating a Heart-Healthy Diet? **14**

2 What *Really* Causes Heart Attacks? **22**

3 Is Being Fat So Bad? **36**

4 Why Not Just Pop a Pill? **40**

PART TWO

The Healthy Heart Miracle Diet, 47

5 The Miracle Approach to Everyday Eating **48**

6 Correct Your Carbs **60**

7 Power Up Your Protein **90**

8 Fix Your Fats **112**

9 The Healthy Heart Miracle Diet 14-Day Meal Plan **140**

10 Maintaining the Miracle **150**

PART THREE

Living the Healthy Heart Miracle Diet, 171

11 The Next Step: Exercise **172**

12 Emotional Rescue **186**

13 Supplements For Your Heart **198**

PART FOUR

Healthy Heart Recipes, 213

Breakfast **214**

Appetizers and Snacks **224**

Salads **236**

Soups **252**

Entrées **262**

Vegetables and Grains **300**

Desserts **328**

Recipe List, 342

Index, 345

Introduction

The Future of Healthy Eating

Major research breakthroughs—the type that change how we collectively think about health—come along infrequently in the world of medicine.

But a sequence of studies released in the past few years has created just such a moment.

There are two parts to this breakthrough new thinking. First is the undoing of a 40-year wrong that may have indirectly caused extraordinary damage to the health of people worldwide. The wrong? Our belief that the number one evil in our diets is fat.

Since the 1970s, the medical establishment has attacked dietary fat as the primary cause of obesity, heart disease, other ailments and chronic conditions common in developed nations. And so two generations of us have it in our heads that the healthiest diet is one in which we eat as little fat as possible.

It's no coincidence that since we shifted our diets towards the low-fat model, our collective health has badly deteriorated. Today, one billion adults around the world are overweight, and 300 million of them are obese (meaning so overweight it's considered a formal medical condition). As a result, heart disease is by far the leading cause of death in these countries.

But let's set aside the big picture and focus on us as individuals. Eat the way that the food industry urges you to, and you feel bloated after meals. Your energy levels surge and then plunge. Over time, your blood pressure goes up, and your waistline expands. Your immune system weakens, making you vulnerable to infections, allergies, colds and flu. An unhealthy diet is the gateway to bad health, pure and simple. And too many of us are struggling with our health.

This is what our current eating habits have wrought. It's time to declare them for what they are: dangerous, out-of-date, and invalid.

So how *should* we eat for good health? You are holding the answer in your hands. The *Healthy Heart Miracle Diet*—supported by a substantial body of new scientific evidence, and the support of an increasing number of leading doctors and researchers—is here to tell you that fatty foods are not the primary cause of the triple epidemic of obesity, heart disease and diabetes.

The bigger culprit? Refined carbohydrates and sweeteners. It is sugar, white bread, corn syrup, cake, cookies, bagels and other refined carbs that are contributing most to our obesity epidemic, and by extension, the fast-rising rates of heart disease and diabetes today.

This is the second part of the breakthrough new thinking about health that could very well change how we all eat from this point forward.

We know—hearing that sugar and carbs are the devils in our diet may not sound so "breakthrough-ish." But think about how we eat. A bowl of sweetened cereal or a bagel in the morning; sandwich bread and potato chips or pretzels at lunch; lots of pasta, potatoes, or rice at dinner; and in between, a shocking amount of sweets, be it cola, candy, cookies, pie or ice cream.

Sweet and tasty, our diet is today. And deadly addictive, too.

Extreme Eating

How did we get here? We'll explain it fully in the pages ahead. But it's in large part the story of how a cure can be worse than the problem.

At the same time the medical world was discovering the negative role of saturated fat in our diet, the food industry was discovering our innate desire for sugar and salt. And they responded by stuffing processed food—including all those supposedly healthy "low-fat" products—with mind- and belly-boggling amounts of these substances. As a result, we shifted our diets from fatty foods to sweet and salty foods. A few decades later, we live in a world where bottled pasta sauce can have more sugar per serving than vanilla ice cream. And where it's possible to get more salt from your breakfast cereal than you can from French fries.

At the same time the medical world was discovering the negative role of saturated fat in our diet, the food industry was discovering our innate desire for sugar and salt.

You'll soon read what the new research reveals about the negative impact refined carbohydrates have on our bodies. It's compelling, fascinating and conclusive evidence that any judge or jury would find damning.

But there's more to this new thinking about food than just body chemistry. In particular, this full-scale food industry assault on our taste buds has the dangerous side effect of making us want more and more food. Today, most of us live on a flavor seesaw: We eat something wonderfully sweet and almost immediately we want to counter it with something salty. After which, it occurs to us that something with a little sugar would hit the spot nicely. And then, wouldn't a bag of potato chips be nice? Washed down with a soda, of course. And so on.

When salt and sugar hit critical levels in the same food, the combination trips satisfaction sensors in our brain that are similar to the ones activated in drug addicts when they get a fix. Think about that: Your fast food breakfast sandwich is like a drug. Since when did it become a good idea to make food an addictive substance?

Healthy Heart Miracle Diet is specifically designed to combat this problem, gently steering you away from these nutritional nightmare foods. You'll substitute deliciously seasoned foods that will fill you up, not leave you craving more. As the salt and sugar content of your food decreases, your palate will come to appreciate previously hidden flavors. Instead of constantly stimulating your hunger, seasonings will leave you sated and happy. There's a bonus: According to the latest research findings, the spices featured in our recipes are good for your heart on their own.

Food Made Healthy

In addition to food's role as a source of almost addictive pleasure, it has become a therapist for many of us. Boss yell at you? Have a candy bar. Stressful commute? Some chips would be nice. Late night and feeling lonely? You deserve some ice cream.

We've all been there. So is it any wonder that given all the positive, heart-warming connections we have with food that we turn to it when we need consoling comfort? Consider all the ways food is intertwined with our emotional lives. It's the centerpiece of nearly every meaningful celebration, from baby showers to birthdays to weddings to funerals. Most holidays revolve around a feast. Unfortunately, the foods we choose—those aptly named comfort foods—aren't doing our hearts or our waistlines any favors.

In the end, food doesn't provide a solution to our emotional challenges. In fact, we often end up feeling guilty or weak when we indulge for emotional reasons. And those feelings can send us right back to the fridge.

Consider all the ways food is intertwined with our emotional lives. It's the centerpiece of nearly every meaningful celebration.

Healthy Heart Miracle Diet can help you break that cycle by letting you recognize the signs of emotional eating and providing you with alternative, healthy outlets for those moments of weakness. Stress release, exercise, and even healthy snacking can see you through.

All this helps you restore a healthier, more natural relationship between you and the food you eat. With *Healthy Heart Miracle Diet*, meals will be primarily to provide the sustenance you need, but in ways that are truly delicious, creative and filling. Among the 102 recipes on the pages ahead are meals to be savored—in the wonderful ingredients, in the time you take in preparing them, in their exquisite flavors, and in the joy of serving them with a flourish. Put them on the table, and you'll hear oohs and aahs. A weekend family breakfast, a picnic lunch in the park, or a special occasion dinner, all will be memorable—guaranteed. But the truly remarkable aspect of these meals is they fit into a smart approach to eating.

Of course, we won't limit you to the recipes in this book. You'll also learn the building blocks for constructing your own *Healthy Heart*

Miracle Diet meals, and also identifying foods at home or on the road that abide by the new principles of healthy eating.

You'll also be pleased at the relatively small amount of change you'll need to make. Too many eating plans ask you to drop everything you like about food and adopt a whole new diet, without acknowledging how difficult it is to make a total change in the way you eat—and expect it to last. With *Healthy Heart Miracle Diet*, you'll be encouraged to replace the foods you love with foods that are similar, so you won't be tempted to fall back on old unhealthy ways.

For example, if you eat cereal for breakfast, you'll find plenty of alternatives that fit nicely into your morning habits *and* your new healthy approach to eating. Our recipes will make following *Healthy Heart Miracle Diet* a snap. You'll get advice on stocking your pantry according to the plan's principles, so that every meal you make will be healthful, simple, nutritious, and delicious. And *Healthy Heart Miracle Diet* will support your new lifestyle with research-tested methods that strengthen your commitment to change.

Activity plays a crucial part in your overall success, but we won't ask you to become a triathlete or even join a gym.

Putting it Together

One of the most reliable ways to insure the "new" you becomes a "permanent" you is to develop an exercise habit. In *Healthy Heart Miracle Diet*, activity plays a crucial part in your overall success. But we won't ask you to become a triathlete or even join a gym. We'll show you how to work regular activity into your daily life, in bite-size pieces or in 30-minute bursts—whatever works best for you. Exercise will help you maintain your weight (or lose weight if that's your goal). It will give your cardiovascular system a workout and help you manage stress, both of which will keep your heart healthy.

We all know the extraordinary benefits of eating a healthier, heart-friendly diet: greater energy, a slimmer body, lower blood pressure, better brain power, and improved moods are just a few. These benefits can be had within a few weeks, and will be yours for the rest of your life—a life that will last longer, thanks to the changes you make! Yes, you'll need to change eating habits that may not be so easy to break. But with *Healthy Heart Miracle Diet*, you'll still be eating wonderful, flavorful food, just slightly different choices than you did before.

At this point, the key question is: Are you ready to make a commitment to a healthy new diet? You couldn't have picked a better time to tackle a new approach to eating, because at this moment, we can finally say with confidence we know what works. Even better, it tastes great.

Everything you need for better health is right here in your hands. The first step? Merely turn the page.

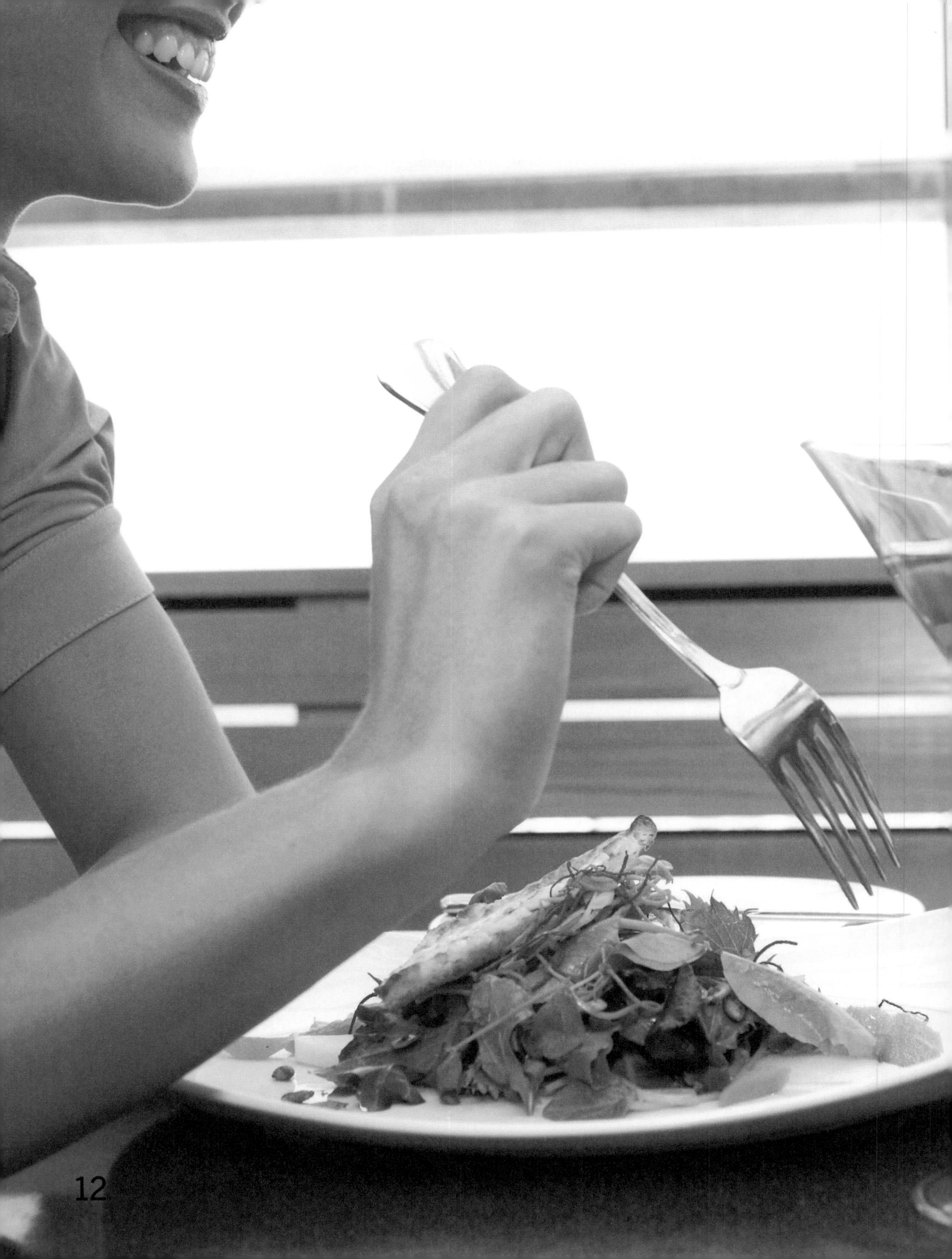

PART ONE

The New View: Heart Disease and Your Diet

Many long-established rules of healthy eating are being proven wrong. You'll be thrilled about everything that's back on the menu.

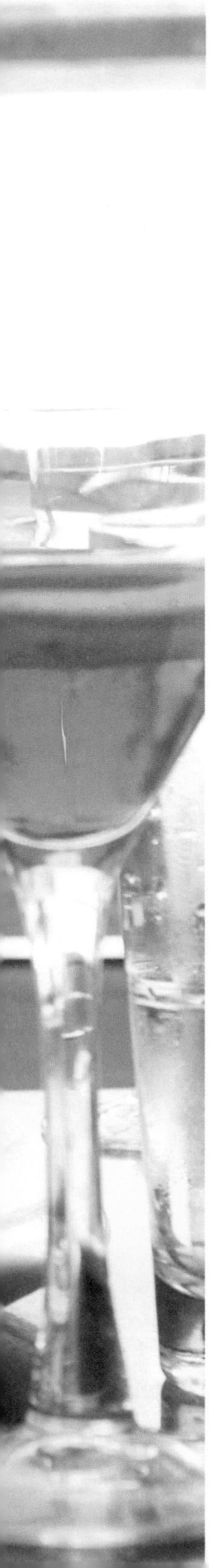

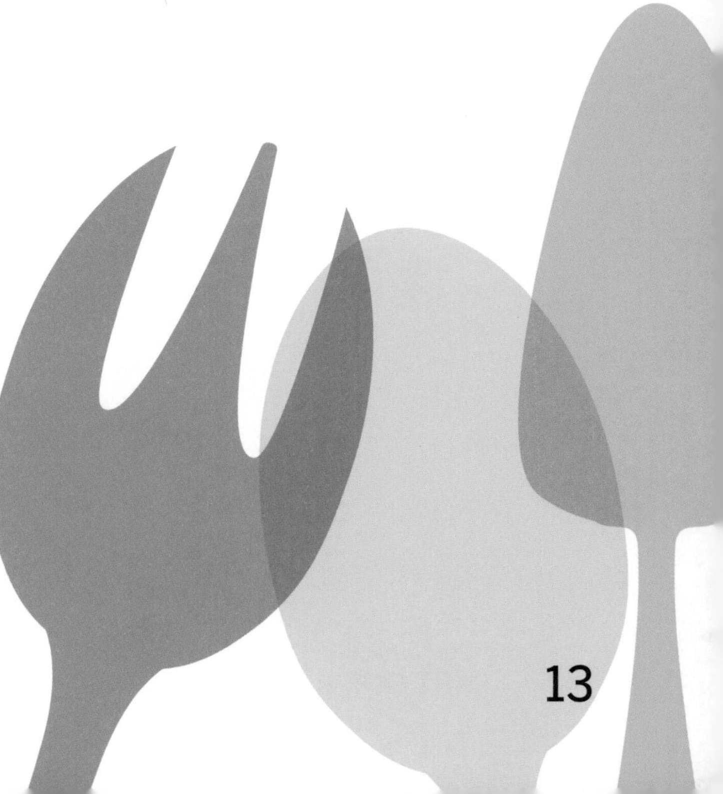

1

Are You Eating a Heart-Healthy Diet?

Are You Sure?

Turns out, the experts had it all wrong: Fat is not the number one evil when it comes to your heart. Believe it or not, the carbs you eat, if you choose the wrong ones, are more likely to kill you.

Ask anyone on the street and they'll tell you that to avoid a heart attack, you have to eat less fat. Your doctor will almost certainly say the same thing. The staying power of this advice is remarkable—and yet the advice itself is remarkably shaky.

For the last 30 years, there has been one clear message when it comes to lowering the risk of cardiovascular disease: Eat a low-fat diet—the less fat the better. In an attempt to follow this advice, people cut back on salad dressing, switched from butter to margarine, and filled up on carbohydrates in the form of bread, rice, and low-fat cookies—all highly questionable moves, as you'll discover later in this book. For their efforts, they began *gaining* weight. And the promised heart protection was AWOL. For example, "lite"-obsessed countries like the United States and England have nearly double the incidence of heart disease of countries notoriously dismissive of low-fat eating, including Italy, Belgium, Poland, Greece, Portugal, and Spain, and nearly triple the incidence of France, where fat in a typical meal is almost double the fat in an average American meal.

So if low-fat diets were supposed to protect us—and fat was supposed to be harmful—what went so terribly wrong? And how can you go right when it comes to eating heart-healthy?

Where Low-Fat Diets Went Wrong

The experts were quick to accept low-fat theories without thoroughly testing the full impact of a low-fat diet. On its surface, the low-fat idea just seemed to make sense. Doctors knew that fat in the blood—namely, cholesterol—was linked to heart attacks and strokes. Therefore, the fat and cholesterol in food *had* to be a problem. How else would levels of cholesterol in the blood rise? From there, it was one long slide down the slippery low-fat slope: A meat-and-potatoes diet was fingered as the likely culprit for everyone's heart woes, and low-fat prescriptions were handed out worldwide.

The experts were quick to accept low-fat theories without thoroughly testing the full impact of a low-fat diet.

Another reason people embraced the low-fat approach is because, gram for gram, fat contains more calories (9) than carbohydrates or protein (4 each). It seemed logical, then, that cutting fat would help not only keep cholesterol down but weight as well.

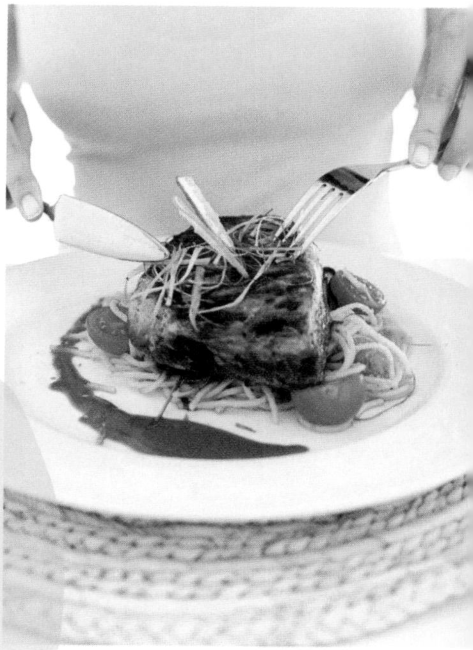

What not everyone realized—and no one explained to the public—is that not all fats are the same: There are good fats and bad fats and, as research has proven, good fats are actually necessary for good health, including heart health. Eating good fats can even help you lose weight. Saying something like this in the mid-1970s, just as the low-fat doctrine really began to catch fire, would have been blasphemy. But in the early 1980s, the results of studies on low-fat diets finally began rolling in, and they weren't exactly what everyone expected.

Anyone who is taking cholesterol-lowering statin drugs won't be surprised to hear that lowering levels of very high cholesterol *with medication* does seem to help stave off heart disease. But eating a low-fat diet barely budges the needle for many. In one trial at the University of California, San Diego, heart specialists tracked 3,806 men who either took a cholesterol drug or followed a low-fat diet. After 10 years, the medication group had suffered 24 percent fewer fatal heart attacks and 19 percent fewer nonfatal heart attacks than the diet-only group. Since all the men in the study had very high cholesterol, this was convincing evidence that lowering it could help prevent heart trouble. However, the findings from the diet-only group were less than reassuring: After 10 years on a low-fat diet, these men saw their risk of suffering a heart attack drop from 8.6 percent to 7 percent, and the risk of dying from heart disease fell from 2 percent to 1.6 percent. Hardly the ringing endorsement low-fat proponents were hoping for.

Cholesterol Is Only Part of the Problem

There was another sticky issue when it came to the obsessive focus on lowering cholesterol. Call it the gorilla in the room: Only about half of all cardiovascular disease can be explained by high cholesterol. In other words, half of the people who suffer heart attacks, strokes, or any other form of heart disease actually have normal—or "healthy"—levels of cholesterol. So even if the widely prescribed low-fat diet did help drop cholesterol levels, it would protect only half of the population at risk for heart problems. But that knowledge wouldn't reach the general public for years. In fact, most people still don't realize that healthy cholesterol levels aren't a guarantee against future heart troubles. This helps explain why cutting fat didn't seem to have a large effect on the numbers of people suffering from heart disease.

Eating Even Less Fat Isn't the Answer Either

Rather than question the low-fat theory itself, some researchers instead questioned whether the advice went far enough in terms of cutting fat. And in small, short-term research in people who had severe heart disease, extremely low fat diets seemed to have startlingly positive effects. In one study of 20 people, a 10 percent fat diet (compared to a norm of 30 to 40 percent) coupled with stress-relief techniques, exercise, and other lifestyle changes actually seemed to reverse blockage in arteries.

The discovery that eating lots of meat and fat didn't send cholesterol levels soaring skyward cast doubt on the whole low-fat hypothesis.

Such findings seemed impressive, but the reality of following this diet was beyond almost everyone but the deathly ill. Who was ready to eliminate all meat, poultry, and fish? All oil? Limit themselves to fat-free cheeses? Besides being unrealistic for most households, limiting fat to this degree may actually be harmful. We've spent so much time thinking fat is bad for us that it's easy to forget that our bodies need it to function. Fat insulates nerves and serves as energy storage, for instance. Another drawback to this approach is that blood pressure can rise along with levels of triglycerides, another potentially harmful blood fat. And levels of "good" HDL cholesterol dipped into what's considered a dangerous, high-risk zone.

Gorging on Burgers Doesn't Work

Around the time the low-fat approach was catching on, a competing theory began to emerge. It held that fat, fat, and more fat was actually what our bodies needed. An early proponent was Dr. Robert Atkins, who developed a very low carb, high-fat, carnivore's-delight diet known as the Atkins Diet. Dr. Atkins believed that carbohydrates were the source of most evil in the diet, and he theorized that they were the reason cholesterol rose and clogged arteries. Although his ultrafatty, meat-heavy diet flew in the face of everything we've heard about fat and heart disease, some potentially healthy things do happen when researchers put people on such a diet.

For one, they actually lose weight—not much, but a bit more, on average, than people who follow low-fat diets. Even more surprising, several studies suggest that people who follow such a diet will experience a drop in triglycerides, and their levels of "good" HDL cholesterol will rise. At least for the short period of time that people can manage to stay on such a diet (the max seems to be about 6 months), their risk of heart disease *drops* while they're gorging on food high in fat and cholesterol. Part of the explanation for this counterintuitive improvement is the fact that people lose weight. Almost anytime you manage to lose weight, your cholesterol will also fall. (And drastically cutting back on carbs also means cutting out a significant number of calories.) Another reason for the improvement is that certain types of carbohydrates *do* spur the rise of blood fats, so it follows that cutting carbs would lower them.

But there are drawbacks to eating this way: Although levels of "good" cholesterol improve, "bad" LDL cholesterol goes up, too. The diet also raises acids in the blood that can leach calcium from your bones and potentially trigger gout.

Although diets high in fat (and protein) and low in carbs aren't really a fix for heart trouble, the discovery that eating so much meat and fat didn't send cholesterol levels soaring skyward cast serious doubt on the whole low-fat hypothesis.

The Day Low Fat Died

In 2006, the bombshell hit. A $415 million research project, known as the Women's Health Initiative, involving 49,000 women released results that all but crushed the low-fat hypothesis. Researchers in the study had asked some of the women to follow a diet that got about 20 percent of its calories from fat. The women, as is typical, had a tough time getting the number that low; they averaged about 24 percent for the first part of the study. Another group was left to its own devices and, consequently, got about 35 percent of their calories from fat. After 8 years of watching their fat calories, the 20 percent group experienced just as many heart attacks—not to mention breast and colon cancers—as the group who ate more than 35 percent of calories from fat. And just like that, the low-fat revolution was effectively over (though some scientists still argue that the low-fat diet in the study was too little, too late).

For low-fat crusaders, the bad news has continued to pile up. In 2009, researchers at the University of Washington reported results from a study in which 71 men and women at high risk for heart disease followed a typical low-fat plan (20 percent of calories from fat) or a moderate fat plan that got 40 percent of calories from fat. (It's a true sign of how far we've come when 40 percent of calories from fat is labeled "moderate.") After just 1 month, the improvements for the group on the "moderate-fat" diet doubled and tripled those of the low-fat group: "Bad" LDL cholesterol fell by an average of 12 points in the moderate-fat group, compared to just 4 points for the low-fat group. The low-fat diet drove down "good" HDL cholesterol by 5 points, while it barely budged for the moderate-fat dieters.

Which is more natural?

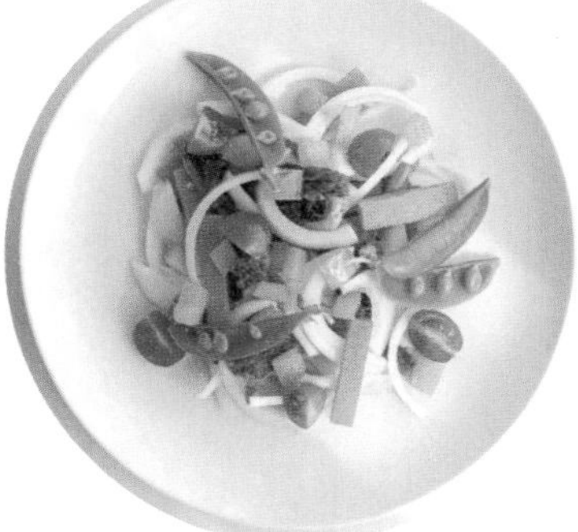

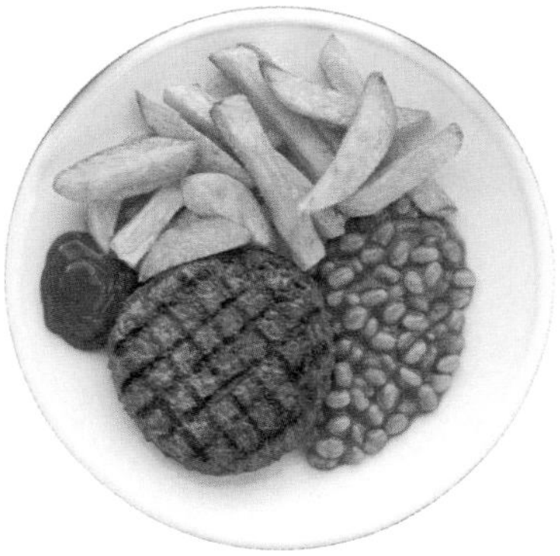

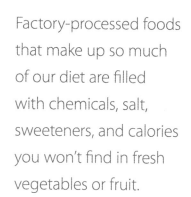

Factory-processed foods that make up so much of our diet are filled with chemicals, salt, sweeteners, and calories you won't find in fresh vegetables or fruit.

And levels of triglycerides fell 29 points on the moderate-fat plan, while *climbing* 11 points for the low-fat dieters.

After 1 month, the improvements for the "moderate-fat" diet group doubled and tripled those of the low-fat group.

The Hidden Culprit: Carbs

Americans' nearly 30-year experiment in low-fat dieting ended up being a rather harsh lesson in unforeseen consequences. When people began eliminating fat from their diets, they replaced it in large part with simple carbohydrates. Pasta became the main course of choice. Nutritionists praised a dinner plate piled high with rice and just a little protein, like fish or chicken, on the side. Food manufacturers rushed to supply shoppers with low-fat and fat-free snacks and desserts like rice cakes, pretzels, and cookies.

What few people realized at the time was that the body digests these simple carbohydrates almost as quickly as it does straight sugar—with dire implications for the heart. While fat, protein, and fiber slow down the process of turning calories into energy, simple carbohydrates are quickly converted to glucose, or blood sugar, which is used to fuel cells.

There are two direct results of eating too many simple carbohydrates. The first is that, shortly after a high-carb meal, there is a big spike and then a decrease in blood sugar, which triggers signals in your belly and brain that make you feel hungry and demand quick energy in the form of more carbohydrates. Ultimately, this glucose spike-and-drop cycle has you consuming more calories than you need.

The other drawback is that all those sugar spikes can start to wear out your sugar-processing machinery. When blood sugar spikes, the pancreas releases insulin to round up the glucose molecules and get them into cells throughout the body, where the sugar can be converted into energy (or fat for long-term storage). Eat too many simple carbs and, over time, your cells may become resistant to insulin's effects, allowing both insulin and glucose to build up in the bloodstream. That's bad news for your artery lining because it triggers inflammation that sharply raises your risk of suffering a heart attack.

Too many simple carbs, not enough good fats—those are two of the main problems with the way many of us currently eat.

Too many simple carbs, not enough good fats—those are two of the main problems with the way many of us currently eat. The Healthy Heart Miracle Diet was designed to correct these problems and more. On this diet, you'll avoid the "bad" carbs that threaten the heart, eat more of the "good" fats that protect it, and get plenty of protein and fiber to keep you full and satisfied. The diet was carefully designed to not only improve your ratio of "good" to "bad" cholesterol but also to protect you against a host of other heart risks that doctors weren't even aware of 20 years ago—risks you'll read about in the next chapter.

How Heart-Healthy Is Your Diet? quiz

Give yourself 3 points for every "A" answer, 2 points for every "B", 1 point for every "C", and zero for any "D" answers.

1. The first beverage I see when I open my refrigerator is:

A. Nonfat or 1% milk
B. Water or seltzer
C. Diet soft drink or fruit juice
D. Regular soft drink

2. I usually prepare pasta:

A. Al dente (firm) with tomato sauce or vegetables
B. Al dente with olive oil and garlic
C. Soft with tomato sauce
D. By heating up a frozen or canned meal

3. My pasta sauce typically comes from:

A. A home recipe with fresh ingredients
B. A home recipe with some fresh and some canned ingredients
C. A jar with 8 grams of sugar or less per serving
D. A jar with more than 8 grams of sugar per serving

4. I mainly eat bread that is:

A. Whole grain
B. Multigrain
C. Brown
D. White

5. When I cook rice at home, I usually choose:

A. Wild
B. Brown
C. White
D. Instant

6. When it comes to red meat, I typically:

A. Eat none, or have a little lean beef or pork once or twice a week
B. Have hamburgers, steak, or meatloaf once a week
C. Have hamburgers, steak, or meatloaf several times a week
D. Eat it daily

7. I eat fish (including canned tuna):

A. At least twice a week
B. Once a week
C. Two or three times a month
D. Almost never or never

8. For breakfast, I usually eat:

A. An egg, some yogurt, or a piece of whole-wheat toast with peanut butter, or oatmeal
B. Some fruit or a whole-grain cereal
C. Sugary cereal, a bagel, muffin, croissant, or frozen waffle, or white toast with jam
D. Nothing

9. If I'm at a party grazing on appetizers, I'm most likely to choose:

A. Hummus or olive spread with veggies or whole-grain crackers
B. Shrimp
C. Chips and salsa
D. Egg rolls or something else fried

10. I eat dairy (yogurt, milk, cheese):

A. Daily, low-fat or nonfat (or a small portion of full-fat cheese)
B. Most days, low-fat or nonfat (or a small portion of full-fat cheese)
C. Most days, full-fat
D. Rarely

11. I typically eat dinner:

A. With my spouse, family, or friends
B. By myself, sitting down at the table
C. In front of the television
D. By myself, wherever I can grab it (sometimes in my car!)

12. I keep fruit:

A. On the counter
B. In a cupboard
C. In the fridge
D. Fruit isn't always on hand

13. I typically eat vegetables:

A. With most meals
B. At dinner
C. Do French fries and mashed potatoes count?
D. When the frozen entrée I microwave contains them

14. I usually cook with:

A. Olive or canola oil
B. Corn, sunflower, or safflower oil
C. Margarine with no hydrogenated oils
D. Butter, or margarine with hydrogenated oils

15. I usually snack on:

A. Nuts
B. Fruit
C. Chips, pretzels, or snack bars
D. Candy

quiz

Your Score

40-45 FOUR STARS

You're eating a heart-healthy diet already—congratulations! But you'll pick up some new hints and tips, not to mention delicious recipes, with the Healthy Heart Miracle Diet to help ensure that your family is protected not only from heart disease but also many other major health concerns.

30-39 THREE STARS

You're doing many things right, but you still have a way to go to fully protect your heart.

20-29 TWO STARS

You're following some of the principles of heart-healthy eating, but you'll learn a lot—and enjoy your meals much more—by adopting the strategies in the Healthy Heart Miracle Diet.

19 OR LOWER: ONE STAR

It's time for a serious intervention. Start by choosing one of the recipes in the back of the book for lunch or dinner today.

Decoding Your Score

If some of the "right" answers above seem confusing, don't be surprised. As you're learning, a lot has changed when it comes to eating right for your heart. Below, you'll find a brief explanation for the scoring. In part 2, you'll read much more about making the right choices when it comes to your diet.

1. **New research shows that dairy foods have surprising health benefits, making low-fat milk your go-to beverage.** Water and seltzer are also great choices. Fruit juice gets relatively low marks because it's a concentrated source of sugar. Diet soft drinks may be calorie-free, but research suggests it knocks your fullness signals off-kilter, ultimately leading you to eat more. And regular soft drinks add a shocking amount of nutrient-free calories to your diet. Some weight experts believe it's the number one contributor to weight gain and diabetes in many countries.

> Fruit juice gets relatively low marks because it's a concentrated source of sugar.

2. **Slightly undercooking pasta will slow down digestion, creating a lower rise in blood sugar.** As you'll discover later in the book, foods that raise blood sugar less than others are better for your heart. A tomato-based sauce provides plenty of heart protective nutrients, especially if you add some other vegetables. Olive oil is a healthy fat and, along with garlic, provides substances that can keep your blood pressure down and your cardiovascular system healthy. Prepackaged meals are generally high in sodium and sugar and low in nutrients.

3. **Cooking with fresh ingredients is one of the nicest things you can do for your heart.** The more preparation you leave to food manufacturers, the higher your intake of substances that can harm your heart. For example, many store-bought sauces are loaded with sugar.

> Cooking with fresh ingredients is one of the nicest things you can do for your heart.

4. **Bread is fine—as long as it contains plenty of fiber.** Fiber slows the digestion of carbohydrates, moderating blood-sugar swings. Only whole-grain bread still has the fibrous shell around the seed, and it contains the most B vitamins, which are also good for your heart. Multigrain breads offer more fiber than white, but to get the most benefit, make sure the package also says *whole* grain. Brown and white breads are essentially the same—all the fiber

has been removed (though you get a point for choosing brown bread because you're attempting to do the right thing!)

5. **White rice isn't junk food—but it's hardly health food, either.** As a refined grain, it's been stripped of most nutrients and, worse, it sends blood sugar soaring, which can raise your cholesterol. Fiber is the reason to choose wild rice or brown. Avoid instant types; they are digested so quickly by your body that they flood your system with cheap energy. Much of the calories instant rice provides end up stored as fat.

6. **Surprisingly, beef, pork, and lamb can all play a valuable role in a heart-healthy diet.** That's largely because they're a great source of protein, which helps you feel full. Of course, the devil is in the details…you'll want to choose lean cuts and keep portions moderate.

7. **People who eat fish twice a week cut their risk of a heart attack by 36 percent.** The more you eat, the better. If you do eat a lot of fish, see chapter 8 for the types that contain the least contaminants.

8. **People who skip breakfast weigh more than those who don't.** The best breakfast contains some protein (yes, oatmeal does) to help keep you full until lunchtime. Because simple carbs are public enemy number one, breakfast can be a minefield if you're not careful. You should avoid sugary cereals and any form of white bread.

9. **Olives and hummus are full of heart-healthy "good" fat, one of the keys to the Healthy Heart Miracle Diet.** Shrimp is another great choice; it provides the same heart-healing fats that other fish have, and its cholesterol has little effect on the levels in your blood. Salsa has plenty of veggies—just don't go crazy with the chips! Avoiding fried foods is a no-brainer.

10. **Dairy gets high grades.** Evidence suggests that dairy foods can help you lose weight, lower your blood pressure, and reduce inflammation in your arteries. But if you eat the full-fat version of most dairy products, you'll be adding a lot of saturated fat to your diet—and that's one fat you want to limit.

11. **How and where you eat may be almost as important as what you eat.** Remarkably, sitting down to a communal meal once a day improves everyone's health. It gives you the kind of social outlet that research has shown is good for your heart. Plus, people tend to eat slower and make more sensible food choices when they eat together.

12. **When it comes to fruit, out of sight means out of mind.** Numerous studies have found that households that keep fruit out in plain sight are more likely to eat it as a snack—and before it spoils. That means you'll get your money's worth out of your trip through the produce aisle instead of regularly tossing the forgotten—rotten—fruit hidden in your fridge's crisper. And you and your family will have filled up on a much more nutritious snack than, say, pretzels or chips.

13. **The carb foods you should eat to your heart's content are colorful vegetables.** These vegetables should be a part of most of your meals, and always on your dinner plate. We'll show you ways to convert this duty into pleasure. French fries and mashed potatoes without the skin, though ever-popular, are far less beneficial than other veggies.

14. **There are plenty of healthy oils you can choose for cooking.** By now you know the benefits of olive oil, but you'll read about other healthy cooking oils in chapter 8. Trans-fat free margarine is a little better than butter, but you'll see that in the Healthy Heart Miracle Diet, there's even a place for butter. In the right amounts, it can provide the flavoring that will leave you satisfied, and the health benefit of not wanting—and eating—more outweighs any damage those few saturated fats might do.

15. **On the Healthy Heart Miracle Diet, you never have to avoid all fats.** Nuts are an excellent snack choice because they contain good fat *and* protein to calm your hunger much better than a bag of chips or candy. Fruit, of course, is also an excellent snack.

2

What *Really* Causes Heart Attacks?

If you think "bad" cholesterol causes most heart attacks, think again. Half of the people who have heart attacks don't even have high cholesterol. The trouble is caused by a more complex cascade of events—all of which the Healthy Heart Miracle Diet helps prevent.

Only half of the people who have heart attacks have high cholesterol. That doesn't mean your cholesterol levels aren't important—they are. But, clearly, cholesterol isn't the whole story. In recent years, scientists have identified other health issues that also play a major role in whether your ticker keeps on ticking or you find yourself clutching your chest and being rushed to the emergency room one day.

Some of these issues work in tandem with cholesterol to raise your risk, while others cause trouble all by themselves. Even if your cholesterol is elevated, focusing on reducing it without paying attention to the other health issues in this chapter can leave you—and your heart—in danger. Read on to discover eight important risk factors for heart disease, beyond cholesterol—and find out how the Healthy Heart Miracle Diet combats every one of them. Meanwhile, know your cholesterol numbers. You should get a cholesterol test every 5 years that includes tallies of your "good" HDL cholesterol, "bad" LDL cholesterol, and triglycerides. (If your cholesterol is high, you may need yearly testing).

The most reliable indicator of heart trouble:

High Blood Pressure

High blood pressure isn't scientifically new, or very sexy. Maybe that's why people tend to underestimate how serious the problem is.

Or maybe they can't picture exactly how it is that high blood pressure harms the heart.

Think about when you run your garden hose: If you partially block the end of the hose with your thumb, the hose will bulge and the water will squirt out around your thumb. Add a spray nozzle and you can increase the pressure enough to knock dirt off lawn furniture or loose paint off the exterior walls of your house if you aren't careful. And all you've done in either case is narrow the opening through which the water must pass.

Your arteries are a lot like that hose. Blood is pumped through them from the heart, and it courses through the body before returning through the veins to the heart and lungs to pick up oxygen and be pumped back out again. But when blood pressure rises for whatever reason—such as narrowing of the arteries—the blood, which can't exactly squirt out through the end of the "hose", is forced up against the artery walls with increasingly brutal force.

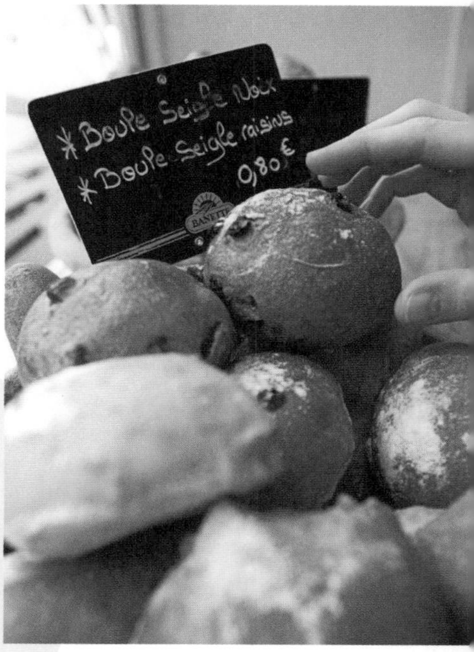

Over time, the pressure can create bulges in the weak parts of artery walls, forcing the body to make repairs that stiffen the walls and reduce the flexibility of the arteries. What's more, as blood under pressure races through your arteries, it can knock loose built-up plaque and detritus, which can then lodge in narrowed passageways, blocking the flow of blood to the heart and triggering a heart attack. Even if high blood pressure doesn't lead to a heart attack, it causes your heart to work harder to push blood through your circulatory system. This taxes your heart muscle, causing your heart to enlarge and weaken, and eventually, the muscle may fail.

All of this helps explain why you can't get anywhere near a doctor's office without someone slapping a blood pressure cuff on your arm. High blood pressure—hypertension—is the easiest heart risk to diagnose and treat. For the last century or so, that simple measurement has helped identify people whose hearts could betray them at any moment. One in three adults worldwide suffers from hypertension. The World Health Organization estimates that, at any given time, 600 million people with high blood pressure are at risk of suffering a heart attack. The risk increases as you age: In developed countries, the average middle-age citizen has a 90 percent chance of developing high blood pressure at some point in their lives.

Why blood pressure rises and stays elevated is still a bit of a mystery. Gaining weight can raise it. So can physical effort—shoveling snow, for example, or exercise of any sort. But such activity is good for you, provided you do it on a regular basis. Pushing your blood pressure up and then letting it fall again seems to help build resilience in the circulatory system and increase the elasticity of your arteries.

High blood pressure–hypertension–is the easiest heart risk to diagnose, treat, and correct.

Chronic stress seems to play a role. Stress hormones can constrict the smooth muscles that envelop the arteries, causing the blood vessels to narrow. This means your heart has to work harder to circulate blood. Stress also raises your heart rate (the number of times your heart beats per minute), which increases blood pressure.

Some people have difficulty processing sodium, which can build up in the body, attracting more and more fluid, and increasing the volume of blood. Because your circulatory system is closed, there's nowhere for that extra fluid to go, so the veins and arteries swell like an overfilled water balloon.

The Numbers:
Normal: Less than 120/80 mmHg
Pre-hypertension: 120/80–139/89 mmHg
High blood pressure: 140/90 mmHg and above

On the Healthy Heart Miracle Diet, you'll effortlessly cut your sodium intake by eating foods closer to their original state.

How the Healthy Heart Miracle Diet Helps

Probably the single biggest benefit of this plan when it comes to taming high blood pressure is the increased physical activity you'll get. Simply walking several times a week will make a serious dent in your blood pressure numbers. Studies suggest that regular exercise can drop the higher number (systolic blood pressure) by 13 points, on average, and the lower number (diastolic blood pressure) by 8.

By following the Healthy Heart Miracle Diet, you'll eat foods closer to their original state—a delicious roast chicken you prepare versus, say, a frozen chicken entrée, for example. That will effortlessly cut back on the sodium in your diet, thought to be a primary cause of hypertension for some people (see "The Great Salt Debate" below.)

The Great Salt Debate

Experts are stuck in a heated argument over how big a danger salt poses when it comes to blood pressure. The truth is, research shows that only about a third of the population is "salt sensitive." When they eat even a little sodium (a component of salt), their blood pressures skyrocket. Because their kidneys do a terrible job of processing sodium, it quickly builds up in the bloodstream, attracting fluid and increasing blood pressure.

But for everyone else, according to the evidence on hand, salt isn't a problem. It's even less of a problem if you cook most of your own food. In a landmark study from 2004, Harvard researchers reported that a low-sodium diet featuring whole grains, fresh produce, and healthy fats reduced blood pressure readings by just one to two points when compared to a high-sodium version of the same diet. "The difference isn't that impressive," says Ronald Krauss, MD, a senior scientist at Children's Hospital Oakland Research Center who has coauthored two editions of the American Heart Association's health guidelines. "You can get all the blood pressure benefits of a healthy diet without having to pay special attention to sodium."

it's a miracle! CUT SALT THROUGH HOME COOKING

The easiest way to stop worrying about salt is to prepare meals primarily with fresh and minimally processed ingredients—essentially, swapping Chef Boyardee for Chef *Moi*. Do that and you will eliminate up to 77 percent of the sodium in your diet, according to the Mayo Clinic. That's how much we get from processed and prepackaged meals, where the mineral is used liberally as a flavoring and preservative. Only about 5 percent of the average person's total sodium consumption is added by them during cooking, and 6 percent at the table. The last 12 percent occurs naturally in foods.

The body fat you can't eee:

Visceral Fat

Just as not all dietary fat is bad, not all body fat is bad—or at least some types are better than others. The extra padding you may carry around on your hips, butt, and thighs doesn't seem to be all that harmful to your health. Think of this fat as long-term storage: The cells in those areas absorb more and more fat when you overeat, but they tend to hang on to it, releasing it only when the body is in desperate need of more energy. For our ancient ancestors, this adaptation meant they could survive food shortages or even famines, and that mothers could breastfeed babies through lean times. But nowadays, it takes a serious gym-and-diet habit to break into that long-term storage, which, like an offsite storage locker, more or less sits off on its own, not bothering the rest of the body.

The fat that collects in your midsection is a completely different animal. A bulge around the belly is a sign that visceral fat—also called intra-abdominal fat—is enveloping and marbling your internal organs, which is every bit as dangerous as it sounds. Visceral fat doesn't just sit there in case it's needed one day. Instead, it churns out hormones that can interfere with insulin, increasing the likelihood that you'll develop diabetes. It also lowers "good" cholesterol. Finally, visceral fat can reenter the bloodstream as blood fats, some of which feed directly into the nearby liver, driving up production of "bad" cholesterol and triglycerides and putting you in danger of suffering a heart attack or stroke.

In 2007, a British study of 24,500 men and women between the ages of 45 and 79 found that a waist considerably larger than one's hips skyrocketed the risk of heart disease and stroke. For men, the risk jumped 55 percent; for women, the likelihood that they would suffer a heart attack leapt by an astounding 91 percent.

The Numbers:

In general, men who have a waist that is the same size or bigger than their hips are at the highest risk of heart disease, diabetes, high blood pressure, and other chronic conditions. For a woman to reach the danger zone, her waist has to be just 0.85 the size of her hips (for 42-inch/106-cm hips, that means a 36-inch/91-cm waist). An easier way to figure out your risk is to measure your belly: Men with waists more than 40 inches (102 cm) and women with waists more than 35 inches (88 cm) are at increased risk of health troubles. For people of Asian descent, the danger zone for men is 37 inches (94 cm) and higher; for women it's 31 inches (78 cm) and higher.

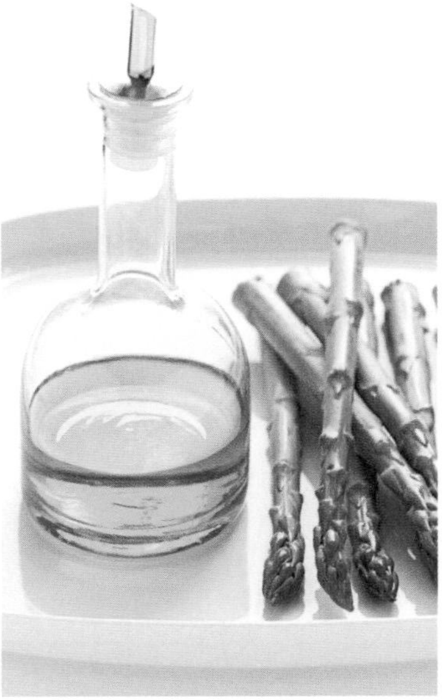

How the Healthy Heart Miracle Diet Helps

The diet fights visceral fat mainly by helping you steer clear of simple carbohydrates and saturated fat. The quick conversion of simple carbohydrates into sugar can leave your body with a surplus of energy, and the easiest place to dump that surplus is the abdomen. Saturated fat also seems to be preferentially converted into visceral fat. On the Healthy Heart Miracle Diet, you'll swap the cookies, crackers, white bread, and other dangerous carbs for whole grains that will help slow down digestion and avoid those quick glucose spikes. And since the extra fiber in these foods is actually indigestible, you'll be cutting calories without even noticing it.

On the Healthy Heart Miracle Diet, you'll also eat more heart-healthy monounsaturated fats, the ones in olive oil and nuts. These have been directly linked to reductions in visceral fat. In 2007, Spanish researchers reported that swapping butter for olive oil in the diets of overweight people helped them shed visceral fat. A low-fat diet made no dent whatsoever in this organ-choking fat.

Remarkably, chronic stress seems to encourage the body to pack on visceral fat. The Healthy Heart Miracle Diet has a fix for that, too, as you'll see in part 3.

The root of much evil:

Inflammation

When you sprain your ankle, it swells. When a cold virus invades your nose, you get congested. Both phenomena are the result of inflammation, a side effect of the healing process. It means that your immune system has recognized an injury or threat and is sending the needed materials to repair muscles and tendons and fight infections.

Inflammation also occurs in places inside your body where you can't see or feel it, and sometimes it goes on for long periods of time, causing its own trouble. For instance, when your arteries are damaged by high blood pressure or by cholesterol particles that burrow their way into artery walls, the body reacts by unleashing immune cells that rush to the area with repair in mind. But if the damage continues, eventually the area gets crowded and the "rescuers" become trapped there and collect in the artery walls, mixing with cholesterol particles and other debris to form fatty streaks called plaque. Scar tissue also forms as the body patches and repatches the same old wounds. Eventually, the scar tissue and the plaque may begin to obstruct the flow of blood by narrowing the passageway and by reducing wall flexibility.

In addition to high cholesterol levels and high blood pressure, another common trigger of chronic inflammation is the visceral fat you just read about. Fat cells in your gut release a constant trickle of inflammatory chemicals into your bloodstream. That's right, a big belly could be directly affecting your heart. Over the last few decades, scientists have begun to realize that chronic inflammation plays a major role in heart disease and stroke, not to mention other conditions such as cancer and diabetes.

One way to measure the amount of inflammatory activity in your body is by testing for a substance called C-reactive protein, or CRP. Your liver manufactures this protein in response to inflammation anywhere in your body. The more inflammation you have, the higher your CRP. Measuring levels of CRP in the blood provides a window into the amount of inflammation occurring in artery walls, according to Paul Ridker, MD, a cardiologist at the Brigham and Women's Hospital in Boston, who also found that testing CRP can help predict heart attacks or strokes in people who have normal LDL cholesterol levels.

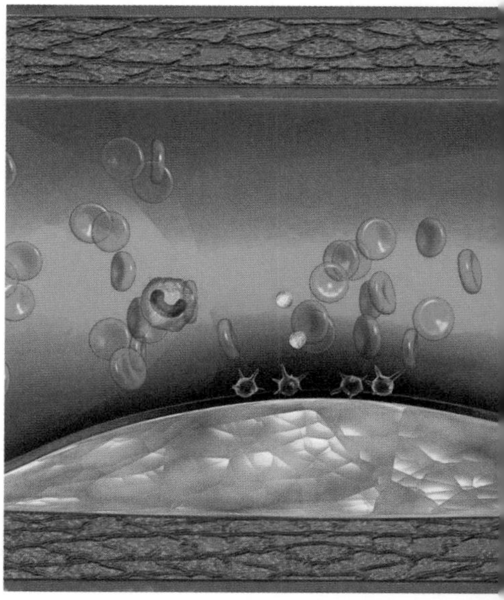

What this reveals, says Dr. Ridker, is that chronic inflammation on its own may be more dangerous than high cholesterol. Even if your cholesterol levels are normal, a CRP test might make sense for you if you have a history of heart attack or stroke in your family. If your cholesterol and blood pressure levels are good and there's no heart disease in your family, you probably don't need one. And if you're already being treated for high cholesterol or heart disease, you certainly don't need one. (Bonus: Statin drugs prescribed to lower cholesterol also fight inflammation.)

The Numbers:
Low risk: Less than 1 mg/L
Average risk: 1–3 mg/L
High risk: 3.1–10 mg/L*

*High levels can also be caused by an acute infection. If your score falls within the high-risk category, wait 3 weeks and repeat the test. Persistent elevations above 10mg/L suggest noncardiovascular inflammation, such as that from rheumatoid arthritis or another inflammatory condition.

How the Healthy Heart Miracle Diet Helps

The type of fats found in fish, avocados, and nuts are particularly effective in blocking inflammation. The omega-3 fatty acids in fish, in particular, are key building blocks for the body's anti-inflammatory compounds, and the Healthy Heart Miracle Diet ensures that you'll get plenty of these important fats. Certain spices, such as turmeric (used in curry), contain anti-inflammatory substances, too, and, in studies, they seem to help tamp down inflammation. The Healthy Heart Miracle Diet employs these spices to not only reduce your heart disease risk but also to add flavor and satisfaction to your meals, helping to eliminate overeating. If you end up dropping some pounds as a result, your risk of suffering damage from inflammation will also fall.

it's a myth. EATING SHRIMP WILL RAISE YOUR CHOLESTEROL

Shrimp is indeed high in cholesterol, but dietary cholesterol doesn't have much impact on the cholesterol levels in your blood. (Saturated fat and simple carbohydrates are bigger villains.) What's more, shrimp contains a little-known nutrient called betaine, also found in spinach, beets, and wheat bran. Greek researchers discovered that people who consume betaine can lower levels of inflammation—a known trigger for heart attacks—by up to 26 percent.

When symptoms start adding up:

Metabolic Syndrome

If your cholesterol levels are healthy but your waistline is bulging, you have several reasons to worry. First, it's likely that you're carrying around too much heart-threatening visceral fat. But the problem might be even worse, especially if you get little or no exercise. Years ago, researchers discovered a cluster of related health problems that tend to occur together and that dramatically increase the risk for heart disease. They stumbled on it when they were studying people with heart disease who had normal levels of cholesterol. As it turned out, many of these patients had symptoms in common: They tended to have large waists, led sedentary lives, and have insulin resistance (an early sign of diabetes). As researchers did more testing on these patients, some other features of the syndrome, dubbed metabolic syndrome, emerged. The patients often had high levels of the blood fats called triglycerides, low levels of HDL ("good") cholesterol, and high blood pressure.

You don't need to have all of these symptoms to get a diagnosis of metabolic syndrome, though. Any three are enough to triple the risk of heart trouble. The bottom line: Even if your "bad" cholesterol levels are in the clear, a large waist and insulin resistance could put you on the fast track to heart disease. If you haven't ever had your fasting glucose level checked, ask your doctor to check it at your next appointment. You'll have to fast for at least 8 hours beforehand, so schedule it for first thing in the morning.

The Numbers:

Visceral fat as measured by waist circumference:

- Men: Greater than 40 inches (102 cm)
- Women: Greater than 35 inches (88 cm)

Fasting blood triglycerides: Greater than or equal to 150 mg/dL (1.67 mmol/L)

Low blood HDL cholesterol:

- Men: Less than 40 mg/dL (1.0 mmol/L)
- Women: Less than 50 mg/dL (1.25 mmol/L)

Blood pressure: Greater than or equal to 130/85 mmHg
Fasting glucose: Greater than or equal to 100 mg/dL

How the Healthy Heart Miracle Diet Helps

The simple exercise plan in the Healthy Heart Miracle Diet may be enough on its own to help battle metabolic syndrome. A 2010 study on elderly British people found that an hour of light exercise three times a week led to significant weight loss and waist shrinkage. The exercisers also improved their insulin sensitivity by 68 percent after just 12 weeks. Regular physical activity also reduces blood pressure.

By choosing healthy fats and eating more fruits and vegetables, you'll also see your "good" HDL cholesterol increase, and opting for high-quality carbohydrates will help tame your triglycerides. And just like that, you're managing the five possible characteristics of metabolic syndrome.

Even if your "bad" cholesterol is in the clear, a large waist could put you on the fast track to heart disease.

Acid in your arteries:

High Homocysteine

Here's yet another reason to eat your spinach: It's full of B vitamins that break down homocysteine, an amino acid that's cropped up as a risk factor for heart disease, stroke, and peripheral vascular disease. As with so many of the natural substances in your body, the dose makes the poison.

Your body synthesizes homocysteine from proteins in the foods you eat. Then, with the help of certain B vitamins, the body uses homocysteine to help build new tissues. The problems start when you don't get enough B vitamins, or when you eat too much protein. If levels of homocysteine rise above normal, the caustic amino acid can corrode the artery wall lining, known as the endothelium, inflaming and scarring arteries.

For reasons that aren't entirely clear, homocysteine may make the platelets in blood more likely to clump together and form clots. When University of Washington researchers tested levels in 386 women, they found that the group of women with the most homocysteine in their blood had double the heart attack risk of women who had the least. Other studies suggest that people with high levels of homocysteine have five times the risk of suffering a stroke compared with people who have low levels.

Most people won't need to have their homocysteine measured, although your doctor could decide it's worthwhile if heart disease is a problem in your family but you have no other known risk factors.

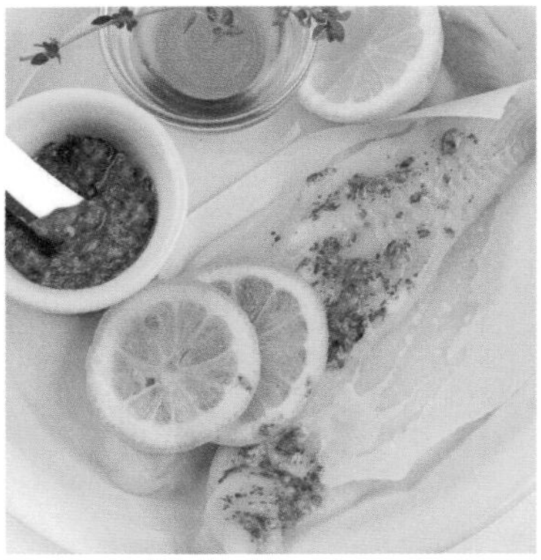

The Numbers:
Normal: 5–15 µmol/L
High: Above 15 µmol/L

How the Healthy Heart Miracle Diet Helps

The older you are, the more you smoke, and the less you move, the higher the likelihood that you'll have elevated homocysteine levels. High cholesterol and blood pressure also tend to go hand in hand with high levels of homocysteine. And too much protein in your diet, such as the levels you reach on a plan like Atkins, can also increase homocysteine.

But this is an easy problem to fix. Following the plan outlined in this book will help balance the protein, carbohydrates, and fat in your diet, which can help tame homocysteine. And the wealth of B-vitamin sources in the Healthy Heart Miracle Diet should also help. In a Harvard study of 80,000 nurses, those with the highest intake of the B vitamin folate (about 696 micrograms a day) had half the risk of heart disease and stroke compared to women who got the least. By following the Healthy Heart Miracle Diet, you'll get plenty of B vitamins from lean meats, fish, nuts, and whole grains.

A breach in the wall:

Endothelial Dysfunction

The endothelium is one of your largest organs, although if you're like most people, you've never heard of it. It's an incredibly sensitive layer of tissue that lines the insides of the miles of arteries and blood vessels snaking through your body. It plays a fundamental role in keeping your heart healthy, though researchers have only begun figuring that out over the last 20 years. Heart experts once thought that the endothelium served only as a barrier between particles in the bloodstream and the walls of an artery. But it turns out that there's a whole lot more going on. The endothelium produces and responds to a variety of substances in your blood, and many of them have a direct effect on the health of your heart.

For instance, it releases the chemical nitric oxide, which combines with another substance in the bloodstream to help relax artery muscles like a soothing balm, so the arteries stay supple and open nice and wide to keep the blood flowing. (Incidentally, nitric oxide is the same chemical that allows blood vessels in the penis to widen, allowing for the increased blood flow necessary for an erection). If the endothelium is unhealthy, it may not produce enough nitric oxide, and the arteries may not dilate fully when they need to, causing narrowing that can eventually lead to blockages. The endothelium also governs the stickiness of blood cells; an unhealthy endothelium will allow the cells to clump together and form a potentially dangerous blood clot. A healthy endothelium, on the other hand, is like Teflon—little sticks to it, including fatty deposits. If it's in good shape, the endothelium can also scavenge for free radicals, the unstable molecules that damage cholesterol particles and make them more likely to stick to artery walls and build up into plaque.

A healthy endothelium, or artery lining, is like Teflon–little sticks to it.

How the Healthy Heart Miracle Diet Helps

Regular exercise helps your endothelium produce nitric oxide, and you'll find easy ways to get more of it on the Healthy Heart Miracle Diet. It's the reason long-distance runners have amazingly healthy arteries with a huge capacity to relax and expand. (Don't worry, no running of any kind is required on the Healthy Heart Miracle Diet.) And you'll eat plenty of the foods (beans, walnuts, fatty fish) that contain the amino acid arginine, a basic ingredient needed to manufacture nitric oxide. You'll also cut back on saturated fat; remarkably, a single meal high in saturated fat can temporarily cut endothelial function by half.

it's a miracle! APPLES SOOTHE YOUR ARTERIES

Apples are a top source of quercetin, a plant chemical that seems to protect the endothelium, or lining of the blood vessels. Damage to the endothelium raises the risk for cardiovascular disease. Other good sources of quercetin include onions, broccoli, and grapes. Antioxidant plant chemicals called epicatechins (in tea, beans, and some fruit) appear to promote healthy endothelial function, too.

The bearer of bad cholesterol:

APO-B

Many experts believe Apo-B is a more accurate indicator of heart-disease risk than "bad" LDL cholesterol. And several studies clearly indicate that high Apo-B levels are far more likely to predict your future heart-disease risk. Your doctor may not use this test yet, especially if you're seeing an internist versus a cardiologist, but he might in the future.

Why? First, the LDL number from your cholesterol report is actually only a guesstimate that's calculated from your HDL and triglyceride numbers. Particularly if your triglycerides are high, that guesstimate may be off. The Apo-B test provides a more direct measure of LDL. What's more, it distinguishes between your levels of "bad" LDL and "very bad" LDL.

Your Apo-B levels are far more likely to predict your future heart-disease risk than your LDL numbers.

That's right, not all bad cholesterol is equally bad. Small LDL particles are more dangerous than big ones—the little buggers can burrow into artery walls more easily than larger, fluffier particles. Only the Apo-B test can indicate how much of which type of LDL you have. If your LDL is moderately high but the particles are mostly the large type, you may not need cholesterol medicine after all, especially if you don't have other risk factors for heart disease. On the other hand, if your cholesterol levels are relatively normal, you might still benefit from mediation if your LDL particles are small.

What is Apo-B? Apolipoproteins are molecules that attach to cholesterol particles and act as ferries to transport them through the bloodstream. "Good" HDL cholesterol is ferried around by apolipoprotein A (Apo-A). "Bad" LDL cholesterol is ferried by apolipoprotein B (Apo-B). For every LDL cholesterol particle, there's one molecule of Apo-B. If your Apo-B count is high, it's likely that you have more, smaller LDL particles than a regular cholesterol test might suggest.

Some experts think that Apo-B may someday overtake cholesterol as the primary measurement for heart disease (it already has in Canada and many other countries around the world). A study from 2003 found that cholesterol tests missed 25 percent of people who needed treatment based on their Apo-B scores. And 15 percent of people who were already taking cholesterol-lowering drugs didn't actually need them based on the Apo-B test. For the researchers, the most worrisome group was people with low LDL and high Apo-B: These people are at very high risk due to the type of LDL they have, but a cholesterol check wouldn't detect their danger. Apo-B is also easier to measure since patients don't have to fast before blood is drawn.

The Numbers:
Normal range: 55–150 mg/dL

How the Healthy Heart Miracle Diet Helps

Just like the LDL cholesterol it transports, Apo-B levels will decrease as you eat more high-quality complex carbohydrates, healthy fats, and fruits and vegetables, and as you begin to build in more activity to your daily life, all of which you'll do on the Healthy Heart

Miracle Diet. And losing weight can help you shift more of your bad cholesterol particles from small (dangerous) to large (more benign).

The other bad fat in your blood:

Triglycerides

Eat too much and the extra calories are converted into blood fats called triglycerides, which are eventually sent to your fat cells for storage. If your triglyceride levels are high, some will be sent to the liver, where it's converted into "bad" cholesterol. Triglycerides aren't a form of cholesterol, though they do make up a part of your overall cholesterol count: A fifth of your total triglycerides is added to LDL and HDL to arrive at the final count. They're also shuttled around on the same "ferries" that carry cholesterol, so it's hard to consider one without considering the other.

For decades, heart experts didn't worry much about triglycerides. Their levels fluctuate wildly depending on what you eat and drink, and research has been mixed on whether the fats actually contribute to heart disease and stroke. One analysis of 29 studies found that having consistently high levels could be linked to a 70 percent increase in the risk of heart trouble. But when the researchers tried to separate the risk increase from that caused by high cholesterol and low HDL levels, the exact threat posed by triglycerides was less clear. That may be because, typically, when your triglycerides are high, so are your LDL levels and your blood pressure. Very few people have high triglycerides and no other heart-disease risk factors.

Still, even small increases in triglycerides could indicate that you're at an increased risk for heart disease as well as diabetes. Being overweight or obese can increase levels; so can drinking too much alcohol or eating too many simple carbohydrates (which also lowers "good" HDL cholesterol). In fact, if your diet contains more than 60 percent carbohydrates from any source, you're more likely to have high triglycerides. Being sedentary and smoking also cause your levels of these blood fats to increase.

Eating too many simple carbohydrates can increase your triglyceride levels and lower your "good" HDL.

A small percentage of people suffer from genetically determined high levels of triglycerides. This is rarely something you have to worry about; your doctor will help you decide whether treatment is necessary. Conditions such as diabetes, hypothyroidism, and kidney disease have also been linked with high triglyceride levels, as have certain medications such as oral contraceptives.

The Numbers:
Normal: Less than 150 mg/dL (1.67 mmol/L)
Borderline-High: 150 (1.67 mmol/L) – 199 mg/dL (2.21 mmol/L)

High: 200 (2.22 mmol/L) – 499 mg/dL (5.54 mmol/L)
Very High: 500 mg/dL (5.55 mmol/L)

How the Healthy Heart Miracle Diet Helps

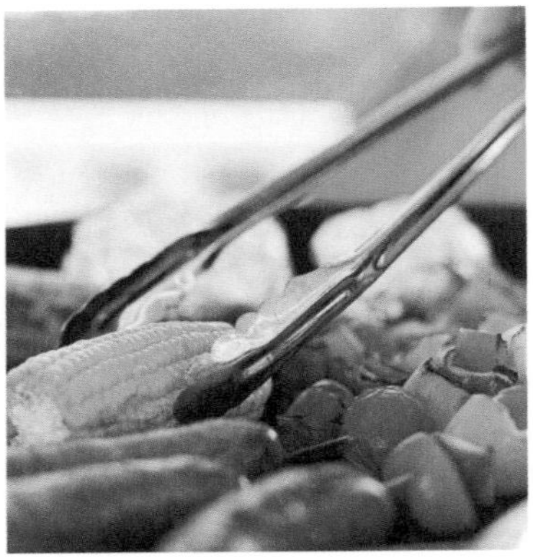

When you swap out refined, simple sugars for quality carbohydrates, your triglycerides will begin dropping almost immediately. And many people who stop eating all the carbohydrates required by the typical low-fat diet (as opposed to the higher-fat Healthy Heart Miracle Diet) will bring their triglyceride counts under control in no time at all. In 2003, the *New England Journal of Medicine* published a study that found that when overweight people followed a low-carbohydrate diet, their triglycerides dropped significantly; whereas people on a low-fat, high-carb diet saw their levels rise. (The low-carb group also lost about 9 more pounds (4.5 kg) over a 6-month period—13 pounds/6.5 kg versus 4 pounds/2 kg.) In the study, people who were diabetic found that a low-carbohydrate diet dramatically improved the way insulin managed blood sugar; the low-fat dieters got no such improvement.

The increased activity you'll get by following the Healthy Heart Miracle Diet will also help tame those blood fats. And if you drop some extra pounds thanks to these changes, your triglycerides will become less of a concern.

What's Your Risk for Heart Attack or Stroke? quiz

Give yourself the number of points indicated for each "yes" answer. Don't give yourself any points if your answer is "no."

1. Are you male? +2

2. Have you ever been diagnosed with a heart condition? +2

3. Has anyone in your family ever been diagnosed with a heart condition? +2

4. Got a calculator? Find your body mass index (BMI). First, multiply your weight in pounds by 703. Divide the result by your height in inches. Then divide the answer again by your height in inches. The result is your BMI. For example, if you're 5'6" (66 inches) tall and weigh 145 pounds, you have a BMI of 23.4 ($145 \times 703 = 101{,}935 \div 66 = 1{,}544.47 \div 66 = 23.4$)

Is the number between 25 and 29.9 (overweight category)? +1

Is the number 30 or higher (obese category)? +3

5. Measure your waist circumference (measured just above your belly button):

Women: Is your waist more than 35 inches (88 cm)? +2

Men: Is your waist more than 40 inches (102 cm)? +4

6. Do you have high blood pressure (greater than 140/90 mmHg)? +2

7. Do you have diabetes or high blood sugar (greater than 126 mg/dL on a fasting glucose test)? +2

8. Is your total cholesterol above 200 mg/dL (2.22 mmol/L)? +2

9. Is your HDL cholesterol less than 40 mg/dL (1.0 mmol/L) for men or less than 50 mg/dL (1.25 mmol/L) for women? +2

10. Do you eat fish at least two times a week? -2

11. Do you get at least five servings of fruits and vegetables a day? (A serving is one medium-size fruit, 1 cup (250 ml) of raw leafy vegetables, or a 1/2 cup (125 ml) of chopped or cooked vegetables.) -2

12. Do you get at least three servings of whole grains daily? (A serving is roughly 1 slice of bread, 1 cup of breakfast cereal, or ½ cup of cooked cereal, rice, or pasta.) -2

13. Do you eat three servings of nuts a week? A serving is 1 ounce (30 g)—about what would fit in the palm of your hand. -1

14. Do you eat butter, red meat, or whole (3.25%) milk two or more times a day? +1

15. Do you eat store-bought baked goods or fried fast foods on most days? +1

16. Do you use vegetable or olive oil for salad dressing or cooking daily? -1

17. Do you have an alcoholic drink once or twice a day? -2

18. Do you smoke? +1 (If you smoke more than a pack a day: +3)

19. If you're a former smoker, did you quit less than 10 years ago? +1

20. Are you regularly around secondhand smoke? +1

21. Do you exercise 30 minutes a day, or 3 hours a week? -2

Your Score

Add up your total points. The lower your number, the lower your risk for heart disease.

MEN

Very high risk Greater than 18

High risk 10-17

Moderate risk 4-9

Low risk Less than 3

WOMEN

Very high risk Greater than 17

High risk 10-16

Moderate risk 4-9

Low risk Less than 3

SOURCE: Adapted from the heart disease questionnaire at www.yourdiseaserisk.wustl.edu © Siteman Cancer Center at Barnes-Jewish Hospital and Washington University School of Medicine.

3

Is Being Fat So Bad?

Pursuing an active, healthy lifestyle is critically important no matter how much you weigh. Stunning research indicates that being overweight but active is better for your health than being a thin couch potato.

If you weigh too much, any doctor worth her salt will tell you to shed some pounds. It's a no-brainer. And yes, maintaining a healthy weight is certainly very good for your heart and your overall health. But as with the story behind cholesterol and heart disease, the story behind weight and heart disease isn't quite as straightforward as it once seemed. It turns out that being fit, or at least physically active, may be more important than being thin.

If the idea that you can be overweight and healthy seems hard to swallow, consider this: In 2008, a survey of the U.S. population published in the journal *Archives of Internal Medicine* indicated that half of the Americans who are considered overweight in terms of their body mass indexes (BMI) have no major risk factors for heart disease, other than the supposed disadvantage of being overweight. They have low LDL ("bad" cholesterol) and high HDL ("good" cholesterol), healthy blood sugar levels (which means a low risk of diabetes), normal blood pressures, and only modest amounts of visceral fat, the fat that accumulates deep in the abdomen, surrounding the internal organs and greatly increasing the risk for heart disease. Surprising? Yes. But not inexplicable. The key thing most of them share in common is an active, healthy lifestyle. Despite carrying some extra pounds, they get out there and exercise, and they try to eat well. Amazingly, what this means is that making the effort to lose weight can be just as beneficial as really losing it.

It also means that not making the effort to eat right and exercise can be dangerous even for people who aren't overweight. In fact, cardiologists at the Mayo Clinic found something shocking when they looked at a group of people whose BMIs were normal but whose cholesterol counts were risky and whose blood sugar control was poor: These "normal weight" people were clinically obese according to another measure, their percentage of body fat. At least a third of their bodies consisted of fat! Even worse, they typically carried the extra fat in their midsections, as deadly visceral fat.

Making the effort to lose weight can be just as beneficial as really losing it.

The researchers pointed to sedentary lifestyles and poor diets as the likely culprits. Lack of exercise would certainly explain the amount of visceral fat these "secretly fat" people carry: Because this fat is so metabolically active, it's among the first to shrink when you start exercising. How is it possible to carry so much visceral fat and still have a normal BMI? It's simple: Muscle weighs more than fat, and this group, the researchers found, had low muscle mass, which was replaced by fat.

None of this is news to Steven Blair, MD, a weight researcher who for years worked with the Cooper Clinic in Dallas, an institute devoted to research on aerobic exercise and weight loss, to tease out the real dangers of being overweight and how exercise might lower those risks. For 30 years, he has been publishing results suggesting that we're focused on the wrong problem. Dr. Blair has tracked more than 80,000 people, measuring their fitness levels and their weight and height, and found that thin and normal-weight people who don't exercise are twice as likely to suffer heart disease, stroke, or an early death due to other causes as overweight people who exercise regularly. And the overweight people who exercise? Their markers of heart health are to be envied: normal cholesterol, high HDL, healthy blood pressures, excellent waist-to-hip ratios. By nearly every measure but one—weight—they are healthy. That's why Dr. Blair, a self-described stocky man himself, would argue that weight, in the company of an otherwise healthy lifestyle, isn't nearly as harmful as the world would have you think.

Thin people who don't exercise are twice as likely to suffer heart disease as overweight people who do.

Any Effort Goes a Long Way

In the Healthy Heart Miracle Diet, the focus is less on changing your weight than on living a healthy life. Rather than you obsessing over the scale (or food, or anything else for that matter), you'll learn simple, enjoyable ways to take pleasure in healthier meals and work more physical activity into your everyday life. Whether or not you lose any weight, every walk you take, every fish meal you eat, every apple you snack on will bring you one step closer to good heart health.

In the Healthy Heart Miracle Diet, the focus is less on changing your weight than on living a healthy life.

Incidentally, you can stop searching for the perfect diet. Bottom line: Despite the hype over every new diet that comes along, the truth is, you can lose weight on just about any plan (though some are more enjoyable—and easier to stick to—than others). Over the last decade, researchers have pitted various weight-loss plans against each other in a number of studies, some running for 6 months, others lasting as long as 6 years. For all their time and effort, they discovered no difference between the competing approaches: Atkins, Ornish, low-fat, low-carb, Paleolithic, and South Beach all came out about even in terms of pounds shed. There was some evidence that a low-carbohydrate/higher protein approach did offer a slight advantage, but even on that plan, dieters lost an average of only 12 pounds (6 kg) over a year-and-a-half.

That may sound depressing, but there's a silver lining that often goes overlooked: Any weight loss at all—or even maintaining your current weight—that comes from good eating habits and getting regular exercise is *very* good for your heart and overall health. Several studies have indicated that losing 10 percent of your body weight confers most of the health benefits that a normal-weight person enjoys, even if you started out overweight and you're still in that category. Even losing just 10 pounds (5 kg) can result in a significant decrease in blood pressure and heart-disease risk.

Again, the important goal is a healthy lifestyle, one that you can sustain not for a week or month or even a year but over a lifetime. Happily, the dietary recommendations in the Healthy Heart Miracle Diet are easy to follow. Unlike low-fat, high-carb diets, it allows plenty of fat to keep you satisfied and plenty of protein to keep you

Are You Secretly Fat?

Get out a soft tape measure—the kind tailors use—to find out. Relaxing your belly, place the tape measure just above your belly button and wrap it around your body so that it's taut but not squeezing you in. If you carry a lot of visceral fat, your waistline will likely be more than 40 inches (102 cm) for men and more than 35 inches (88 cm) for women.

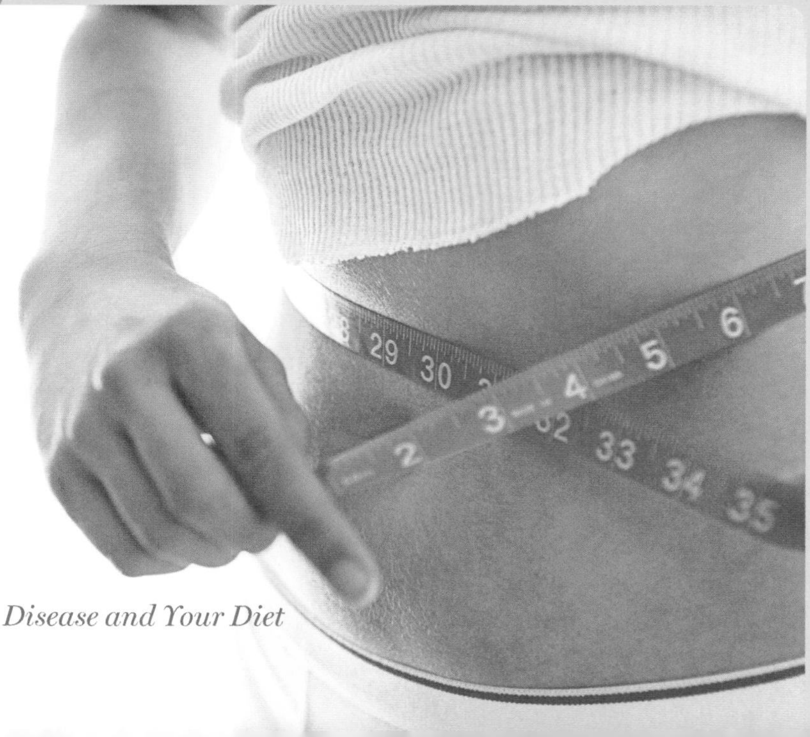

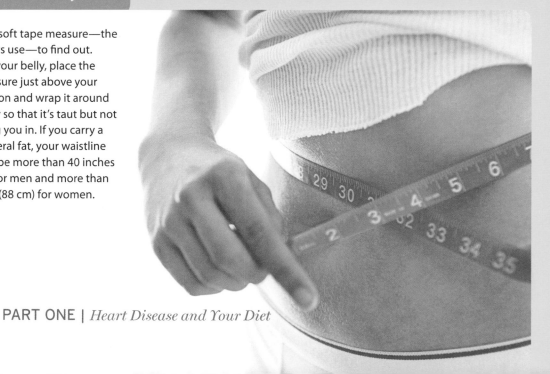

Could a Few Extra Pounds Actually Protect You?

If you're having trouble losing weight, here's one finding that should let you rest easier. A 2005 study published in the *Journal of the American Medical Association* analyzed mortality data of people in different weight categories and found that there were fewer early deaths among overweight people than in any other weight group, including the normal-weight folks. That's right: The overweight group outlasted the thin, the normal, and the obese.

When the researchers analyzed what killed the subjects in the study, they found that the overweight group was no more likely to die of heart disease, cancer, or diabetes than the normal-weight group (who were the second healthiest, followed by obese, and then the underweight crew). Though no one's sure why, one explanation is that some of the thin people in the study may have been thin because of a developing but undiagnosed disease such as cancer. It's possible that at the end of life, having some extra padding can help you weather a hospital stay and get back on your feet. Or maybe it's that people who carry a few too many pounds may be prompted to pay more attention to what they eat and how often they exercise. At any rate, it seems that a little "insulation" isn't an automatic death sentence.

full. By cutting back on refined and sugary carbohydrates, you'll find that you have far fewer food cravings. If you are trying to shed pounds, know that it's much easier to sustain weight loss if you're getting some exercise on most days, which you'll do on this plan (no gym membership required—all you need are some decent walking shoes). You'll also find plenty of research-proven weight-loss techniques in later chapters. And, of course, more than 100 delicious recipes to help you put the eating advice into action.

4

Why Not Just Pop a Pill?

If cholesterol isn't the sole culprit behind heart attacks, then cholesterol-lowering drugs can't be the sole solution. Even aspirin isn't a cure-all. But up to 80 percent of heart disease cases can be prevented through modest lifestyle changes like eating better and exercising.

Swallowing a pill is so simple that it's nearly everyone's favorite fix for whatever ails them. Why hit the treadmill or dine on salmon instead of bacon cheeseburgers when modern medicine can make up for a poor diet and lack of activity? That's simple: Because it can't.

While drugs do save countless lives—and it's important to take the medications your doctor has prescribed—what many people fail to understand is that the promise of a pill often outstrips the reality.

Lifestyle Trumps Medicine

For starters, there's only so much damage a drug can undo. Once gunky plaque has built up in your arteries and high blood pressure has thoroughly stressed your heart and blood vessels, drugs will provide only so much insurance against a heart attack or stroke. No drug can make hardened arteries more pliable or wash away existing plaque. While medications can help prevent these problems from getting worse, they can't actually reverse heart disease. That's something only you can accomplish by making tweaks—delicious ones if you follow our plan!—to your diet and getting yourself off the couch and out of your chair.

Follow the Healthy Heart Miracle Diet approach to eating and daily exercising (as little as a walk around the block) and you may drop your blood pressure several points beyond what you can expect from medication, raise your "good" HDL cholesterol, and improve your body's ability to use insulin (which lowers your risk of diabetes), not to mention boost your mood, lower your stress, and help you sleep better at night.

There's only so much damage a drug can undo.

Even if pills do save you from a heart disease disaster, they all come with caveats. Just finding the medication that works for your particular risk factors takes some trial and error. Then there are side effects, most of which are mild but some of which can be serious.

The truth is, certain drugs can plain old make you feel worse. For instance, beta blockers, used to lower blood pressure and slow the heart rate so the heart needs less oxygen, can make you feel tired or even depressed. Many drugs used to lower blood pressure can make you feel dizzy. Others can give you a dry mouth or upset your stomach. And, of course, pharmaceutical companies aren't exactly giving their products away; depending on your needs, you can spend a big chunk of your monthly income on medications.

No one is suggesting that you run to your pill cabinet and throw out your meds. Far from it. Drugs that prevent clots, lower cholesterol, and bring down blood pressure are important weapons in the fight against heart disease, if you need them. But the battle doesn't end there. In fact, don't think of pills as permanent solutions; instead, think of them as stopgap measures that will lower your risk while you're making other efforts to do the same.

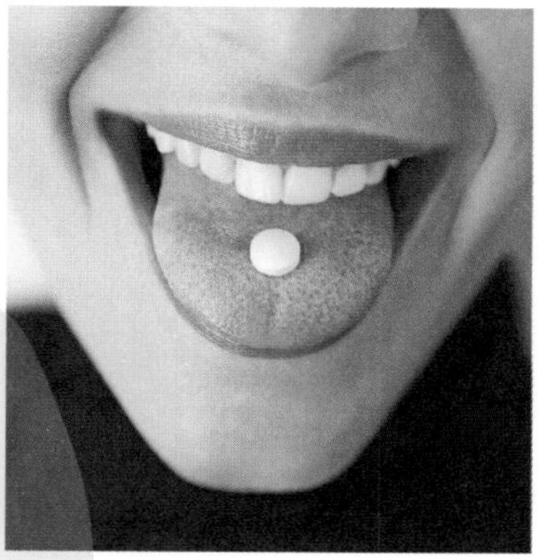

Can lifestyle changes really compete with powerful drugs in terms of lowering your heart-attack risk? The surprising answer is "yes." Several studies suggest that improving your everyday habits can lower cholesterol, blood pressure, and other heart risk factors as much as or more than medication. Research from the Harvard School of Public Health suggests that up to 80 percent of heart disease (and 90 percent of type 2 diabetes) could be prevented through modest lifestyle changes like eating better and exercising.

Don't think of pills as permanent solutions; instead, think of them as stopgap measures.

Research published in 2009 provides a nice illustration of how dramatic the benefits of a plan like the Healthy Heart Miracle Diet can be. For 8 years, German researchers tracked 23,153 volunteers between the ages of 35 and 65. They gave them each one point for each of four healthy lifestyle factors: never smoking, having a body mass index lower than 30 (this includes people who are overweight but not obese), being active for at least 30 minutes a day, and eating a healthy diet that featured fruits and vegetables, whole grains, and lean protein. The findings were impressive: People who met all four of the healthy criteria were an astounding 81 percent less likely to suffer a heart attack, and half as likely to suffer a stroke, as those who didn't. They were also 93 percent less likely to develop diabetes and a third less likely to suffer from cancer. Overall, their risk of developing a chronic disease was 78 percent less.

Improving your everyday habits can lower heart risk factors as much as or more than medication.

The healthy people in this study were not hard-core triathletes or carrot-munching vegans. They weren't model-thin, either—in fact, nearly half fell into the overweight category. All they did was find 30 minutes in their day to be active, follow a diet like the Healthy Heart Miracle Diet, avoid cigarettes, and maintain their weight. And the best part? This approach has zero side effects, unless you count a happier, healthier life.

Weighing the Risks and Benefits

Drugs save lives. There's little argument there, and some people—for instance, those who are genetically predisposed to very high blood pressure or cholesterol—will need to take one or more medications for life. There are dozens of different types of heart medicines used to lower blood pressure and cholesterol, stabilize heart rhythm, thin the blood, dilate the arteries to prevent angina (chest pain), and more. Here's the lowdown on three of the most common treatments—statins, blood pressure drugs, and aspirin—and what they offer.

it's a myth. STATINS ERASE YOUR RISK

While most statins lower cholesterol, they don't erase your heart risk completely. That's especially true for people with diabetes, metabolic syndrome, and low HDL ("good") cholesterol. Even on a maximum dosage, only about 25 percent of people will find that their heart risk drops out of the danger zone. That means that 75 percent of patients prescribed a statin will have to take extra measures—including making lifestyle changes and taking drugs that target different blood fats or high blood pressure—to bring their risk out of the red.

Statins

Statins are a stunning success story: They quickly reduce "bad" LDL cholesterol by blocking an enzyme in the liver that helps manufacture the sticky stuff. At the same time, they promote the manufacture of "good" HDL cholesterol. There's little doubt in anyone's mind that people with high cholesterol can benefit from these drugs. In fact, they reduce the chance of a first heart attack or stroke by 25 to 35 percent, and they cut the risk of a repeat occurrence by 40 percent.

Besides improving patients' cholesterol ratios, statins also seem to limit the oxidation of cholesterol in the blood. Oxidation occurs when cholesterol particles are attacked by unstable molecules known as free radicals. This process makes the cholesterol more likely to stick to artery walls. Statins also reduce inflammation in the arteries. In a recent Harvard Medical School study, people over age 60 with high levels of inflammation (based on a test for an inflammation marker called C-reactive protein, or CRP) who took a statin saw inflammation cool and their heart attack risk fall by 80 percent. Because of the drugs' ability to reduce inflammation, some doctors are even suggesting the drugs for older or at-risk people with normal cholesterol levels.

However, their side effects aren't to be taken lightly. Your doctor should monitor you closely while you're on this prescription. Several studies suggest that the drugs can slightly increase the risk of diabetes. Statins can also be hard on the kidneys of people who already have diabetes. Other side effects include muscle soreness or tiredness, and in rare cases the soreness can progress to a life-threatening form of muscle damage. Because the drugs are active in the liver, they occasionally trigger liver damage. Milder concerns include diarrhea or constipation and rashes or facial flushing. Although no studies prove it conclusively, some people taking statins have reported that their memory seemed to suffer.

There's little doubt that people with high cholesterol can benefit from statin drugs. But their side effects aren't to be taken lightly.

Doctors have narrowed down the groups who seem to be most likely to have problems with statins to women, people taking multiple cholesterol-lowering medications, people small in stature, people 65 and older, people with kidney or liver disease, and those with diabetes. But even with the increased risk, the drugs may still offer enough benefit to justify taking them; your doctor will be able to help you sort out the pros and cons.

Blood Pressure Drugs

Doctors usually prescribe a combination of medications to lower blood pressure. The frontline treatments are diuretics to trigger water loss. (They're similar to "water pills" that have been sold as over-the-counter weight-loss pills.) The pills are cheap but effective because they reduce the volume of fluid in your circulatory system, easing pressure on your heart and artery walls.

If your pressure doesn't drop enough, your doctor may prescribe an ACE inhibitor, such as enalapril (Vasotec) and ramipril (Altace), that helps relax the muscles that constrict artery walls or beta blockers, such as propranolol (Inderal) and acebutolol (Sectral), that slow your heartbeat. The good news is that one or more of these treatments almost always works: Your blood pressure will drop.

But again, there is a trade-off. Diuretics may cause the loss of important minerals like potassium and calcium, which help protect your heart, and you may need to take supplements to make up the difference. ACE inhibitors can worsen the trouble by causing further loss of potassium. Beta blockers may lead to weight gain, in part because they slow your metabolism. And because they keep your heart rate low, they can make you tired and therefore interfere with your efforts to exercise. Yes, your blood pressure will drop, but at the price of potentially raising other heart risk factors.

The more medicines you swallow, the higher the possibility that the drugs could interact badly with each other.

A bigger issue is that you're now taking a cocktail of treatments: The more types of medicine you swallow, the higher the possibility that the drugs—along with the vitamins or herbs you take—could interact badly with each other. Most doctors are very careful to track patients' medications, but the danger still exists.

Aspirin

It reduces inflammation. It eases pain. It makes blood platelets less sticky, preventing them from clumping together and forming clots that can cause strokes and heart attacks. Taking aspirin can potentially protect you against heart attacks and stroke in so many ways that swallowing a daily baby aspirin (for most people, a baby aspirin is just as effective as an adult aspirin) seems like an obvious choice.

But even at half a dose, aspirin can be hard on your stomach. It can trigger minor internal bleeding in some people; in others it can lead to stomach ulcers. And then there's the risk that if you suffer a hemorrhagic stroke (the less common type that leads to bleeding in the brain), the anticlotting properties of aspirin will make the bleeding much worse and the damage to the brain will be more extensive.

People with a history of ulcers or problems taking aspirin have always been warned against this therapy, even if they have a risk of heart trouble. But even those who can tolerate aspirin may want to think twice about taking it daily to prevent a heart attack or stroke. In 2009, British researchers found that aspirin therapy could lower heart-attack risk by about 20 percent, but it didn't protect against stroke. And the heart-attack protection came at a price: There was some indication that the very people who have the most to gain by taking aspirin also had the highest risk of developing gastric bleeding.

The bottom line is that if you've had a heart attack or a stroke, daily aspirin can help prevent a second event. But people at low to normal risk of a heart attack probably don't need it. If you're risk is higher, you might. Either way, talk with your doctor about the risks and benefits of aspirin therapy in your particular case. And before you start taking aspirin, be sure you're committed to it. People who stop aspirin suddenly can experience a rebound effect where they're *more* likely to develop blood clots and suffer a heart attack or stroke.

One final note on aspirin: If you think you're having a heart attack, after you or someone else calls 911, chew and swallow a regular-strength, 325-milligram aspirin. A study in the medical journal *Circulation* suggests that 10,000 more people each year would survive heart attacks by following this advice. The same is not true if you suspect a stroke: A small percentage of strokes are due to hemorrhaging, and aspirin could make the bleeding worse.

Could Your Future Be Medication-Free?

Could following the Healthy Heart Miracle Diet put you on the path to a drug-free future? It's possible, though there are a lot of variables to consider. Some of your risk factors for heart disease may be beyond your control. A family history of heart disease can mean that you'll always need the combination of a healthy lifestyle *and* medications to keep your risk out of the danger zone. And once you pass age 55, your heart risk can climb even if you're diligent in maintaining healthy habits. But nothing is inevitable: If you don't have a family history of heart disease or high blood pressure or cholesterol, you may never need heart meds!

People at low to average risk of a heart attack probably should pass on aspirin therapy.

Even if you're currently taking drugs for your heart, you may be able to transition off them if you're so motivated. Smoking, weight gain, sedentary living—these factors are all within your ability to control, and changing any of them can have a huge impact on your heart risk. If your desire is to be free of daily medication, talk with your doctor to see if the goal is realistic. At the very least, a concerted effort to eat better and exercise can make you eligible to take lower doses of your drugs.

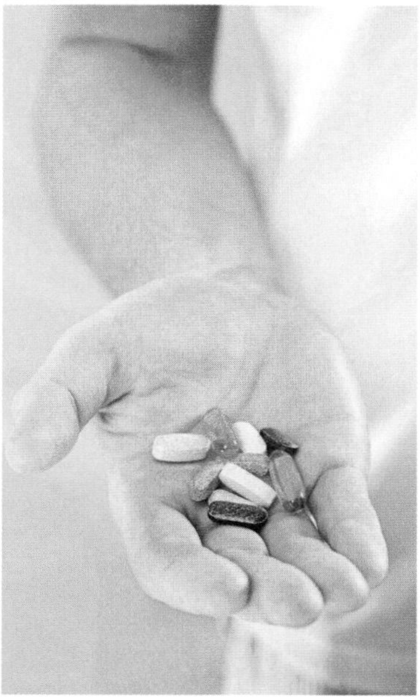

If your doctor thinks it's wise, set up a plan to taper off of your medications. You should check in with him every 3 months to evaluate your progress. Say that you're on blood pressure medication and your blood pressure is still in the pre-hypertension range (120/80 to 139/89 mmHg). Your first goal will be to introduce lifestyle changes to see if you can get your blood pressure consistently below 120/80 mmHg. (You can find blood pressure cuffs at most drugstores that will allow you to track your progress at home.) Once you've achieved that goal, you and your doctor can begin lowering your dose of medication while tracking your blood pressure to make sure that it stays in the normal zone. Keep it up, and one day you could wake up medication- and worry-free.

You can take a similar approach to weaning yourself off of cholesterol drugs. All it takes is commitment on your part and regular communication with your doctor. And the Healthy Heart Miracle Diet, of course!

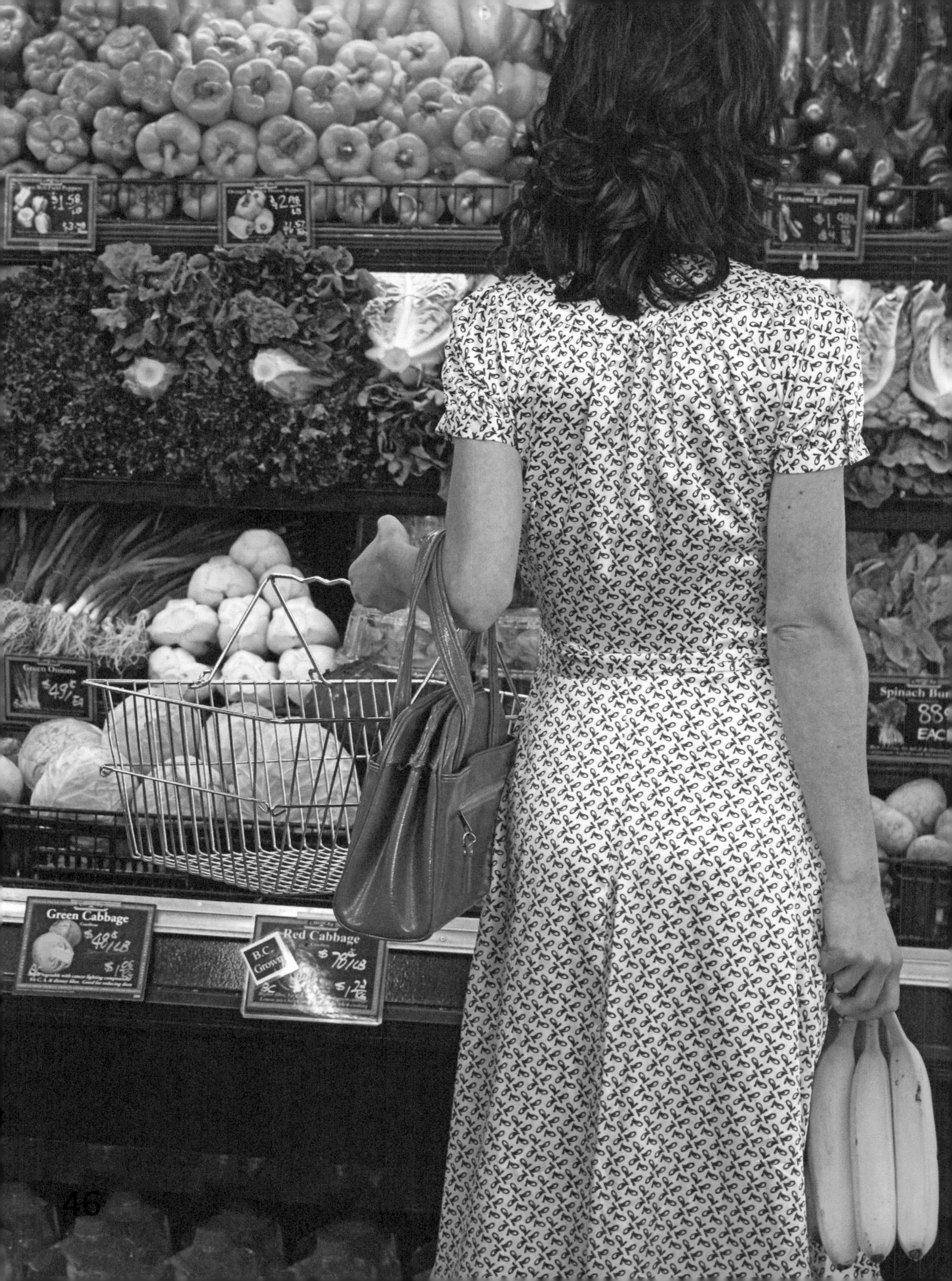
Green Onions
Green Cabbage
Red Cabbage
B.C. Grown
Spinach

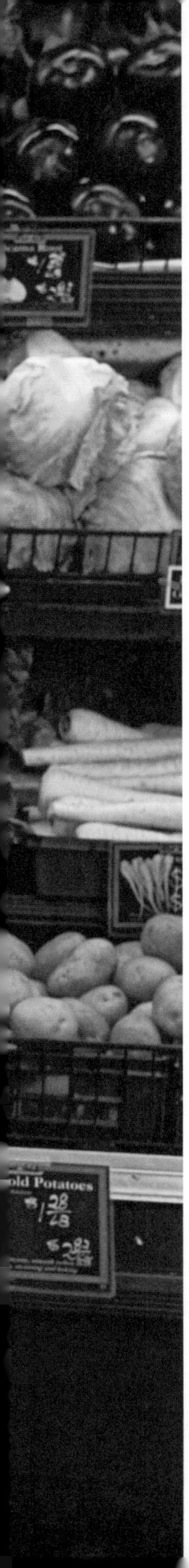

PART TWO

The Healthy Heart Miracle Diet

What to eat, when to eat, even *why* to eat: We make it all easy for you with delicious, natural, healthy food choices in just the right amounts.

5

The Miracle Approach to Everyday Eating

Before you change *what* you eat, you may need to change *why* you eat. Returning to the simple joys of eating real food to fill a hungry belly could be the most important dietary transformation you make.

Very soon, you'll read about the Healthy Heart Miracle Diet's simple but revolutionary three-step approach to eating a truly heart-healthy diet and significantly lowering your risk for heart attacks and strokes. But even before we get into *what* to eat, let's spend a little time thinking about *why* we eat. Because the truth is, if we all simply ate less to begin with, rates of heart disease would automatically begin to plummet. (Why don't French women get fat? It's simple: They don't overeat.)

Of course, we all eat out of genuine hunger, at least some of the time. And if that were the only reason we put food in our mouths—and if we stopped eating when we were full—we could pretty much say goodbye to obesity and diabetes, both of which ratchet up heart-disease risk. But these days, most people don't gravitate to the pantry or fridge because their stomachs are growling and their bodies are crying for calories. A host of other reasons drive them there—and once they arrive, all bets are off.

Ever had an overwhelming craving for a specific food, such as fudge-striped cookies or mint cookie ice cream? That's a sign that your emotions may be playing a part in your eating habits. What about an overpowering desire to eat something—anything—salty or sweet? That's a good indication that the modern food industry has taken over your taste buds and driven you to eat far more food than your body actually needs just to get your "fix" of salt and sugar. Both phenomena make it more difficult to lose weight and can thwart your well-intentioned efforts to follow the eating strategies of the Healthy Heart Miracle Diet. Learning to tame these urges will make it that much easier to choose the healthy foods and make—and thoroughly enjoy—the dietary changes recommended.

In this chapter, you'll take a closer look at two common motivations for overeating and ways you can control them. Begin by taking the quiz "What Kind of Eater Are You?" below, then read on to discover 1) what you can do to break free of hidden habits that are holding you back and 2) remember what it's like to want food—everyday healthy food—simply to fill an empty stomach.

What Kind of Eater Are You?

quiz

Many of us eat not out of hunger but for emotional rescue or to balance the extremes of flavors in packaged foods and fast foods. Your first step is to recognize what's making you head for the kitchen, the vending machine, the convenience store, or the drive-thru. Take this quiz to learn if you're an "Emotional Eater" or an "Extreme Eater," then read on to discover effective strategies for bringing your eating back in line.

Circle every statement with which you agree.

1. When I don't have much to do, I often find myself in the kitchen looking for something to nosh on.

2. A bag of chips just isn't satisfying unless I have a soft drink with it.

3. After a stressful day, or when I'm feeling blue, I often soothe myself with a food treat.

4. Whether I feel hungry or not, I can't imagine getting through the afternoon without a snack of some sort.

5. The dishes I make at home seem kind of flavorless compared to store-bought or restaurant meals.

6. I know my breakfast isn't all that healthy, but if I don't start my day with a sugary cereal (or toaster tart, or doughnut, or greasy breakfast sandwich), I just don't feel like my day will go right.

7. Eating fruits and vegetables is often a chore because they're kind of flavorless.

8. I typically eat at least one meal a day while watching TV.

9. I have a hard time drinking coffee unless I have something sweet with it, like a cereal bar or a doughnut.

10. Hunger strikes me suddenly, and I have to satisfy it in a hurry.

11. When my urge to eat hits, it's for very specific foods.

12. My cravings tend to be more general, like for something salty or sweet.

Your Score

Give yourself two points for every statement you circled, then tally how many were BLUE and how many were GREEN.

18-24 points: Both your emotions and your love of extremely salty and sweet flavors are dictating what, when, and how much you eat. You'll find the tips on the following pages very useful for exerting more control over your diet and food choices.

10-16 points: You're eating for reasons that aren't completely in your control. If you agreed with mostly BLUE statements, then emotions are likely undermining your healthy eating efforts. Mostly GREEN? Then it's a desire for extremely sweet and salty foods that drives your eating choices—and drives up your total calories consumed.

4-8 points: Not bad, but you're still making some eating choices for the wrong reasons. Check to see which color the statements were that you agreed with: Chances are, it was predominantly one color.

0-2 points: Congratulations! You're mostly eating for the right reasons, and therefore making the dietary tweaks suggested in the Healthy Heart Miracle Diet should be a breeze.

Emotional Eaters

Once upon a time, it was enough to have a meal taste good, provide sustenance, and not be too tough to prepare or clean up afterward. In other words, we were content to feed ourselves. But now we look to food to pick us up when we're sad, help pass the time when we're bored, relax us when we're stressed, and gratify us when we feel deprived. In other words, we feel compelled to eat at any moment, for any reason.

Boss yell at you? Have some candy. Late night and feeling lonely? You need some ice cream. Stressful week? A cheeseburger with fries seems the perfect solution. It's no surprise that we associate food with happiness and love. It's the centerpiece of nearly every holiday and special occasion. What kid's birthday is complete without cake and ice cream? Even a wedding isn't a wedding without the requisite multitiered confection. And every family has their must-haves at Thanksgiving, starting with stuffing and candied yams and ending with a choice of pies à la mode.

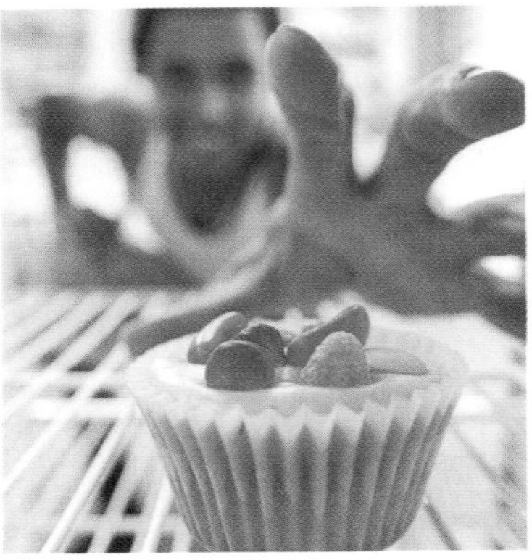

Those Darned Carb Cravings

If we craved spinach or carrots for comfort and joy, there would be no problem. But it's the sweet stuff and the simple starches—mashed potatoes, crackers, crusty white rolls—that many of us desire, and these foods aren't doing our hearts or waistlines any favors (much more on this in the next chapter). Why do we gravitate toward, say, macaroni and cheese instead of green salads? Thank biology. The simple carbohydrates in pasta, crackers, cookies, chips, and French fries trigger the release of serotonin, the same natural antidepressant that some drugs target to get us back on an even emotional keel.

Women seem especially sensitive to carbohydrates' mood-lifting powers. In a recent study at the University of Chicago, researchers offered women an "A" or "B" version of identically flavored fruit punches. Unbeknownst to the women, the beverages differed in one significant but undetectable way: One was high in carbohydrates, the other in protein. The women sampled each, and then the researchers conducted a long interview, asking the participants about sad or stressful events. Throughout this emotional Q and A, the women were offered a choice between the drinks: The more distressed the women became, the more likely they were to pick the carbohydrate drink. The women also rated the carb version as more flavorful than the protein one, even though an independent test panel couldn't distinguish between the two. Is it any wonder, then, that people often "self-medicate" with simple carbohydrates when they're feeling blue?

Unfortunately, overloading on those same carbohydrates shocks your system, paving the way for diabetes, inflamed artery walls, and the precipitous rise of triglycerides and "bad" cholesterol. And that's not all. You read in part 1 about the heart dangers of visceral fat, the stuff that pads the internal organs in your abdomen. One sure way to accumulate visceral fat is to eat plenty of simple carbs. They flood your circulatory system with glucose, or blood sugar, much of which is converted into fat that is stored in your midsection, coating and marbling your organs and raising your risk of heart disease.

As you'll read in the next chapter, scarfing down simple carbs also makes you hungry again in no time, causing you to reach for more food. It's a double whammy. And here's the rub: Like going on a shopping binge, going on a carb binge lifts your mood only temporarily; you may even feel guilty afterward for overindulging. And, of course, you'll want to soothe that guilt by heading back to the kitchen for still more of the bad stuff.

Like going on a shopping binge, going on a carb binge lifts your mood only temporarily.

Rx for Emotional Eaters

Changing the way you respond to stress and emotional trouble in your life is tough. Some experts compare it to a smoker trying to break the psychological cues that make him reach for a cigarette. Start by identifying the feelings that make you want to eat when you don't really need to, just as a smoker must look for the behaviors that make him reach for a cigarette.

One way to do it is to keep a notebook or pad of paper in the kitchen. After you put your food on a plate or in a bowl, take a minute to jot down what you're feeling before you take a bite. Are you anxious? Angry? Sad, bored, or resentful? Make a note of it, then eat. About halfway through the snack or meal in front of you, stop and write down how you feel now. If you're seeing a dramatic improvement after starting to eat, you've nailed down the emotions that are driving your eating.

Food can't solve the problems in your life. It can temporarily make you feel better—but so can other strategies. Below, you'll find solutions that can help you get through the moment of wanting to eat, after which you should be home free.

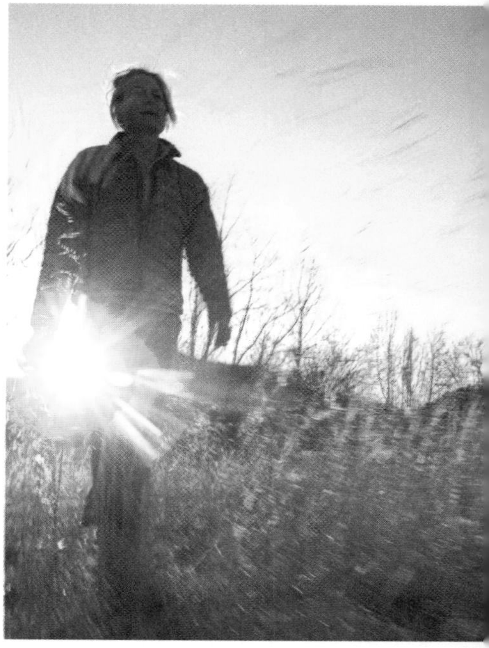

Go for a walk. If you're bored, stressed, or even angry, a short walk in the great outdoors will likely do much more for your state of mind than a bowl or bag of food. Chances are your craving will be gone or greatly diminished by the time you get back.

Chew gum. Sometimes what drives you to the refrigerator is just a need to move your jaw as if you're chewing something, and it can be satisfied by a chewing a stick of gum. Keep several packs of sugar-free gum around the house and the office so that anytime you feel the urge to eat, you can pop a stick in your mouth. You'll either quickly forget the urge to eat or the hunger will continue, signaling that you're genuinely hungry and it's time for a smart snack.

Photograph your food. Most cell phones come with a camera these days, and you can employ it to control your eating. University of Wisconsin-Madison researchers had 43 people take a snapshot of what they were going to eat before they ate it, and that simple act had a very sobering effect on their indulgences. When the participants looked at the photographs, they did a double take, realizing the portions were too big, that the meal lacked vegetables, or that the snack was something they didn't actually need. One of the study subjects said, "Who wants to take a picture of a jumbo bag of M&Ms?"

Don't eat to relax; instead, relax and then eat. When you come home from a long, busy day, chances are you may be tempted to grab crackers, chips—whatever's readily available to shove into your mouth—to "tide you over" until dinner. But a lot of this "hunger" is, in fact, nerves or tension. Next time, try this instead: When you come home, immediately devote 20 minutes to doing something relaxing. Play on the floor with the kids, spend some time stretching, take a warm shower, weed your garden, or pick flowers for the dinner table. Suddenly, you're not so starving, are you?

The same strategy works during the day. Anytime you feel stress pushing you to the vending machine or the fridge, give yourself a time-out. If you're sitting at your desk, try taking five slow, deep breaths. Count to four as you breathe in, and then exhale for a count of four while rolling your head and dropping your shoulders. You may find that pause to relax is enough to quell your urge to eat. If not, get up, get a glass of water, and take a 10-minute stroll. The water will satisfy your oral urge to put something in your mouth, and the physical activity will distract and relax you.

When you come home, immediately devote 20 minutes to doing something relaxing.

Avoid eating alone. Sure, sometimes it can't be helped. But if you plan to eat as many meals as you can with family or friends, you'll enjoy your food more, you'll eat more slowly, and you'll feel fuller afterward. Plus, the social contact will help tame stress, another source of emotional eating. Diet researchers have found that people who sit down for at least one meal a day with family (usually dinner) are more likely to be thinner, eat healthier, and have lower risks of major diseases like cancer and heart disease. (By the way, if your family sits around the television, the benefits are lost.) You may be less likely to overeat at your next meal, as well. Canadian food researchers had a group of people eat lunch either in twos at a table or standing alone at a kitchen counter. Although everyone got the same amount of food, at their next meal, the people who ate alone at the counter ate 30 percent more than the people who sat together.

Eat only at the table. There's a whole body of research that suggests that when you eat on the couch, at your desk, in the car, or standing at the sink, your brain doesn't always register the fact that you've had a meal, and that can lead to feelings of deprivation and overeating later in the day. Even when you're just having a snack, take the time to put it on a plate and then have a seat at the table with a glass of water or seltzer to eat. Taking time to get out a plate and utensils (or a napkin) will give you a chance to reflect on whether you're really hungry or just looking to satisfy some other type of urge. It also forces you to focus on the food you're consuming so it registers in your brain.

Measure it out. Don't let yourself eat anything straight from a box or a bag. If you want potato chips, put a handful on a plate, put the bag back in the cupboard, and then sit down to eat.

State your intentions. You're sad or lonely or bored, and you're about to tuck into a large bowl of ice cream. Okay, fine. But first admit what you're doing out loud by saying "I'm not hungry, but I'm going to eat this anyway." Brian Wansink, a food and diet researcher at Cornell University, has asked volunteers to try this method with great success. Simply taking time to think about what you're about to do may be enough to dissuade you from doing it. If it doesn't, the inherent contradiction in eating when you're not hungry—and admitting as much—should eventually wear down your desire for whatever food is your weakness.

When you eat on the couch or at your desk, your brain doesn't always register the fact that you've had a meal.

Say yes—to the right foods. When you're trying to change the way you eat, you can start to feel like you're constantly denying yourself. But with a slight shift in perspective, you can actually feel like you're indulging instead. Focus on a few healthy foods that you really like. Consciously remind yourself how much you enjoy these foods—then "indulge" in one of them when you feel the urge to eat. Think fresh blueberries in a bowl of milk, a spoonful of creamy peanut butter on a celery stick, a ripe juicy pear paired with a piece of sharp cheese.

Extreme Eaters

Over the last several decades, food producers have discovered that we all have a seemingly insatiable desire for sugar and salt. They've responded by stuffing our food with mind-boggling and heart-wrecking amounts of these substances. We live in a world where bottled pasta sauce can have more sugar per serving than vanilla ice cream. It's possible to get more salt from breakfast cereals than we do from French fries. This full-scale assault on our taste buds has the dangerous side effect of making us want more and more food.

We live in a world where bottled pasta sauce can have more sugar per serving than vanilla ice cream.

That's because processed foods place us on a flavor seesaw: We eat something terrifically sweet, and almost immediately we want to counter it with something salty. Part of what's happening is that sugar and salt are both distinct appetite stimulants; the scientific term for this is sensory specific satiety. What that means is that you can feel completely full from eating something salty, yet your sweet-related hunger sensors can still be craving satisfaction. (Sensory specific satiety helps explain how we're able to magically have room for dessert after a big meal).

Sweetness and saltiness also indicate to the brain that certain nutritional needs are being met. When sweet sensors are activated, your brain may register that sweet-related nutrients are being digested, such as the vitamins you might find in fruit. For nutritional balance, the brain may then activate nerves that communicate the need for salty foods. This plays out when you crave some jelly beans or a soft drink after eating a bag of potato chips. We are more likely to seesaw back and forth between sugar and salt cravings when we eat processed and fast foods because they're so much sweeter and saltier (sometimes in the same item) than more natural foods. A nectarine won't excite sweet sensors to nearly the degree that some candy or a soft drink will.

In a separate phenomenon, foods that contain high levels of both salt and sugar can trip satisfaction sensors in our brain that are similar to the ones activated in drug addicts when they get a fix. Think about that: Your fast-food breakfast sandwich is like a drug, as is your favorite peanut butter cup.

Rx for Extreme Eaters

If you've become accustomed to the salt and sugar blast from fast food and prepackaged meals, your biggest challenge will be retraining your overwhelmed taste buds to remind you how to taste—and enjoy—subtler flavors again. You'll be happy you did it: Within a few days of following the tips below and reining in your intake of extreme flavors, you'll discover that healthy food is bursting with a wide variety of flavors, not just sweet and salty. And savoring them all will go a long way toward satiating your hunger as well as pleasing your palate.

Extreme eaters need to retrain their overwhelmed taste buds to remind them how to taste–and enjoy–subtler flavors again.

Wean yourself off fast food. If you typically eat a fast-food lunch with a soft drink, start by having the meal with water or unsweetened iced tea. Even if you drink a diet beverage, make the change. The dramatic sweetness of diet beverages still flips the craving switches in your brain and can cause you to overeat.

Once you've adjusted to water, try substituting salad for fries. Most fast-food chains offer some sort of greens. The last challenge will be the burger, and it's a tough nut to crack. A fast-food burger is loaded with both sugar and salt. You could switch to a grilled chicken sandwich, but the sodium content is much higher than you'd expect—higher, in some cases, than in a cheeseburger. And at this point you might be ready to start packing your lunch instead. Make your own sandwich with turkey or lean ham, lettuce, tomato, pickle—and go ahead and throw on some mayo if that helps you make the adjustment.

Make your own dinner. The convenience of microwavable food is nice, but the price you pay is remarkable. Not only is it vastly more expensive to buy prepackaged food versus making a meal from scratch, the processed stuff is just loaded with chemicals and fake flavorings that you don't need. And although time savings is the one big reason people give for choosing prepackaged, heat-and-serve meals, that time advantage is mostly a myth, according to University of California, Los Angeles researchers. They tracked the time it took families to get takeout or prepare heat-and-serve meals and compared it to the time other households spent preparing home-cooked meals. The difference? A home-cooked meal took 5 to 10 more minutes of hands-on time, on average.

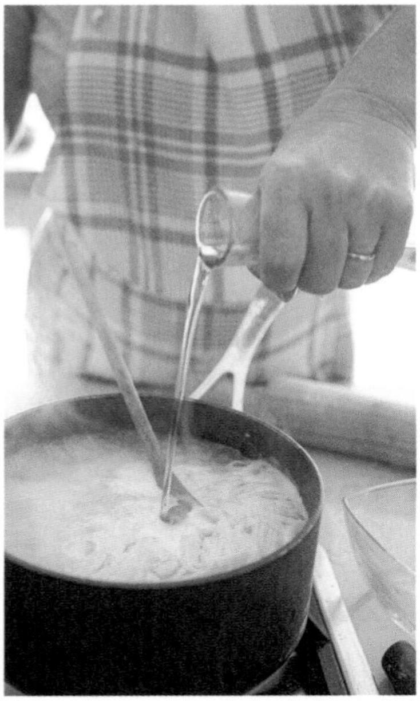

Start simple. For greens, buy prewashed salad mixes. Then look for easy recipes like this one for tomato sauce and pasta from noted Italian cook Marcella Hazan. Just open a 24-ounce (796 mL) can of chopped tomatoes and pour it in a saucepan. Peel and cut one onion in half and add to the pan, along with 6 tablespoons olive oil. Turn the heat on low and simmer for 45 minutes. Discard the onions, add salt and pepper to taste, and serve over the noodles of your choice. You will not believe how flavorful this sauce is, and it will encourage you to seek out similar recipes. (You'll find plenty in Part 4, Healthy Heart Recipes.) With a few simple meals like this committed to memory, putting a satisfying meal on the table becomes a breeze.

Add your own salt and sugar. You'd have a tough time dumping on as much as food manufacturers and fast-food chains manage to squeeze into their products, so you'll actually eat less salt and sugar this way. Try this trick: Buy unsweetened and low-salt versions of your favorite foods, then sprinkle on what you think is missing. The advantage to putting the seasoning on the surface of the food is that it will hit your tongue first, thereby reassuring you (and your brain) that you're getting the flavor you want. At first, sprinkle on as much as you need to satisfy your taste buds. But over the next few weeks, reduce the amount you add. Pretty soon, you'll find that you can get by with a fraction of the salt or sugar you thought you needed.

Buy unsweetened and low-salt versions of your favorite foods, then sprinkle on what you think is missing.

Substitute less-extreme snacks. For a sweet fix, have a clementine or tangerine instead of candy. They're easy to peel and easy to pack, so try taking some along with you to work or on errands. Need a salt fix? Try celery with peanut butter—again, you can make a few stalks in the morning and take them with you in a ziplock plastic bag. The less extreme flavors are less likely to send you chasing the opposite sensation.

Snack on one piece of dark chocolate. Not exactly a hardship, right? A study from the University of Copenhagen in Denmark found that people who ate dark chocolate, with its bitter-and-sweet taste, eliminated both their sweet and salt cravings in one go. After eating a bar of either dark or milk chocolate, study volunteers recorded their feelings of hunger and/or cravings for the next 5 hours. After eating dark chocolate, the volunteers reported no cravings, while the milk chocolate–eaters began to feel hungry and desire salty foods within an hour or two. The dark chocolate group also ate about 15 percent less pizza at a later meal compared to the milk chocolate–eaters.

Learn to enjoy just a taste. For some people, going cold turkey by quitting sugar altogether for a week or two is a surefire way to end their sugar cravings. Afterward, allow yourself to enjoy sugar in much more moderate doses. Instead of eating a whole chocolate bar, enjoy one of the individually wrapped single-serving squares of chocolate that are popular on the market now. Instead of eating a modern-size brownie (today's brownie recipes serve 8, whereas the same recipe from 1936 served 12), cut a smaller piece, and slowly savor every bite. With ice cream, try a single modest-size scoop—about the size of a golf ball. Focus on quality over quantity.

If a food isn't supposed to be sweet, a serving should have less than 4 grams of sugar.

Spot hidden sugar. If one of the first four ingredients in a product is sugar or some other form of sweetener, you're holding an extremely sweet product; unless it's a form of dessert, you'll want to pass on it. This is especially true for things that shouldn't be sweet to start with: Salad dressings, pasta sauces, soups, and peanut butter. Plenty of seemingly healthy products like yogurt, instant oatmeal, and smoothies can contain loads of sugar as well. If a food isn't supposed to be sweet, a serving should have less than 4 grams of sugar (check the nutrition label under carbohydrates). If it is sweet, still try to get less than 10 grams of sugar per serving. Sugar often hides on labels as white grape juice, dehydrated cane juice, honey, and anything that has "syrup" in its name or ends in "-ose" (such as dextrose or fructose) or contains the words "malt" (as in maltodextrin).

Satisfy salt cravings with nuts. You'll learn more in later chapters about how nuts play an important role in keeping your heart healthy. In the meantime, if you need a salt fix, try a handful of nuts instead of potato chips, popcorn, or fries. Yes, nuts can be salty, but the dose

it's a miracle! AN EASY WAY TO RESIST TEMPTATION

Is chocolate your weakness? Ice cream your downfall? Try this simple trick from psychology researchers at New York University. When you're tempted to indulge, sit down and write an if-then statement along the lines of "If I eat ice cream, then I will go for a walk." Simple, but according to the research, it works. The researchers asked 84 volunteers to either compose such statements or try to resist a food temptation in their usual fashion. People who wrote the statements were half as likely to indulge. Keep this up for 3 weeks—about the time it takes to make a new behavior stick—and you'll have conquered your weakness!

of healthy oils and protein they provide will satiate you and won't leave you hungry for more food.

Nuts in the shell are a nearly perfect snack. Shelling pistachios, peanuts, or sunflower seeds spreads out the amount of time it takes to eat your treat. That gives your brain time to register the calories you're taking in, and your snack will feel more satisfying just because you spent some time and effort in consuming it.

Make Every Meal a Feast

In some cultures, meals are wolfed down between other tasks. Even when these meals leave you full, they may leave you fundamentally unsatisfied. (Have you ever eaten lunch at your desk, only to forget what you ate an hour or two later?) Sometimes, we eat our food so fast, and focus on it so little, we don't even taste or enjoy it. In other cultures, mealtime is an experience that involves gathering around a table to talk, relax, socialize—and yes, eat some food. Not surprisingly, people in cultures that embrace the latter strategy tend to be thinner, with lower rates of heart disease. That's because relaxing and socializing are both good for the heart, as you'll learn later in the book—and because when food isn't the main focus, a smaller, healthier meal is all the more enjoyable, and you can leave the table happy even if you have a little room left in your stomach.

The take-home message: Any meal, almost regardless of what foods it contains, can be a feast if you eat it slowly and with people you enjoy. Embrace these strategies to making all of your meals more satisfying, no matter what you're eating.

Eat with others. This isn't always possible, but it's possible more often than you think. Does everyone get up and leave the house at the same time? Rise 10 minutes earlier and have the family sit down together to cereal with berries or an egg on whole-wheat toast. If you spend your day at an office, a lunch shared with workmates will be more pleasant and relaxing than one you eat alone at your desk. Most important, schedule dinner for a time when everyone can be there. Is "everyone" just you? Invite a friend or neighbor for a casual, come-as-you-are dinner.

Create a pleasant atmosphere. Take a look at your dining room or the place where you typically eat your meals. Are there places for your eyes to rest other than on your plate? Are there windows that look out onto nature or the street? Make sure the curtains are open. Adorn the walls with favorite paintings or photographs. And put out cut flowers in a vase every so often. Try playing some soft music. The more attractive your eating environment, the more likely you are to linger in that room, putting down your fork to look and listen.

Any meal, almost regardless of what foods it contains, can be a feast if you eat it slowly and with people you enjoy.

Set the scene for conversation. Turn off the TV and the cell phones; no reading material or earphones allowed. If your family is unaccustomed to conversation during mealtime, you can get the ball rolling by warning everyone that they'll have to share one anecdote from their day—funny, insightful, or mundane. And let the audience know that they need to be active listeners, querying the speaker about the details of the experience.

Put your fork down between bites. One of the biggest pluses to slowing down is that it gives your brain and gut time to register that energy is on the way. By taking your time, you give your body a chance to release natural appetite suppressants.

Warm your dinner plates. One hazard of lingering over food is the possibility that it will get cold before you finish. Keep food warm longer by putting your ceramic or china plates in the oven for a minute or two before you set the table. The oven doesn't have to be very hot—if you just put it at its lowest setting, say 175°F (79°C), and take the plates out as soon as the oven reaches that temperature, they'll be plenty warm. If you're using the oven to make dinner, save energy by turning it off when the dish is finished and pop in the plates for 2 minutes. The warm plates will keep your meal warm while you savor your food and company.

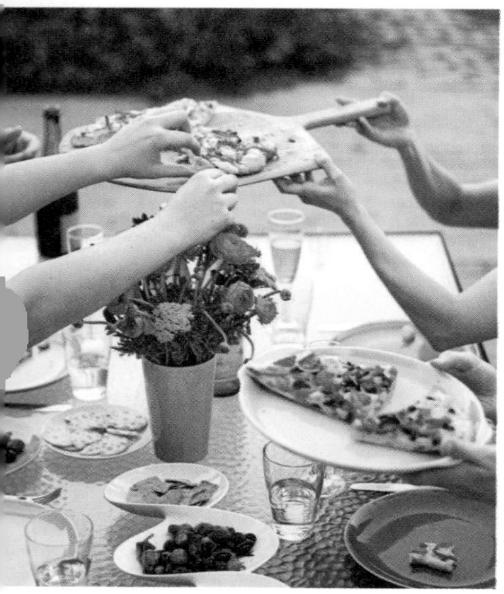

Serve hot food first, salad second. Another easy way to enjoy your food while it's hot is to have the hot course first, and serve a salad second. An advantage to reversing the order of your meal is that after one serving of the main event, you move to the low-calorie, bulky, and filling greens. That gives your high-calorie main course time to reach your stomach and register in your brain, helping fill you up with fewer calories. You're much less likely to want a second helping.

Looking Ahead

Once hunger—the basic physiological need for calories—is dictating your eating, you'll find it infinitely easier to choose the right kinds of food. These are the kinds of food shown by huge bodies of research to protect your heart and your brain from heart attack and stroke, so you can live long enough to enjoy countless more joyous, delicious meals around the table with friends and family.

If you start to cut down on sugary processed foods as a result of reading this chapter, you're already well on your way to achieving the goal of the next chapter, "Correct Your Carbs." There, you'll learn that by avoiding fast-burning carb foods that leave you hungry again in no time, you'll feel less hunger and suffer fewer cravings for the wrong foods, leaving much more room on your plate and in your stomach for the right ones.

One of the more gratifying aspects of following the Healthy Heart Miracle Diet is that food will end up playing a more reasonable role in your life. You won't be one of those people trying to find satisfaction in a vending machine or emotional fulfillment in a cheeseburger. (That's a lot to ask of a Big Mac.) In the following chapters, our meal-by-meal and snack-by-snack guidance will show you just how much enjoyment can be had from wholesome, nutritious foods. And the recipes in part 3 will have your family oohing and aahing, too.

6

Correct Your Carbs

Changing the carbs you eat could be the single most important step you take to lower your risk of heart disease. And when you cut back on "danger" carbs, you'll find that eating well—and losing weight—will suddenly be a snap.

It's no accident that your first step on the Healthy Heart Miracle Diet—and on the road to better heart health—is to fix what ails the carbohydrate portion of your diet. That's right: Correcting your carbs comes even before you think about touching the burgers, the cheese, and ice cream you eat.

That's because when you get the carb part right, the rest will fall into place. You'll find that you're less hungry between meals (and even *at* meals), that your cravings have all but disappeared, and that,

YOUR CARB PLAN at a Glance

1	Eat fewer carbohydrates in general—except for fruits and vegetables—especially at breakfast.
2	Replace simple, refined carbs, including "white" foods, fruit juice, and soda, with whole grains and produce.
3	Purge your kitchen of "danger" carbs to reduce temptation.

almost magically, it's easier to lose weight, not to mention lower your cholesterol.

For a good idea of what's wrong with the carbs we eat today, picture this common scenario: The alarm clock sends you stumbling to the shower. Then, if you're lucky, you have a chance to grab a breakfast bar or half a bagel, and maybe a glass of orange juice, before you begin your day. By 10 a.m., despite having eaten breakfast, somehow you're ravenous. And chances are, you're craving something sugary or heavy on carbs. Maybe you give in to a doughnut at work. But at lunch, again, you're starving. A sandwich on a big white roll or giant tortilla quells your hunger pangs, but at 3 p.m., your eyes are starting to droop and you doubt you can make it through. A bag of chips, a candy bar, and maybe a soda help you limp your way to the evening. But before dinner is even started, you've hit the snack cupboard because of cravings or a gnawing hunger and an alarming lack of energy.

Our love affair with "bad" carbohydrates may be one of the main reasons that people gain weight and develop heart disease.

Some version of this story—either the whole thing or some small part—plays out in many of our lives every single day. We gorge on simple, refined carbohydrates—including sugar, white breads and baked goods, and sweet drinks—and pay the price in the form of increased hunger, lack of energy, and a higher risk of heart problems. More and more, researchers are beginning to think our love affair with "bad" carbohydrates is one of the main reasons that people gain weight and develop heart disease. On the Healthy Heart

quiz

Can You Spot the "Danger" Carbs?

No foods are entirely good or bad. But as you'll discover in this chapter, consuming too many carbohydrate foods and drinks that digest quickly and raise blood sugar in a hurry can wreak havoc on your heart over time. Can you spot the 6 "danger carbs" on this list of 12 items? Some may surprise you. See page 62 for the answer.

1. 100% fruit juice
2. Multigrain bread
3. White rice
4. Berries
5. Baked potatoes (with the skin)
6. Fruit-filled cereal bars
7. Mashed potatoes without the skin
8. Pasta
9. Chickpeas
10. Rice- or corn-based breakfast cereal
11. Dried apricots
12. Popcorn

Miracle Diet, you'll break the cycle by learning to spot and avoid these carbs and replace them with carbs that will help keep you full and dramatically reduce your heart risk.

How Simple Carbs Wreak Their Havoc

Avoiding troublesome carbohydrates isn't as simple as saying no to doughnuts and cake. An innocent-seeming piece of white toast and jam at breakfast can be as bad as a glazed old-fashioned. The jam is loaded with sugar, and the bread—if it's made with white flour—may as well be sugar, given the way it behaves in your body. You prefer bagels? Your gut handles them the same way, speedily breaking down the simple carbs into sugar and pouring it into your bloodstream. Breakfast cereal? Unless it contains plenty of fiber, the results are again the same. Even an innocent glass of orange juice is mostly sugar.

Start your day with "danger" carbs, and you've essentially set your body at the top of a blood sugar roller-coaster.

Start your day with any of these or similar carbs, and you've essentially set your body at the top of a roller-coaster of dizzying ascents and plunges throughout the day. Your energy and hunger will spike and dip, and that will help keep food foremost in your mind as you go about your business. Your cravings will dictate what you eat for the rest of the day.

Why are simple carbohydrates such a concern? Your body quickly converts them into glucose, a sugar your body relies on for energy. (The faster and higher a serving of food raises glucose levels in the blood, the higher its *glycemic load.*) There's nothing wrong with glucose—unless a huge amount hits your bloodstream all at once. Then you have a problem on your hands.

Desperate hunger. A sudden spike in glucose causes the body to churn out a flood of insulin (the hormone that manages glucose) to move all that sugary stuff out of the bloodstream and into cells. The insulin works, and works fast, sending blood glucose levels crashing. This spike-and-plunge cycle can suppress hormones that help control hunger, tricking your body into thinking that it needs more calories. That's the reason you feel hungry again within a couple of hours of eating a high-carb meal.

The extreme energy rush you get from a big bowl of sugary cereal, a pile of pancakes, or a sandwich on a giant white roll with fries on the side can feel like an energy crash after your glucose levels have simply returned to normal. The sense that all your energy has been pulled out from under you often drives people to guzzle a soda or grab another quick-energy, high-sugar food. That's right, most likely your brain will steer you toward more sweet, simple carbohydrates. Then the whole process begins anew.

quiz

Answers to quiz on page 61: 100% fruit juice; Multigrain bread; White rice; Fruit-filled cereal bars; Mashed potatoes without the skin; and Rice- or corn-based breakfast cereal.

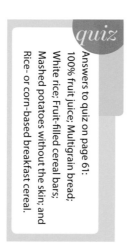

A bulging belly. The body usually keeps a 24-hour supply of glucose on hand in the bloodstream to meet immediate demands for energy. But a morning bagel supplies far more quick energy than you'll need to get in the car, drive to work, and sit at your desk until lunchtime. The rest of the glucose is sent off for long-term storage as fat, and a lot of it ends up in your abdomen as heart-threatening visceral fat. If you read chapter 2, you know where that story can end: with you in the hospital.

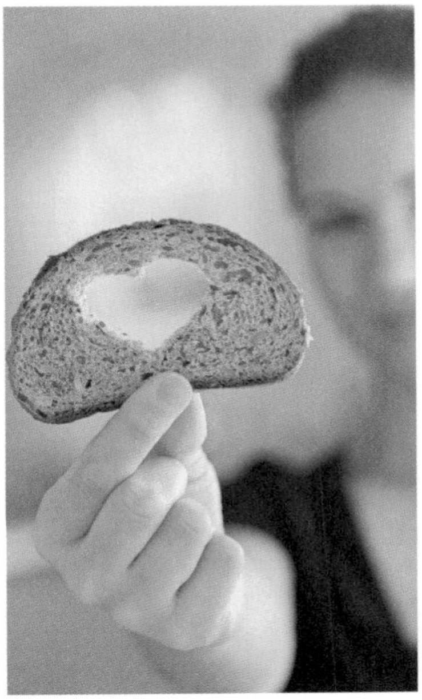

Inflamed arteries. Remember that healthy arteries are your body's best defense against heart disease and heart attacks. A steady diet of "bad" carbs put those arteries at risk, in part because it raises insulin levels. An unfortunate characteristic of insulin is that, like sugar, it is mildly corrosive to artery walls. In the amounts that most people need to process normal amounts of glucose, the corrosiveness isn't much of a problem. But repeated spikes in insulin levels cause a lot of wear and tear on arteries that can lead to inflammation and narrowed blood vessels.

When you consume too many danger carbs for days and weeks, months and years, the problem gets even bigger. That's because in some people, insulin stops doing its job as well as it once did, and the pancreas must generate more and more of the hormone to handle even small amounts of blood sugar. This phenomenon is known as insulin resistance, and it's an early sign of type 2 diabetes. More insulin equals even more artery damage.

Bad marks on your cholesterol tests. One hallmark of a high-carb diet is that it elevates triglycerides, blood fats that have been linked to higher risk of heart problems and diabetes. High triglycerides are also one of the five indications of metabolic syndrome, along with insulin resistance, belly fat, high blood pressure, and low levels of "good" HDL cholesterol. And, by the way, a high-carbohydrate diet—even one consisting of mostly good carbs—can drive down levels of HDL cholesterol.

When you begin eliminating the bad carbs and eating the right ones, almost overnight, the dangerous dynamics in your arteries shift.

The Healthy Heart Miracle Diet Solution

A diet filled with the wrong kind of carbs is clearly dangerous. A 2007 study of 15,714 Dutch women found that eating a diet loaded with simple carbohydrates increased their risk of heart attacks and strokes by 47 percent.

What's remarkable about correcting your carbs is the dramatic reversal in heart risk it brings. When you begin eliminating the bad ones and eating the good ones, almost overnight, the dangerous dynamics in your arteries shift: Inflammation decreases, and along with it, so do blood pressure levels and blood fats. Even better, your cravings diminish, making better food choices easier if not exactly effortless. The fat that has built up in your belly gets burned up for energy, and that spare tire deflates. It may take a few weeks or months for the biggest benefits to add up, but you'll start to see a difference in your appetite and cravings right away.

Purge the Bad

It's time to scour your shelves, read ingredient lists, and eliminate all the "bad" carbohydrates from your house so that you won't be tempted to take a ride on the blood sugar roller-coaster. The basic plan: If it's white (white bread, white rice, anything made with white flour), don't bite. Plan to toss or donate foods that fall outside the Healthy Heart Miracle Diet style of eating. And next time you hit the grocery store, stock up on the stuff you *should* be eating. Ready to get started?

Identify Your Danger Carbs

Everyone has a weakness that they turn to in times of a desperate carb craving. Yours might be mashed potatoes, French fries, a bag of barbecue chips, or crusty French bread. Identify your downfalls from the left column, and substitute them, one at a time, for the swap in the right column, which will satisfy that craving and won't lead to overeating later.

Danger Carb	The Swap
Mashed potatoes	Sweet potatoes
French bread	Real (bakery) sourdough bread
French fries	Sweet potato fries
White rice	Pearled barley
Sweet cereal or cornflakes	Whole grain cereal
Waffles, pancakes	Whole-wheat French toast
Bagels	Whole-grain English muffins
Dried bananas	Dried apricots
Fruit-filled snack bars	Fresh fruit
Soda	Flavored seltzer
Chips	Rye crackers

Bread

If you're eating white bread, you might as well be eating pure sugar, since the effect on blood sugar is similar. So let's begin with your bread box (or wherever it is you keep your bread). Take a look at the ingredient label. What's first? If it doesn't include the word "whole," you'll need to replace it, even if the front of the package makes the bread sound healthy with meaningless words like "wheat" (word to the wise: almost all bread, including white bread, is made from wheat). Without the word "whole" in front of "wheat," you're looking at processed flour to which some brown coloring may have been added. Multigrain bread? It doesn't much matter how many different grains a bread contains if none of them is a whole grain.

"Enriched wheat flour" also sounds promising, but is again a ploy: All flour at the very least is enriched with folic acid as mandated by federal law. (The folic acid helps protect against birth defects.) Manufacturers will often add back some of the nutrients stripped away by processing, but fiber is still missing and, without it, your bread is veering into doughnut territory.

Even if your bread is made from whole grain, check where sugar falls on the ingredient list. If it's one of the first four ingredients, that's too high; it means you're getting a substantial amount of unnecessary sweetener in your bread. Remember the sweet/salt seesaw from chapter 5? One way you end up bouncing back and forth between those flavors is to have them show up in unexpected places, like your bread. It's time to retrain your taste buds to appreciate the earthy goodness of grains in their naked state.

MIRACLE **ADVICE:**

- Buy whole-grain bread with the word "whole" in the first ingredient.
- Look for at least 3 grams of fiber per serving.

- The coarser the bread, the better. That texture indicates that the best parts of the bread have been preserved, including the flavor. Even whole wheat probably raises blood sugar more when it's finely ground than when it's coarser.
- If you see sugar in any form in the first four ingredients, just say no.

it's a miracle! THE WHITE BREAD YOU *CAN* EAT

If you can love a good slice of sourdough, you're in luck: The glycemic load of these loaves is on a par with some whole-wheat breads, and 40 percent lower than basic white bread. Look for a crusty, artisanal loaf—those are the ones most likely to use fermented sourdough yeast, which contains acids that slow the bread's digestion. Many local artisanal bakers are turning to old-fashioned methods of baking bread, using either fermented yeasts or organic salts and lactic or citric acids when leavening their loaves, and all of these methods seem to lower the glycemic load of a bread. Unfortunately, regular store-bought sourdough bread isn't the same; its sourness may be the result of sour flavoring.

Cereal

No surprise here: Sugar is the big concern. You're actually better off buying an unsweetened cereal and spooning on the white stuff yourself, because you would have trouble adding as much sugar as manufacturers manage to pack into the typical serving.

Nutritionists recommend that you limit your intake of added sugars—those that don't occur naturally in food—to 25 percent of your total calories, so that's a good guideline for your cereal. Multiply the grams of sugar per serving by 4 (since sugar has 4 calories per gram); the result should not be more than one-fourth of the total calories per serving.

Sugar isn't the only problem to watch for. If you favor cornflakes or rice cereal for breakfast, the relative lack of fiber can send your blood sugar soaring. (Corn and rice both convert to glucose very quickly in the body.) For a truly filling heart-healthy choice, look for cereal that is both high in fiber and low in sugar.

MIRACLE **ADVICE:**

- Look for whole-grain cereal that provides 4 grams or more of fiber per serving.
- Total sugar should be less than 25 percent of calories.

Pasta

Noodle-lovers will be pleased with this news: The glycemic load of pasta is fairly low—provided you prepare it al dente, which means the texture is firm and offers slight resistance when you chew it, as opposed to melt-in-your-mouth soft. The other way your pasta can pass muster is if it's served with homemade tomato sauce (or jarred sauce with very little added sugar) and plenty of vegetables like squash, broccoli, carrots, peas, bell peppers, and onions.

REMEMBER THIS

If It Isn't Supposed to Be Sweet, It Shouldn't Contain Sugar

One easy way to correct carb overloading is to scan ingredient lists for sugar in products that aren't supposed to be sweet. Spaghetti sauce? Salad dressing? Bread crumbs? Hamburger buns? Crackers? All of these store-bought items can be full of sugar in the form of high-fructose corn sweetener, honey (which is still a simple sugar), fructose, maltose, dextrose, sucrose—almost anything that ends in "-ose" equals sugar. Without too much searching, you'll be able to find options at your grocery store that aren't laden with sugar.

Interestingly, the thicker a pasta is, the lower its glycemic load. So farfalle, penne, fettucine, and lasagna noodles are better choices than spaghetti, angel hair, and spaghettini, for example. Any meat, cheese, or olive oil you add to your dish will slow the digestion of the carbs and blunt any blood sugar spike (much more on this important concept in the next two chapters).

If you want to get more fiber and stay even lower on the glycemic scale, give whole-wheat pasta a try. Yes, the texture is different, and the flavor is stronger. But many people like it, especially once they get used to it. Some brands are better than others, so keep trying until you find one that works for you. Or you can try one of the half-and-half pastas available: By mixing whole-wheat and white flours, noodle-makers have developed a pasta that cooks and mostly tastes like the one you're accustomed to, but that still delivers fiber and more of wheat's nutrients.

Want even more fiber, more protein, and a lower glycemic load? There are products on the market that aim to deliver. For instance, you can buy pasta made with Jerusalem artichoke flour for a truly low glycemic index. And some pasta companies have mixed the grains in their pasta to achieve higher levels of protein and even healthy fats. If you like the flavor, these pastas will add plenty of good nutrients and fiber to your noodle dishes.

MIRACLE **ADVICE:**

- Choose thick noodles over thin.
- Cook noodles al dente; don't eat them mushy.
- Switch to whole-wheat pasta or consider half whole-wheat, half white.
- Serve pasta with plenty of vegetables.

The Shorter the Ingredient List, the Better

Think about all the single-ingredient foods that are good for you. Broccoli. Apples. Carrots. Roasted chicken. Grilled fish. Then there are two-ingredient ones like oil-and-vinegar salad dressing, or spinach sautéed in olive oil. Choosing between different types of cereal? The best ones have a relatively short list of ingredients: Whole grain, maybe some nuts, seeds, or dried fruit, and a little bit of sweetener. By choosing foods with minimal ingredients, you avoid all the extra sweeteners, added salt, and multiple chemicals that alter flavor to the point where it's not clear what you're actually eating or supposed to be tasting. Simple foods taste good. We've lost sight of that with all the processed foods we're surrounded by. Eating something real will let you enjoy meals again, and they'll satisfy you more.

it's a *miracle!* VINEGAR AND LEMON KEEP BLOOD SUGAR LOW

Experts like to say that there are no magic foods, but new research suggests that vinegar and lemon juice come pretty close. Add just a tablespoon to any meal containing carbohydrate and it could lower the glycemic rating by 20 to 40 percent. Chalk it up to acidity, which seems to slow the digestion of carbs. Red and white vinegars can both pull off this stunt, though red-wine and balsamic vinegars are the types most likely to complement your cooking. A tablespoon for salad dressing (mixed with some olive oil) is a simple way to add vinegar. Many Italian dishes call for balsamic vinegar in the sauce. Lemon and lime can add flavor to numerous dishes, like chicken piccata, asparagus with lemon, fish with lemon, and lime in guacamole. No obvious way to work in these flavors? There's another source of vinegar in your kitchen: Tabasco, or any of the other similar hot sauces.

Rice

White rice may look like a grain, but in your body, it acts much more like sugar. Like white flour, it doesn't start white; only a rigorous milling and polishing can deliver those familiar milky grains, much in the same way whole wheat is converted to white flour. And, as with wheat, that processing strips away fiber and nutrients. White rice loses up to 90 percent of its heart healthy B vitamins, half of its supply of the mineral manganese (which helps the body convert protein and carbohydrates into energy), 60 percent of its iron, and all of its fiber and essential fatty acids. That's a pretty high price to pay for rice that cooks a little faster. Eating brown rice will ensure that you get all those nutrients, and you'll find it far more filling.

But even brown rice has a relatively high glycemic load, and it doesn't work with every meal. When you're serving vegetables or a chicken-and-tofu stir-fry, brown rice will complement the meal nicely. But on its own, as a side dish, you may find its nutty flavor and chewy consistency a bit too much. Luckily, there are some good options that won't jack up your blood sugar as dramatically as white rice. For instance, wild rice blends actually include some seeds and other grains that substantially lower the glycemic load.

You'll also run across so-called converted white rice. The rice is steamed under pressure before the husk is removed, and that forces some of the husk's nutrients into the center of the grain, preserving it for when you cook. As a result, converted rice does offer a slight nutritional advantage over other types of white rice. It's still missing all the fiber and essential fats of brown rice, but it has a lower glycemic load than regular white rice, so it's a slightly better choice.

MIRACLE **ADVICE:**

- Choose brown rice over white.
- When brown won't do, wild rice is a good side dish option.
- Keep barley on hand as a great low-glycemic substitute for rice.

it's a myth. YOU CAN NEVER EAT POTATOES AGAIN

French fries and most mashed potatoes are loaded with fast-digesting carbohydrates and can drive up blood sugar in a hurry. But you don't have to give up tubers completely. If you mash potatoes, leave the skins on. Baking them? Eat the outside, too. The potato skin contains many good nutrients such as vitamin C and potassium, not to mention fiber that slows down their digestion. Russet potatoes even deliver a wallop of antioxidants. They're also high on the glycemic load scale, but varieties such as new and red potatoes actually have a fairly low score and fit well within the Healthy Heart Miracle Diet. Sweet potatoes are another excellent choice because of their low glycemic index (despite their sweet taste). Another way to keep your mashed potatoes low on the glycemic load scale is to mix in some greens such as spinach, kale, or chard. Cook the greens first and mix them with the mashed potatoes just before serving.

Soft Drinks

Toss it all—regular, diet, even so-called natural soda pop. You don't need it, your heart doesn't need it, and your waistline definitely doesn't need it. More than any other dietary change over the last 40 years, the spiraling consumption of soft drinks can be most directly linked to out-of-control weight gain worldwide. Here's a prediction: Within the next 10 years, most of us will come to view soft drinks the way we view cigarettes—as a major threat to health.

Many obesity experts refer to colas as liquid candy, and the comparison is apt. In countries where soft drinks are popular, the drinks are the number one source of added sugar in the diet; citizens consume up to 50 gallons (190 L) of the stuff yearly. Besides the empty calories you don't need, there's another problem: The hunger sensors in your gut and brain don't register all of these liquid calories. In other words, you could drink hundreds of calories' worth of soft drinks and still be almost as hungry as you were before. Even if you opt for diet soft drinks, you're not out of the woods. When rats are given artificial sweeteners, they actually eat more food and gain more weight than rats that get real sugar.

Training yourself to expect the extreme sweetness of soda pop also dulls the flavors in food: The subtle yet rich taste of fruits, grains, and vegetables all pale by comparison. What's more, if you're drinking a lot of soft drinks, you're probably not drinking heart-healthy beverages such as milk and tea.

If you love cola, giving it up could be the toughest challenge you face in following the Healthy Heart Miracle Diet. But there is absolutely no case you can make for continuing to drink it if you care about your heart health.

Don't worry, you can still have bubbly beverages. Try seltzer flavored with lemon, lime, or fruit juice. Or switch to plain old water. Some beverage companies have done a nice job convincing you that water isn't good enough for your body, yet it's actually the perfect drink. After a week or two of switching over to these low-calorie, healthy alternatives, you won't look back.

MIRACLE **ADVICE:**

- Toss the pop. You don't need it and, soon enough, you won't miss it.
- Drink chilled water, unsweetened iced tea, seltzer with a few splashes of fruit juice, or seltzer with a spritz of lemon or lime.
- If you drink soda for the caffeine, substitute more-healthful coffee or tea.

Juice

Yes, fruit juice sounds healthy. It seems healthy. After all, it's made from fruit. So what's the problem?

Compared to the actual fruit, a cup of the juice can have as much as twice the calories but none of the fiber. The fiber in fruit is the reason fruit's natural sugar doesn't cause glucose and insulin spikes in your blood. Drink 1 cup (250 mL) of orange juice and you'll get 100 calories and less than 0.5 gram of fiber. Eat an orange and you'll get seven times the fiber (3.5 grams) and only 65 calories. Which one do you think will fill you up faster? Now take apple juice. The fiber is practically nonexistent, while an apple has 4 grams. And the juice has nearly twice the calories.

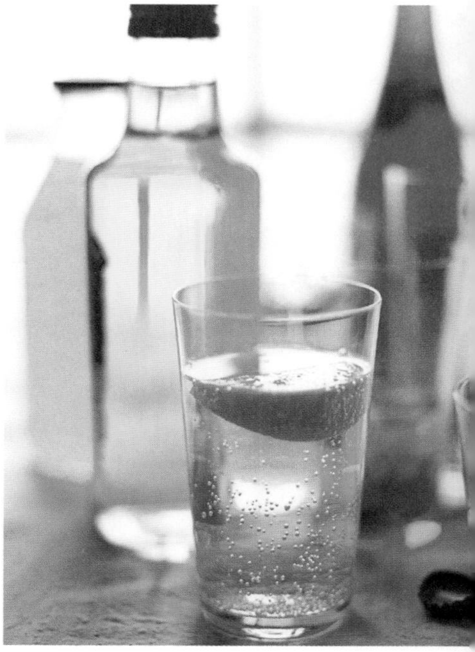

Like the calories in soda, the calories in juice don't satisfy hunger very well. One study found that people who drank about 150 calories' worth of juice or cola with their meals took in 105 more total calories, on average, than people who drank water. The problem is that your body deals with thirst differently than it does hunger. Whether you drink a glass of water or cola, the blood volume and fluid content of cells increases, and nerve impulses indicate that you're no longer thirsty. When you eat, it's the solids in your intestines and stomach that trigger the message that you no longer need food. Add calories to your fluids, and your brain will completely miss them. You'll end up eating almost as much as you would if you were drinking water.

You don't have to throw out your fruit juice, as long as it's 100 percent juice. (Juice "drinks" are, essentially, uncarbonated sodas: loads of sugar and loads of calories, with no redeeming value.) But do drink less of it. In fact, instead of pouring out a glass of high-calorie orange juice, think of using just 1/4 cup (50 mL) to 1/2 cup (125 mL) as a flavoring for seltzer. You'll still get that kick of orange sweetness and some vitamin C, and you'll be able to save calories for much more nutritious and filling foods. After a few days of drinking this concoction, regular juice will seem unbearably cloying. If you prefer straight juice, limit yourself to just 4 ounces (1/2 cup/125 mL).

MIRACLE **ADVICE:**

- Drink 100% fruit juice, but don't guzzle it. Stick to just 4 ounces (1/2 cup/125 mL) or add 1/4 to 1/2 cup (60 mL to 125 mL) of fruit juice to seltzer or club soda over ice.

Packaged Snacks

When we reach for a snack, most of us reach for carbohydrates—crackers, cereal bars, pretzels, chips. It's really no accident: These foods provide quick energy and, because they increase release of the feel-good brain chemical serotonin, they can temporarily boost mood—the two most common reasons we reach for a snack in the first place. There's nothing terribly wrong with having a carb snack (though you'll do yourself a big favor if your snack contains some protein), as long as it meets a few basic requirements—but many don't. The vast majority of the carb snacks we eat are loaded with white flour, sugar, or both. That includes a whole lot of snacks masquerading as "healthy," especially cereal bars and granola bars. Even pretzels, which diet experts once urged us to eat in place of fattier snacks, are pure white flour and contain more calories than you might realize.

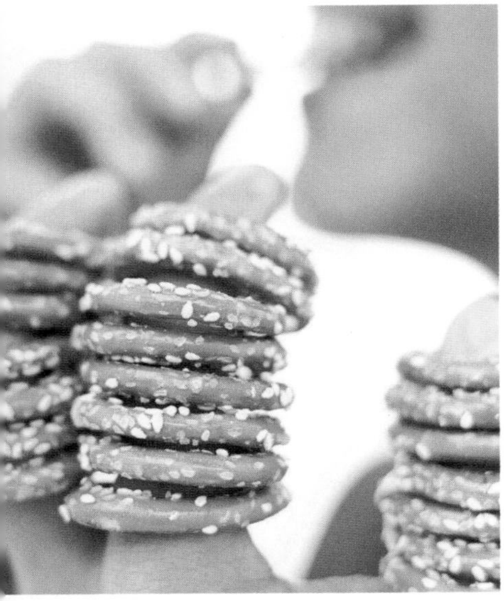

The best advice: Stop eating packaged snacks. Reach for fresh fruit, nuts, or cut-up vegetables instead. If you are going to eat crackers, snack bars, and the like, the trick is to find ones that provide fiber without a lot of white flour or sugar. There is a wide selection of baked, whole-grain crackers these days. You can also find whole-grain pretzels. (Hanover brand sourdough pretzels are made with real aged sourdough, lowering the glycemic load and making them a good fit for the Healthy Heart Miracle Diet.)

Chips are trickier. Corn chips tend to be lower in glycemic load and higher in fiber than potato chips, though you'll want to read the labels to make sure that you're getting real corn and some fiber before you buy. The same is true of pita chips, which also come in whole-grain versions. Chips even offer a surprise benefit over low-fiber, low-fat snacks: Their vegetable oil slows digestion (just make sure it's not hydrogenated oil). Since most chips are overly salted, look for low-sodium versions.

The trickiest part of any snack is making sure that it's something you can eat in a measured amount without wanting to go back for more. If you can't stop eating a particular snack, don't buy it in the first place.

MIRACLE **ADVICE:**

- Seek out carb snacks that contain whole grain and 1 to 4 grams of fiber.
- Limit snacks to 100 to 200 calories.

- Choose snacks that limit calories from added sugar to less than 25 percent of total calories. For a 100 to 200 calorie snack, that's 4 to 8 grams of sugar.

Add More of the Good

So, you're purging your pantry of refined simple carbohydrates. You're eating fewer French fries, muffins, bagels, and sugary granola bars. You're drinking less fruit juice. You've switched to whole-grain bread, whole-grain cereal, and brown rice. But where should the rest of your carbs come from? (On the Healthy Heart Miracle Diet, you're aiming to get about 40 to 45 percent of your calories from carbohydrates.) Read on to discover.

Fruits and Veggies: Have as Many as You Want

That's right, all fruits and vegetables contain mostly carbohydrates, though people tend to forget that fact. And you'll want to fill your plate with as many as possible. In fact, of the 40 to 45 percent of your daily calories that you should get from carbohydrates, at least half should come from fruits and vegetables. (Most of the rest will come from high-fiber grains and beans.)

Unless you've been living under a rock for the last half of a century, you probably already know the one unchanging truth regarding heart disease, high blood pressure, and stroke: Eating plenty of produce can dramatically lower your risk. Studies in Europe and North America have found that eating the amount of produce recommended in the Healthy Heart Miracle Diet can reduce your risk of heart disease by 20 to 40 percent and your risk of stroke by as much as 25 percent. Regular consumption of green, red, blue, orange, and purple produce can lower blood pressure and help ward off diabetes.

it's a myth. AVOID TROPICAL FRUITS

Mangoes, pineapples, papayas, and guavas are so sweet and rich that many people assume they can't be good for you. Yes, ounce for ounce, they can be higher in calories than apples and oranges, but the difference isn't enough to worry about. Plus, it's much better to get extra calories from fruit than from, say, potato chips. What's more, tropical fruit is especially high in nutrients that can protect your heart. Half a mango provides all the beta-carotene you need for an entire day, half of your vitamin C requirements, and plenty of B vitamins—and all of these are antioxidants that can help keep bad cholesterol from damaging your arteries. A serving of papaya delivers more vitamin C than an orange, and it's one of the best produce sources of vitamin A (in the form of beta-carotene) and potassium (which helps protect against strokes). Tropical fruit also contains respectable amounts of fiber to balance their sugar when it hits your digestive system.

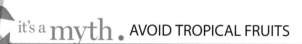

Fruits and vegetables do contain natural sugars, but those sugars come with plenty of other good stuff like vitamins, minerals, antioxidants, and fiber. Those vitamins and minerals can do wonders in terms of lowering your heart risk, and antioxidants help battle the process by which artery walls bulge, scar, harden, and develop plaque that can erupt and cause heart attacks.

Simply by adding more produce to your diet, you'll be taking a huge step toward correcting your carbs. Fill up on apples, bananas, carrots, and celery, and you won't need to remember much more about good and bad carbs, because there will be less room on your dinner plate for French fries and less room in your belly at snack time for chips or candy.

Simply by adding more produce to your diet, you'll be taking a huge step toward correcting your carbs.

Eating more fruits and vegetables is also your best way of getting enough heart-protective fiber. Fiber is a wondrous substance, especially considering that you can't digest it. It comes in two types, soluble (it dissolves in water) and insoluble (it doesn't). Both pass right through your system undigested. But they take their time wending their way through your intestinal tract. Along the way, they slow and even block the absorption of sugar, some fats (including cholesterol), and some calories. At the same time, the bulk they add to food convinces your gut and brain that you've eaten a substantial number of calories.

Soluble fiber is especially helpful when it comes to controlling blood sugar. When it does its dissolving trick, it turns into a gummy substance that serves as a temporary barrier between the starches in food and your digestive system. That barrier slows down the conversion of carbohydrates into sugar, allowing a gentle rise in blood sugar that helps tamp down inflammation in your arteries. That, in turn, lowers your blood pressure and your risk of heart disease. Barley and oats are excellent sources of soluble fiber, as are beans, but some fruits and vegetables are good sources, too.

Best Produce for Soluble Fiber

Brussels sprouts (1 cup cooked)	4 grams per serving
Citrus fruit (oranges, grapefruit)	2 grams
Pear	2 grams
Prunes	1.5 grams
Apples	1 gram
Broccoli	1 gram
Bananas	1 gram
Carrots	1 gram
Nectarines, peaches	1 gram

Currently, most people get less than half the daily fiber they need. Women under 50 should aim for 25 grams of fiber a day; those over 50 need less—21 grams daily. Men under 50 need 38 grams daily, while those over 50 need about 30 grams. Getting the recommended amount isn't easy unless you make produce a part of every meal and most snacks. Apples, pears, and berries deliver 5 or more grams per serving, as do broccoli, peas, and many dark, leafy greens.

For all these reasons, on the Healthy Heart Miracle Diet, you're encouraged to eat as many fruits and vegetables as you want—provided they're as close to their natural state as possible. That means eating fresh fruit and minimally cooked vegetables. It also means limiting canned produce (which is often packed minus the skin, an important source of fiber) and opting for either fresh or frozen to get the most fiber and nutrients. With most carbohydrate

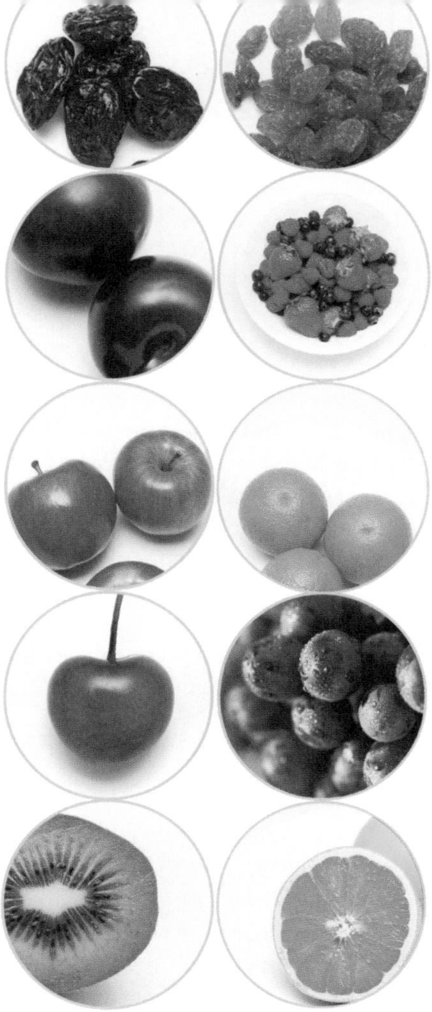

Top Antioxidant Fruits and Vegetables

Fruits	Vegetables
1. Prunes	1. Kale
2. Raisins	2. Spinach
3. Berries	3 Brussels sprouts
4. Plums	4. Alfalfa sprouts
5. Apples	5. Broccoli flowers
6. Oranges	6. Beets
7. Red grapes	7. Red bell peppers
8. Cherries	8. Onions
9. Kiwi fruit	9. Corn
10. Grapefruit	10. Eggplant

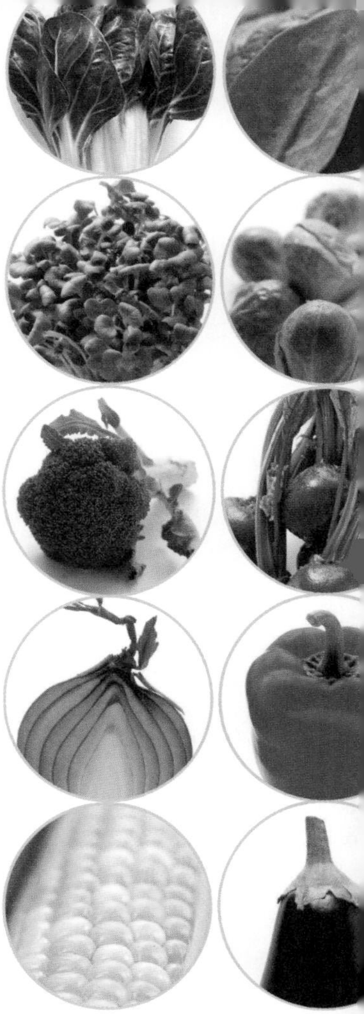

foods and even food in general, the more processing and handling a food undergoes, the more nutrients and healthful substances are stripped away.

What About All That Sugar in Fruit?

It's true: Fruit is naturally sweet. That's one reason we humans like it so much. The fiber is its saving grace and the antidote to those natural sugars, so, in general, don't worry about eating too much—*fresh* fruit, that is. Many canned fruits are packed in heavy syrup. All that extra sugar makes these products as bad as some types of candy. Dried fruit also has a higher concentration of sugar—and, as a result, calories—than fresh fruit since most of the fluid has been removed. But it still contains plenty of fiber and is a good substitute for the fresh version, with a couple of caveats. A full serving is just 1/4 cup (125 g) since the nutrients and fiber are more concentrated along with the calories. In nutritional comparisons, dried apricots and peaches come out as the most nutritious because of their mix of vitamins, minerals, and high fiber. Dried currants and figs also score well. Raisins are okay to eat but their glycemic load is higher than that of other dried fruits, so be especially careful to keep your portions small. Dried bananas are often coated in a glaze and fried, and are therefore best avoided.

Eat Your Fill of Low-Glycemic Grains

On the Healthy Heart Miracle Diet, you're avoiding white rice and white bread, in part because they lack fiber and in part because they digest quickly and send blood sugar soaring. Even brown rice and some whole-grain cereals, despite their fiber, can trigger glucose spikes (one reason we're going to ask you to pour only one serving of cereal in the morning). You still want to include plenty of whole grains in your diet, which are shown to lower blood pressure and reduce your risk of heart disease and stroke. The solution is to add some grains to your diet that might be new to you—but once you discover them, you'll wonder why you didn't eat them before.

Barley

It's not just for mushroom and barley soup! Pearled barley is a hugely underappreciated cereal grain and a smart addition to your diet, thanks to its low glycemic load. Even though it's had the hull, bran, and germ ground away, it still contains plenty of soluble fiber, which runs throughout the grain. It can substitute for white rice in many recipes. Use it in soups and grain salads instead of white rice, in

Not All Calories Are Equal

Same calories, same carbohydrates—but that's where the similarities end. That tablespoon of sugar is just adding empty calories to your cereal or soda. The fruit contains 8 grams of fiber to help ward off hunger and slow digestion, and antioxidants that block damage to your arteries. Plus, the berries taste amazing, and your mind and body will register them as "real" food.

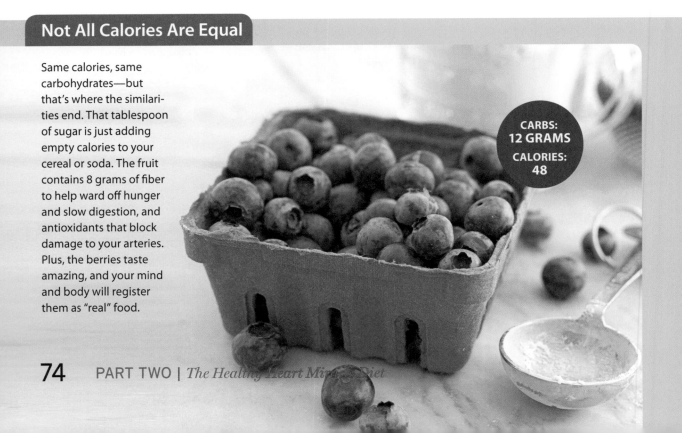

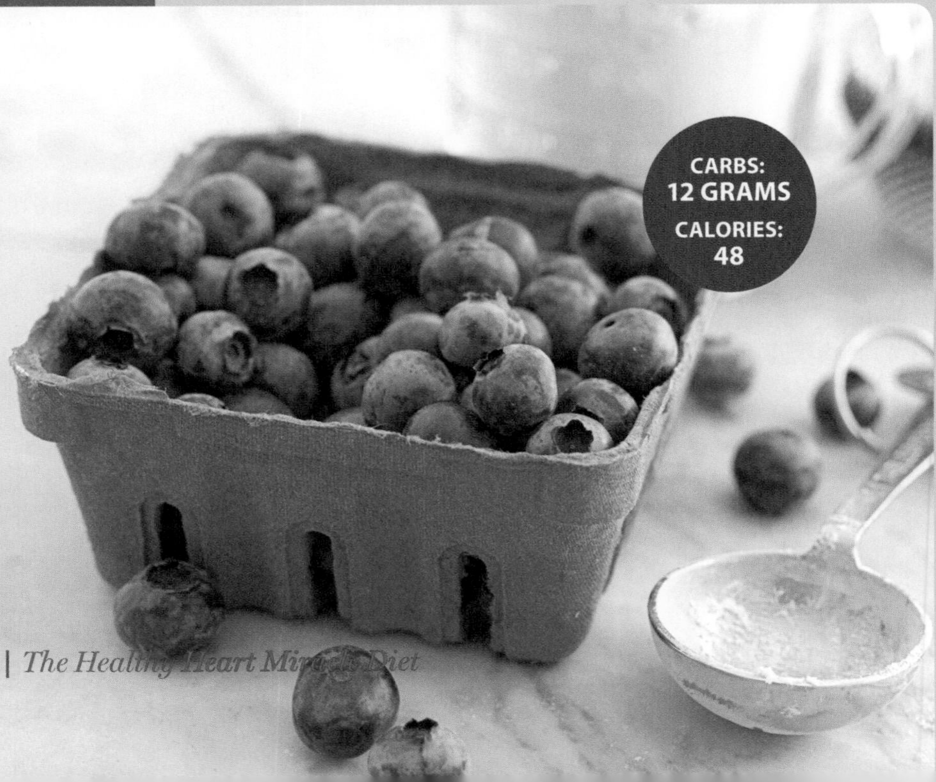

risotto instead of Arborio rice (a blood-sugar disaster waiting to happen), or in place of white rice in an oven-baked rice dish. If you want to use barley with the bran—barley groats or hulled barley, or the slightly more refined version, Scotch or pot barley—you'll want to soak it overnight and then cook it for 1 to 1 1/2 hours in 4 to 5 cups (1 to 1.25 L) of water for each cup (250 mL) of barley). It will have a stronger, nuttier flavor and work well on its own with stock or mixed with vegetables.

Bulgur

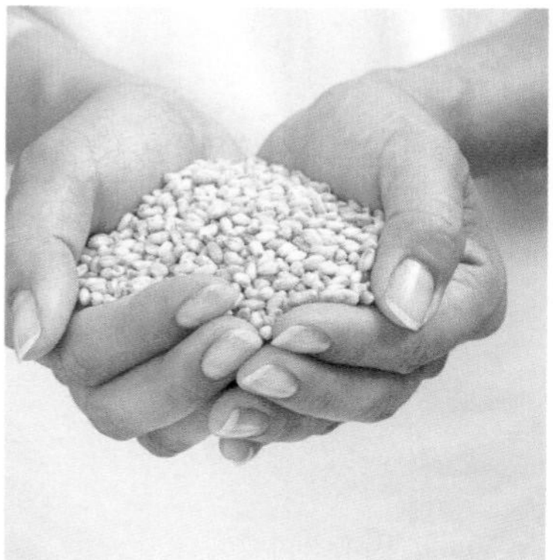

Bulgur is simply wheat that's been partially cooked by boiling or steaming and then dried or cracked. Its mild, nutlike flavor goes well in many dishes or can stand on it's own as a substitute for rice. It also makes a great hot breakfast cereal. Because bulgur is partly cooked before it's sent to market, it's incredibly easy to prepare: Just pour boiling water over it and let it sit. That means it's an easy way to add good carbs to your diet. Because bulgur is the entire grain of wheat, it contains not only plenty of fiber but also vitamin E and other nutrients.

Bulgur comes in fine, medium, and coarse grinds. The coarse is good for dinner side dishes and salads. Pour 2 1/2 cups (625 mL) boiling water over a cup of bulgur, mix in a 1/2 teaspoon (2 mL) salt, and then cover and let soak for about a half-hour. The bulgur will absorb most of the liquid. (Put in a fine mesh colander and press out any excess liquid.) Mix it into a stir-fry or make a refreshing summer salad by tossing it with pine nuts, fresh parsley, cut-up pieces of dried apricots, and an oil and vinegar dressing. Or toast it in a table-spoon of butter in a saucepan for a minute or so and then pour in a couple cups of chicken stock, bring to a boil, and cook until the stock is absorbed (about 30 minutes). This makes a nice side dish.

Quinoa

This grain (pronounced KEEN-wah) hails from South America. Its light flavor mixes well with toasted nuts such as walnuts or pecans. You can serve it alone in place of rice or pilaf, use it to thicken soups, or sprinkle it over salads (or even your breakfast cereal). It's unusually high-protein content (more than double that of some grains) means that it's particularly filling. Quinoa has been gaining favor because of the fact that it's gluten-free (some people have trouble digesting the glutens in wheat). A rich source of fiber, the grain also delivers the same healthy oils found in other grains, along with a good concentration of vitamins and minerals.

The small grains cook quickly in water—use 2 cups (500 mL) liquid (water or stock) for each cup of grain—taking less than 15 minutes. When preparing quinoa, try toasting the uncooked grains briefly in a deep skillet with olive oil and garlic; add 2 cups chicken stock, bring to a boil, and then reduce the heat until the stock is absorbed, 12 to 15 minutes. Fluff with a fork and serve, or let it cool to toss with salads.

Shopping for Good Carbs

The grocery store can be a minefield when you're trying to eat right. Most are carefully laid out to encourage you to spend—and eat—more. Most of the stuff you don't need, such as junk food and sweets, will be waiting to waylay you on your way to the staples like bread and milk. And by the way, all highest-price version of foods will be at eye level; you'll have to bend over to see the more reasonably priced items.

One of the most obvious grocery-shopping mistakes is to arrive hungry. All the stuff that's ready to eat, especially the high-carb, high-calorie snacks, will beckon as you roll your cart around the store. So have a snack before you go, or shop after a meal. When you get there, keep these tips in mind.

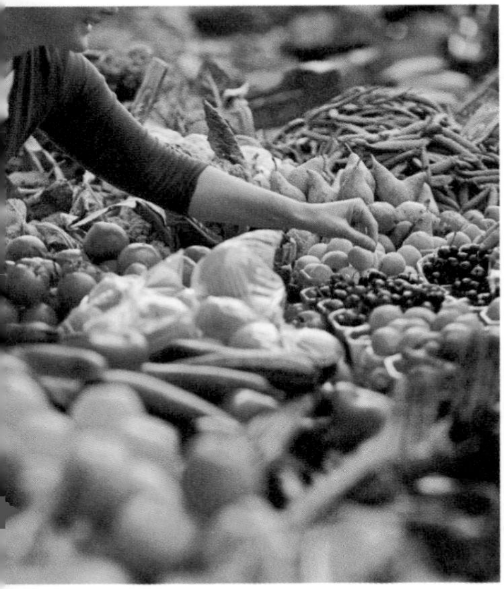

1. Head to the store with vegetable and grain recipes in hand. It's impossible to come home with the ingredients you need to make healthy vegetable dishes and grain salads and sides if you don't know what those ingredients are. Without recipes in hand, you'll likely end up with the same old romaine lettuce and box of rice mix in your cart. See the recipes in part 4, and "Great Greens" on page 84 for inspiration.

2. Start in the produce section, and fill half your cart there. Many of the carbs you eat should come from fruits and vegetables. Fortunately, most grocery stores are set up so that you walk into the produce section first. Start there, and plan to spend some time picking out the best-looking fresh fruit. Challenge yourself to try at least one vegetable you gave up on in childhood. Tastes change radically, and a new spice or cooking technique can make foods like Brussels sprouts and cabbage taste completely different.

3. Choose a variety of colors. How's this for handy? The best way to ensure that you're getting the full complement of vitamins and minerals in your diet is to make sure that your produce selections represent all the colors of the rainbow. Yellow bell peppers, green apples, red potatoes, orange carrots, blueberries, white onions—you get the picture. The more color in your cart, the better for your health.

4. Dive into the bins. More and more stores are including bins of whole grains like brown rice, bulgur, quinoa, and whole-wheat flour.

Make use of these to expand your grain repertoire. Often the grains in these bins will be fresher and less inexpensive than the bagged versions in the aisles, and the variety may inspire you to try new types.

5. Get more vegetables from the freezer section. The methods for fast-freezing produce are so efficient that, nutritionally speaking, there isn't a big difference between fresh and frozen versions these days. (In fact, the only way to get fresh produce that has a substantial nutritional advantage over frozen is to buy it at a local farmers' market.) With vegetables in your freezer, you'll always have them on hand when you run out of fresh (or don't have time to chop them).

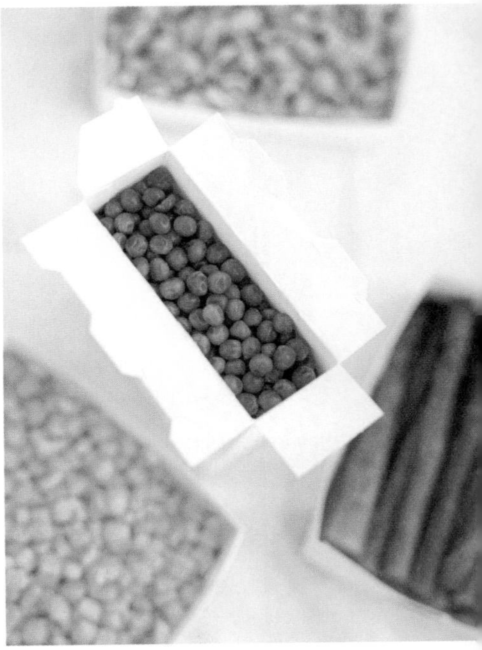

6. Grab a few cans of fruit. Yes, canned fruit is often packed in syrup and loses much of the flavor of fresh. But if you buy the kind that's packed in its own juice without added sugar, the ease of popping open a can of pineapple and tossing it into a salad can't be beat.

7. Skip the beverage aisle. Honestly, there's nothing you'll need here, unless it's seltzer. If you head down the aisle to pick up your bubbly water, leave your cart at the end, pick up what you need and carry it back to your cart. You'll get a little more exercise and you won't be tempted to slide a six-pack of something sugary into your cart. And by leaving your cart at the end, you won't have any hands free to pick up any of the chips and other high-carb, salty snacks that are usually placed opposite the beverages.

CORRECT YOUR CARBS: Your Meal-by-Meal Plan

Now that you've learned what it takes to correct your carbs—by avoiding fast-digesting danger carbs and adding more fruits, vegetables, and whole grains to your diet—it's time to put your new carb plan into practice, meal by meal. If you're the type who likes to make one change at a time, feel free to start the Healthy Heart Miracle Diet by correcting your carbs at just one meal (breakfast is easy to start with). When you're ready, move on to another meal, or change your snacks. People who make changes gradually are more likely to stick with them.

In chapter 10, you'll find a two-week meal plan that shows you exactly what to eat for 14 days. The meals there feature some of the recipes in part 4, but you should feel free to dig into those recipes at any time (like right now!). You'll find plenty that fit the bill for correcting your carbs.

YOUR CARB PLAN at Breakfast

1	Have breakfast every day.
2	Avoid white breads, bagels, and muffins, breakfast bars, and sugary cereals, and choose high-fiber whole-grain versions instead.
3	If you have toast, have 1 slice. If you have a bagel, make it a mini-bagel (3–4-inches across).
4	If you have cereal, don't eat more than one and a half times the serving size listed on the box. Fill the rest of the bowl with berries.
5	Drink no more than 4 ounces (125 ml) of 100% fruit juice.

Breakfast

What does breakfast look like to you? Are you accustomed to sitting down to a big bowl of cereal or a full-size bagel? A store-bought muffin? A breakfast bar? As you may have figured out, eating simple carbs first thing in the morning is like stepping on a banana peel as you get out of bed. You'll find you're slipping into poor food choices for the rest of the day.

Or maybe you feel like you don't have time for the morning meal. Does it seem like skipping breakfast is an easy way to cut calories? There are some serious flaws in that logic that may not be immediately apparent. Sure, that's one meal of calories you just eliminated. But people who skip breakfast tend to more than make up for the missed calories later in the day, while those who *do* eat breakfast tend, on average, to make much better food choices throughout their day and have healthier diets overall.

When you don't eat first thing in the morning, you aren't just missing a meal, you're denying your body sustenance that it desperately needs following 8 or more hours of fasting. Research suggests that not giving your body calories first thing in the morning will hamper your concentration and focus throughout the morning. Even worse, it means that you're more likely to overeat when you finally do sit down to some food. And your body will be craving quick energy, raising your desire for those simple carbohydrates that are so easy to digest but so harmful to your arteries. Finally, when you skip meals, your metabolism slows, meaning you burn fewer calories throughout the day; the excess is sent to long-term storage in the form of fat. It's no wonder, then, that people who eat breakfast every day are more likely to lose weight and keep it off.

If you don't feel particularly hungry first thing in the morning, take some time to see if you can come up with a breakfast food that sounds appealing. If foods like toast and cereal don't work for you, glance at the next chapter, where you'll discover that eating protein foods such as yogurt and eggs is an especially good way to start the day.

Eating simple carbs first thing in the morning is like stepping on a banana peel as you get out of bed.

Good Carbs at Breakfast

If you want to start your day with a carb-based breakfast (as opposed to eating eggs or yogurt), that's fine—as long as you choose the right carbs and don't overdo it.

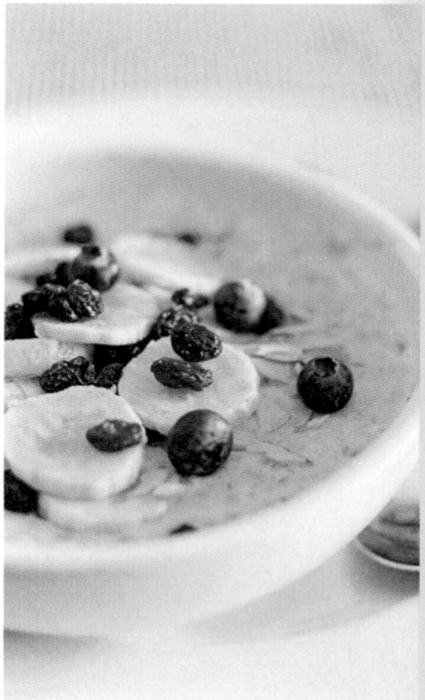

Make cereal the perfect meal. Assuming you read the "Purge the Bad" section earlier in this chapter, you now know what good cereal looks like (plenty of fiber, not too much sugar). A smart cereal choice makes a fine breakfast and helps you get some whole grains into your day. Just don't overdo it; even some high-fiber cereals have a fairly high glycemic load and may leave you hungry again soon if you eat too much. (Note: Bran is one of the lowest glycemic choices.) Pour a small bowl and fill the rest with a handful of berries, apple cubes, or banana slices to get some fruit servings into your day and fill you up on fewer calories.

Go for oatmeal. For a warm breakfast, oatmeal made from rolled (not instant) oats is an excellent way to start the day. A good source of soluble fiber, oatmeal tends to expand in your gut, making you feel fuller than you would expect. Better still, soluble fiber converts to a sort of gel that slows digestion and traps some of the fats in food, causing them to pass through your gut undigested. In heart research, eating a bowl of slow-cooked oats daily dropped "bad" LDL cholesterol counts while preserving the "good" HDL cholesterol. Cold oat bran cereal had a similar effect.

Avoid the instant. A word about instant oatmeal: The convenience is appealing, and it's not a terrible choice in a pinch, but if you're at home, take the extra 5 minutes to make the real kind. To get a food to the point where mixing it with hot water makes it ready to eat requires processing and precooking it to a degree that makes the food much easier to digest. That means it converts to sugar faster. The other issue with most instant foods is that they're loaded up with sugar, sodium, and other flavorings. Make your own, add your own flavorings, and you'll enjoy it much more. With hot cereal, mix in fresh or dried fruit and sprinkle on some brown sugar. Be in charge of creating your own flavor explosion.

Avoiding "instant" goes for farina, too (such as Cream of Wheat). It sounds healthy, but its glycemic load is high. Instead, look for a whole-grain hot cereal.

Pour a *little* fat with your milk. You'll need something to pour over your cereal, especially if it's cold. For people who already drink nonfat milk and eat nonfat yogurt, congratulations. But you don't have to eliminate all fat from your dairy products on the Healthy Heart Miracle Diet. After all, a little fat can slow the digestion of carbs, and it can make meals feel more satisfying because hunger sensors in the gut and brain are more likely to be appeased by the presence of some fat. And the fatty acids in dairy fall into the healthy fats category (see chapter 8 for more on dairy). That makes 1 percent milk a fine choice.

Breakfast Suggestions

Mains	Sides	Beverages
Half of an oat bran bagel with cream cheese	½ cup berries or mixed fruit	Hot tea or coffee
1 piece of whole-wheat toast with butter and fruit preserves	1 piece of fruit (apple, orange, banana, peach)	Up to 4 ounces (125 ml) of 100% fruit juice
Cold or hot whole-grain cereal with 1 percent milk	1/4 cup (50 ml) of dried fruit	
Low-fat plain yogurt with ¼ cup (50 ml) whole-grain granola		

What About Coffee?

For java junkies, the news could not be better. A study that tracked 3,000 men and women for 20 years could detect no link whatsoever between coffee drinking and heart risk, and the study participants drank up to four cups daily. A study of women found that drinking coffee actually lowered a woman's risk of developing diabetes. And results of research that followed 129,000 women and men for 20 years found that daily cups of joe dropped the risk of heart disease by a third.

How could coffee pull off this trick? It's relatively high in antioxidants. In fact, diet research suggests that coffee is the number one source of antioxidants in many people's diets (though that probably has more to do with how little produce these people eat). If you remember, antioxidants—especially the type found in java—seem to tamp down inflammation in the arteries. Coffee also contains chlorogenic acids, which may lower blood sugar.

There is a caveat to all this: Unfiltered coffee contains diterpenes—substances that seem to raise bad cholesterol. If you drink several cups of coffee daily that are made with a French press or an espresso machine, or you use a metal filter in your drip machine, you could be getting high amounts of these cholesterol-raising substances. One cup a day won't be much of a concern, but if you drink a couple of cups a day, consider switching to paper-filtered drip coffee or instant (the freeze-drying process removes diterpenes) and you'll be fine.

Lunch

Bread tends to be the biggest stumbling block at lunch. A sandwich on a big white roll or even a large tortilla wrap may be tempting, but you'll regret it later when your energy sinks.

Construct a carb-friendly sandwich. If you're at a deli, choose the grainy whole-wheat or the fresh sourdough bread. Portion size will be key here: By choosing bread that comes in smaller slices, you can really cut back on calories and carbs. If the bread you want comes in large rolls or hefty slices, ask the person at the counter to wrap half of the sandwich in plastic before putting it in the bag; now you have lunch for two days instead of one.

The right way to construct that sandwich includes plenty of vegetables, such as tomatoes and dark green, leafy lettuce. Also think pickles (if you're not watching your salt intake); because they contain vinegar, they will help lower the glycemic load of your meal. Mustard is a better choice for a condiment than mayonnaise, but if a sandwich seems dry without mayo, just request that they spread it thinly.

Don't be fooled by wraps. They may look like a healthy alternative to a sandwich, but tortillas can be stuffed with a startling amount of meat and cheese. And the tortilla itself may be thin but it delivers up to 350 calories and just a couple of grams of fiber compared to the 140 calories and 4 grams of fiber you get from two slices of whole-wheat or oat bran bread. Better to stick with the sandwich or, if you choose a wrap, eat just half today and save half for tomorrow.

Lose the bread altogether. You don't always have to swap bad bread for good bread. An easy way to cut back on carbs, in general, is to roll your lunch meat and place it over a salad instead of stuffing it between two slices of bread.

Go with the grain. Grain salads, that is. Tabbouleh, for instance, is incredibly easy to put together the night before. This Middle-Eastern salad is made with bulgur, chopped parsley, cucumbers, tomatoes, olive oil, and lemon juice. In part 4, you'll find several delicious grain salads from which to choose.

YOUR CARB PLAN at Lunch

1	If you have a sandwich, make sure your bread is whole grain.
2	Beware of carb traps like "healthy" wraps; tortillas are loaded with carbs and calories.
3	Gets your carbs in the form of veggies by dumping your "sandwich" over leafy greens.
4	Use lunch as an excuse to have another piece of fruit.

A sandwich on a big white roll or tortilla wrap may be tempting, but you'll regret it later.

Lunch Suggestions

Mains	Sides	Beverages
A sandwich on whole wheat or rye with plenty of added vegetables	Salad of dark leafy greens, oil and vinegar dressing (avoid light dressings which can be loaded with sugar)	Water or seltzer (mix with 4 ounces (125 ml) fruit juice, if you prefer)
Turkey and Swiss (or any other protein choice) over greens	Steamed vegetables	Unsweetened iced tea
One slice of cheese or vegetable pizza	Piece of fruit or fruit salad	
Vegetables over brown rice		
Bean soup		

REMEMBER THIS

Don't Eat at Your Desk

Lunch is the meal you're most likely to eat on the go, whether that's in front of a spreadsheet or running between errands. But eating this way is likely to leave you feeling deprived. Even if your body registers that it's had sustenance, you're likely to think later that you deserve a food reward for your diligence. That's when the high-carb treat lure is most likely to upset your day. A candy (chocolate) bar at 2 p.m. leads to a bag of chips at 4 p.m., followed by a predinner snack at 6 p.m. Avoid the trap: Make time in your day to stop and enjoy what you're eating. Savor the taste and the way the flavors mix on your tongue. That's the way to find true satisfaction from your food.

Treat yourself to pizza. For fast and easy good carb choices, a slice (not two) of cheese or vegetarian thin-crust pizza is a surprisingly good option. The glycemic load is low, and the cheese will help fill you up. If you can find a place that offers whole-wheat or cornmeal crust, your pizza will leave you even more satisfied.

Lean on leftovers. One of the fastest, easiest, and most satisfying ways to enjoy a healthy lunch is to eat a healthy dinner—the leftovers, that is. Meals like vegetarian chili or chicken stir-fry make excellent lunches the next day.

Avoid the steam table. These are the hot foods sitting under sneeze shields at delis. Leaving aside the murky origins of this food (how many days has the macaroni and cheese been there, anyway?), the other problem with the choices on the table is that they've been cooking for hours. Not only does the prolonged heat degrade the nutrients and break down the fiber in the food, it makes your meal so soft that it's nearly predigested. Your gut will have to do very little work in converting the food to glucose, and that means your blood sugar will rise rapidly. Hit the cold salad fixings instead.

Dinner

On the Healthy Heart Miracle Diet, your main course at dinner will typically feature protein, not carbohydrates. As you may have gathered by now, protein is going to play a significant role in correcting your diet. But carbohydrates aren't something to avoid at all costs. Choose wisely, and they'll help turn your dinner into a heart-healthy feast. (Make the wrong decision, and your arteries and gut will pay the price.)

Think green, not white. One of the common dinner pitfalls is thinking of potatoes as a vegetable. Technically, they are vegetables, of course. And there's nothing wrong with eating them now and then. But if you rely on potatoes as your vegetable of choice most of the time, that's bad news for your heart. Potatoes raise blood sugar more than green vegetables do. And without some color—greens, oranges, or purples—on your plate, you'll be missing out on countless plant chemicals that protect your health (and a whole lot of fiber, too). Thinking about eating greens—how to cook them and how to make the family like them—can be daunting. But with a few simple tricks up your sleeve, you can turn just about any vegetable into something your family will ask for. Start with the tips on page 84 this chapter, "Great Greens".

Add a whole-grain side dish. We've been knocking simple carbohydrates throughout this book, but it's important to keep in mind that *whole-grain* carbohydrates are a boon, not a bust. Let them play a complementary role at dinner. Brown rice is fine, but the possibilities are endless. Amaranth, barley, quinoa, bulgur—most of these can stand in for white rice or replace the potato on your plate. In part 4, you'll find recipes that include many of these grains, but you can also just cook them in chicken or vegetable stock as you would rice, following the package instructions.

YOUR CARB PLAN at Dinner

1	Enjoy a whole-grain side dish with most meals.
2	Heap on the quick-to-fix greens—dinner is your best chance to fill your vegetable quota.
3	Replace white rice and French fries with vegetables or lower-glycemic grains.

Dinner Suggestions

Mains	Sides	Beverages
Pasta primavera	Any colorful vegetables	Seltzer
Thai Noodle Salad	Any whole-grain side dish (brown rice, quinoa, etc.)	Mineral water
Barley or quinoa pilaf with vegetables	Mixed green salad with Balsamic vinaigrette or Italian dressing	Wine
Ratatouille	Potatoes with skin (mashed or baked)	Beer
Bean-based stew or chili	Bean salad	
Vegetable stir-fry (add nuts or tofu for protein)		

Beyond Salad: *Great Greens*

On the Healthy Heart Miracle Diet, you will get less of your carbs from French fries and white bread and more of them from vegetables. That doesn't mean you have to eat broccoli every night, or even put a lot of time or thought into creating vegetable side dishes. It's simple and easy to prepare a variety of greens in a matter of minutes, while the main dish is cooking.

A basic principle to remember: While there's no point, healthwise, in smothering your vegetables with butter or cheese sauce, using a little butter, salt, and sugar or a splash of maple syrup isn't a bad thing when cooking greens. If it makes the dish more palatable and you're more likely to eat it, then it's worth it.

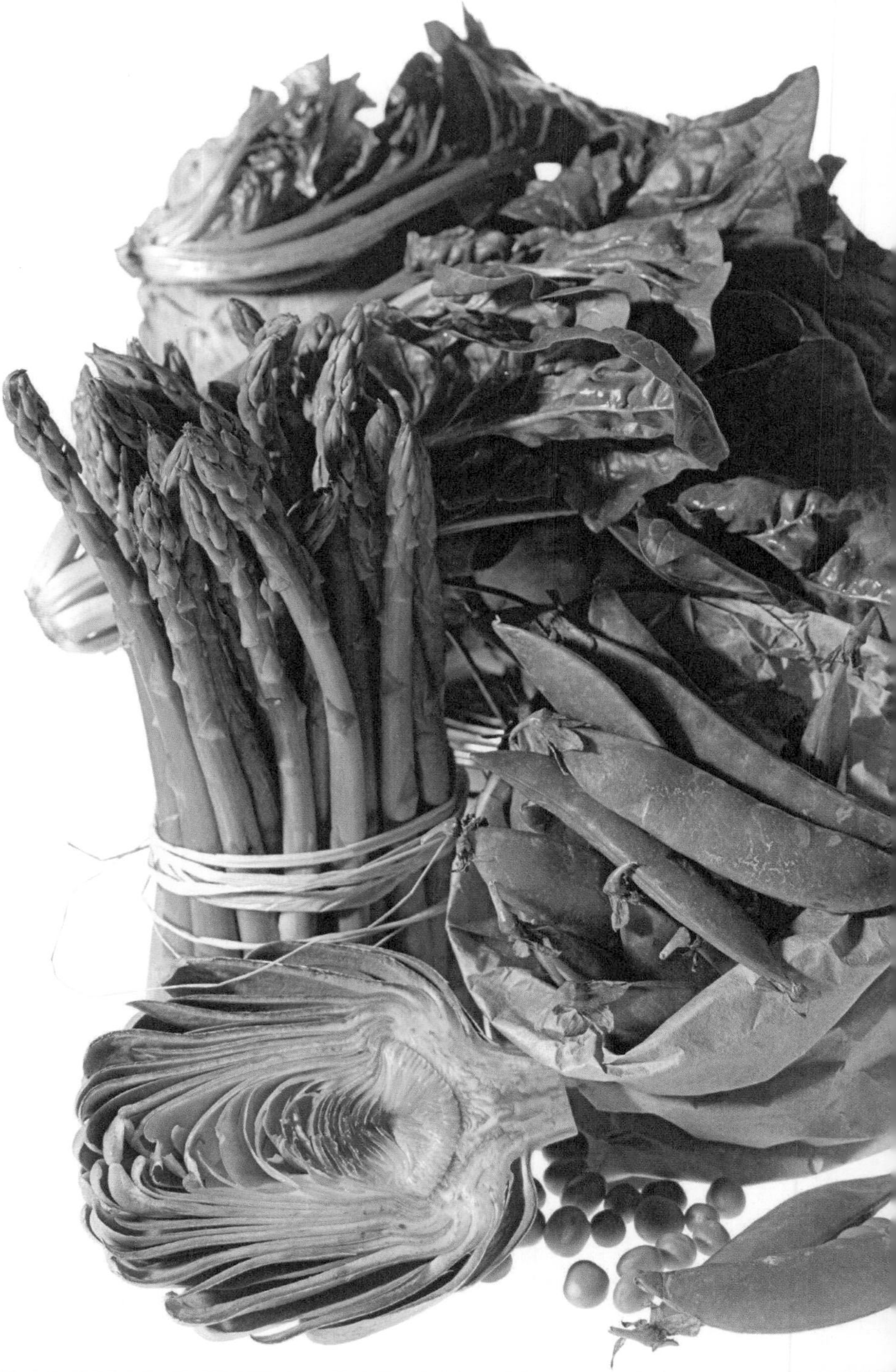

Fibrous leafy greens with thick stalks such as bok choy, collard greens, kale, Swiss chard, mustard greens, turnip greens

amount: 1 to 2 pounds (500 g to 1 kg) will serve four people.

prep: After washing and draining the leaves, cut away the stems by folding each leaf in half lengthwise on a cutting board and running a paring knife along the inside of the exposed stalk. In some recipes, the stalks can be put to good use (they are a great source of fiber), but they take about twice as long to cook; the method here is just for the leaves. If you want to cook the stalks as well, slice them crosswise into 1/2-inch (1 cm) pieces and plan on throwing them into the pan for about 5 minutes before adding the leaves. (Or you can save the stalks to use in a soup or stew.)

cook: Tear the leaves up, and remember that they'll cook down to a fraction of their original size, so don't be worried about having a big pile. Then splash some olive oil and pressed garlic (just press the whole clove—no need for peeling and dicing) in a large saucepan. Once the oil is hot, throw in the leaves—as many as you can fit. Let them cook down, and then add some more, stirring all the while. Once you have all the leaves in the pan, splash in some chicken broth and soy sauce, and 1/2 teaspoon (2 mL) sugar. Let simmer until the leaves are soft and wilted, about 10 minutes.

Asparagus

amount: 1 pound will serve three or four people.

prep: This recipe works especially well if the oven is already hot from cooking your main course. After you pull out your main course, turn the oven to 500°F (260°C). Wash a pound of asparagus and snap off the bottoms of the stalks. Toss the stalks with 1 tablespoon olive oil, a clove or two of crushed garlic, and some salt and pepper, then spread them out in a single layer on a baking sheet.

cook: Cook in the oven for 9 minutes. This dish can be served piping hot or at room temperature.

Soft greens such as arugula, spinach, baby beet

amount: About 2 pounds of leaves will serve four (figure 5 to 8 ounces (140 to 225 g) of fresh leaves per serving).

prep: Wash the leaves well and trim the stems. Shake the leaves to get rid of excess water, then stack and cut them into ribbons.

cook: In a large skillet, season the leaves with salt and cook them over medium heat for about 5 minutes. Toss them with olive oil, lemon juice, and pressed garlic in a large bowl and serve.

Green beans, peas

amount: 1 pound will serve three or four people.

prep: Bring about 3 quarts (2.8 L) of salted water to boil (use about a teaspoon of salt).

cook: Drop the beans or peas in the water for 6 minutes (until they're just a little softer than crisp—go for a texture you and your family will enjoy). While the beans are cooking, mix 2 tablespoons (25 mL) olive oil with 1 teaspoon (4 mL) each of parsley, tarragon, and lemon juice.

When the beans are done, drain them and toss together with the olive oil mixture in a salad bowl. Add salt and pepper, to taste, and serve.

An even quicker method is to heat a skillet over medium-high heat, add the olive oil and then, before the oil can burn, toss in the beans and sear them, stirring frequently until they just begin to soften. Sprinkle with red-pepper flakes and serve.

REMEMBER THIS

Cook Once, Eat Twice

What's delicious and good for you at dinner is equally delicious and good for you at lunch the next day. Always make extra, especially if the dish freezes well. That way, you'll never be caught without a healthy meal in the house.

Think of pasta as a vehicle for vegetables. Pasta is pretty much as good, or bad, for you as what you eat with it. The pasta itself isn't a problem; it's not a big blood-sugar offender, and if you choose whole-wheat pasta, you're getting a good dose of fiber with your meal. In short, there's no need to avoid it—unless you insist on overcooking it, covering it with cream sauce, loading it with cheese, or eating prepared pasta meals out of a box. It's quick, it's easy, and it's inexpensive. To make it really worthwhile health-wise, add some steamed broccoli, chopped tomatoes, or just about any other vegetable and top it with a swirl of olive oil. Or cook any vegetable you like and puree it in a blender. Serve over hot pasta and top with herbs and spices of your choice.

Don't Skimp on Seasonings

So often, when people switch to healthier diets, they also eliminate fat, salt, and other perceived nutritional ills. But a healthy diet doesn't have to taste bland—in fact, it shouldn't, or you'll give it up. If it takes a dab of butter on your green beans to get you to eat them, by all means, add it (though if you try olive oil, you may find that it tastes just as good). But don't stop there.

Any chef worth his freshly ground pepper will tell you that herbs and spices bring dishes to life. And researchers agree that they can add to *your* life as well. Most spices are packed with antioxidants, substances that can help keep cholesterol from clogging arteries (not to mention help ward off cancer). A tablespoon of dried oregano has the same antioxidant power as an apple. Some herbs, such as ginger and turmeric, also tamp down inflammation.

Top Healing Spices

A study published in the *American Journal of Clinical Nutrition* found that these are the top 10 antioxidant-packed dried or ground herbs and spices.

1. **Cloves**	6. **Basil**
2. **Oregano**	7. **Yellow mustard seed**
3. **Ginger**	8. **Curry powder**
4. **Cinnamon**	9. **Paprika**
5. **Turmeric**	10. **Chili powder**

The more you use, the better. Make a marinara sauce with oregano, basil, and parsley. Use ginger to season fish, in barbecue sauces for beef or chicken, or in vegetable and noodle dishes. Or serve a curry dish; they typically rely on turmeric, curry powder, paprika, and chili powder—all powerfully healing spices.

Snacks

Snacks are where carbs can do the most damage during your day. Snack on the right carbs and controlling your hunger will be a breeze. Make the wrong choices and your weight will balloon and your arteries will swell and narrow.

Avoid seemingly healthy choices made from simple carbs. The trouble is that most ready-to-go snacks are simple carbohydrates: a bag of pretzels, a box of sweets, a handful of cheesy fish-shaped crackers—even healthy-seeming choices like rice cakes or fruit bars are loaded with the kind of carbs that will jack up your blood sugar and prime you for an energy crash later (followed by gnawing hunger pangs and more eating).

If you want carbs, pair them with protein. Have a slice of cheese with your whole-grain crackers, or a smear of peanut butter. You'll learn why in the next chapter.

Keep calories under 200. What's key for snacks is that you make sure you're not eating too much. This is just something to get you to the next meal. As a very general rule of thumb (there are some exceptions), a snack should fit in one cupped hand.

Eat out of different kind of bag. Bring a ziplock plastic bag from home filled with fruit (grapes, apple wedges, orange quarters) or vegetables (carrot sticks, grape tomatoes, cucumber wedges). Even dried fruit is a good choice, though the sweeter it tastes, the more sugar it has. Dried dates and bananas are very high on the glycemic load scale, while dried apricots and apples have a low glycemic load. Keep your serving size of any dried fruit to 1/4 cup.

YOUR CARB PLAN at Snack Time

1	Make sure you're really hungry before eating any snack.
2	Try to avoid snacking on simple carbohydrates—turn to fruit, vegetables, or whole-grain carb choices instead.
3	Control portions by planning ahead.

Calorie-Free Snacking

Sometimes, when we think we're craving food, it's boredom or habit that's taking over our impulses. With nothing but a long afternoon of chores or work stretching out in front of you, a chance to get up, stretch your legs, and get a snack is tempting. But putting something caloric in your mouth is only one part of that ritual, and it's the easiest to manipulate. What you're craving more than anything else is a break and a small reward. So keep the parts of your afternoon ritual that support your health—the break, the walk to stretch your legs—and change the part that doesn't. Here are five ideas for replacing that reflex to reach for a snack you may not need. If you still want a snack following your attempt to overcome your hunger, then go ahead and have one. But keep trying the above techniques around snack time. Eventually, you may establish a new routine that will be calorie-free.

1. Drink some water. Psychologists have found that we often mistake thirst for hunger. Keep a bottle of water handy and take swigs of it regularly. You may find that quenching your thirst helps douse your desire to eat.

2. Make a cup of tea. If you need an energy boost to make it through the day, go with black; otherwise pick green or herbal tea. Not only is tea calorie-free, real tea (not herbal) is loaded with the type of antioxidants that can protect your heart.

3. Chew some sugarless gum. Getting your jaw going can fool your brain into thinking that you've had something to eat. And research has found that chomping on gum can help increase your focus on the tasks at hand.

Snack Suggestions

Fresh fruit
Cut-up vegetables
Dried apricots
Air-popped popcorn
Sourdough pretzels
Dark chocolate-covered almonds

4. Try a relaxation technique. Tension can trigger the need for a quick bite. There are many ways to practice quick relaxation. Here's one that you can try anywhere, anytime: Sit or stand with your back straight, eyes forward, and slowly breathe in through your nose to the count of five. Hold it for a moment, then exhale for the same amount of time. Repeat this five times, and notice as your shoulders and neck relax. Roll your head to help release the muscle tension.

5. Distract yourself. Try making a phone call you've put off (with a cell phone, you can combine this with a stroll around the block). Or give yourself a break from what you're doing and complete a crossword puzzle or Sudoku. Once your mind is occupied elsewhere, you may find that the urge to eat has evaporated.

Dessert

YOUR CARB PLAN at Dessert

1	Eat dessert only occasionally, not every night.
2	For sweetness, look to fruit.
3	Slow down and savor every bite so you can be happy with a small portion.

There's little point in making healthy changes to your diet if you can't eat that way for life. We should—we need to—enjoy our food. If you like sweets, that means treating yourself to dessert now and then.

A few luscious bites will do. Especially if you've enjoyed a nice relaxing meal with family or friends, you shouldn't need a huge serving of cake or pie to make you happy. Treat yourself to a few tastes, and leave it at that. Dense, fudge-like chocolate cake? Serve yourself a small slice and fill up the rest of your plate with beautiful fresh berries.

Develop a repertoire of fruit-based desserts. A baked apple or pear served with a splash of maple syrup, a fresh fruit cobbler, even a bowl of berries with a dollop of crème fraîche or plain yogurt and maybe some diced candied ginger—all are deliciously sweet without a lot of refined sugar.

Hunt for whole grains. Most baked goods are made with white flour, but they don't have to be. Many of the desserts in part 4 cut down the amount of white flour and use heart-friendlier whole-wheat flour, oats, or other ingredients instead.

Like chocolate? Go to the dark side. You've no doubt heard some of the news, but chocoholics won't mind hearing it again: Eating small amounts of dark chocolate on a regular basis can actually lower your heart disease risk. You'll read more about dark chocolate in chapter 8. But for now, know that dark chocolate shavings over that bowl of berries is a perfectly heart-healthy dessert, and so are baked goods made with cocoa powder, which contains most of chocolate's antioxidants. Milk chocolate's benefits are offset by the extra sugar and milk fats.

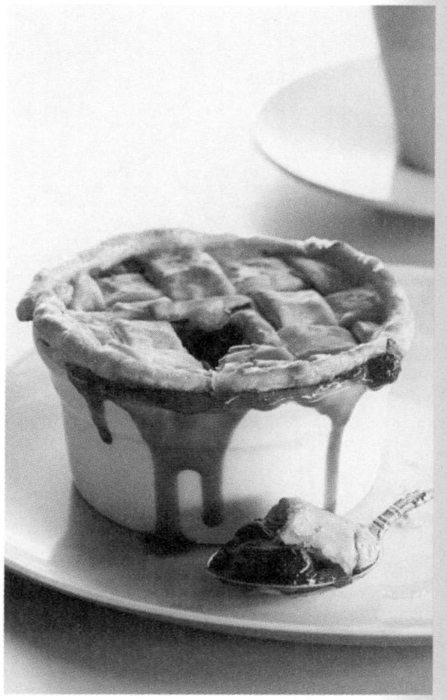

Go for the good stuff. Don't waste calories and carbs on store-bought cakes and baked goods that simply aren't that special and undoubtedly contain ingredients you don't want or need. If you're a chocolate-lover, purchase high-quality dark bars and break off just a few squares. Eat them slowly, savoring the rich, complex flavor. You'll find that those few squares will be enough (especially if you accompany them with a cup of coffee or some red wine). Is ice cream a favorite? Buy the premium kind and then serve up a golf ball-size scoop. Sit down at the table like you would for dinner and savor your serving. You'll be amazed when you finish and you're not craving more.

Dessert Suggestions

- Baked apple, pear, or peach drizzled with maple syrup or sprinkled with sugar
- Bowl of berries with a dollop of real whipped cream or crème fraîche or some dark chocolate shavings
- Fresh fruit cobbler
- Small piece of a dark chocolate treat, preferably with berries on top

7

Power Up Your Protein

Nutrition experts have insisted for years that a typical diet provides more than enough protein. But now there's evidence that increasing protein to the levels you'll get by following the Healthy Heart Miracle Diet can dramatically improve your heart risk profile—and help you lose weight.

During the low-fat craze of the last several decades, fat was out, carbohydrates were in, and protein was all but forgotten. If you were to ask a dietitian about protein, she would have told you that most of us get more than enough of the stuff (and some would still say so now). Protein, in general, got a bum rap, since many of the protein foods in a Western-style diet (think hamburgers and fried chicken) are also full of saturated fat. Yet research shows that protein may be key to keeping your heart healthy and your weight in check.

YOUR PROTEIN PLAN at a Glance

1	Aim to include a source of protein at every meal, especially breakfast.
2	Choose snacks that are protein-based.
3	Favor beans, poultry, lean meats, and fish over fatty steaks and burgers.

When researchers studied various populations, they discovered that people who consumed the most protein of any kind had the lowest heart disease risk. But eating plant-based protein foods (beans, grains, and nuts) may be even better. A 20-year study involving 80,000 women found that eating a low-carb diet high in vegetable protein could lower the risk of heart disease by 30 percent compared to a high-carb, lower protein diet. And when researchers tracked the effects of several different diets on 164 adults with mildly elevated blood pressures, they discovered that a high-protein diet produced superior improvements in blood pressure, LDL ("bad") cholesterol, and triglycerides compared to a typical high-carbohydrate diet.

The Healthy Heart Miracle Diet recommends getting 20 to 25 percent of your calories from protein, compared to the 15 to 20 percent that many Westerners average. Making up the difference is as simple as starting your day with an egg instead of a mini-bagel and a cup of 1% milk instead of orange juice, snacking on a handful of almonds instead of an ounce of potato chips, and enjoying a side of a half-cup of black beans instead of a half-cup of white rice.

With a judicious amount of lean protein-based foods in your diet, you'll be shocked at how much easier it is to feel satisfied after a meal. And eating more protein should help you eat fewer simple carbs.

How Protein Helps Your Heart

One of the benefits of eating more protein is that, by default, you'll be eating fewer simple carbohydrates, which can inflame arteries and spur overeating. Research shows that diets that replace some carbohydrates with protein help people protect their hearts in other ways, too.

Lower cholesterol and triglycerides. Some amazing things happen when researchers feed people with heart or weight troubles higher protein diets. A large trial known as the OmniHeart (Optimal Macronutrient Intake Trial for Heart Health) Study confirmed that replacing some carbohydrates with either protein or monounsaturated fat improved cholesterol levels and lowered the blood fats known as triglycerides.

In other research, Australian researchers put 215 people with high triglycerides on a high-protein or standard-protein diet for 3 months. The high-protein-eaters cut their triglyceride levels in half and experienced double the drop in cholesterol compared with volunteers following the standard-protein plan. And although both groups lost about 15 pounds over the 3 months, the high-protein group lost more heart-threatening visceral fat—2 to 4 pounds (1 to

Which plate has the correct amount of protein?

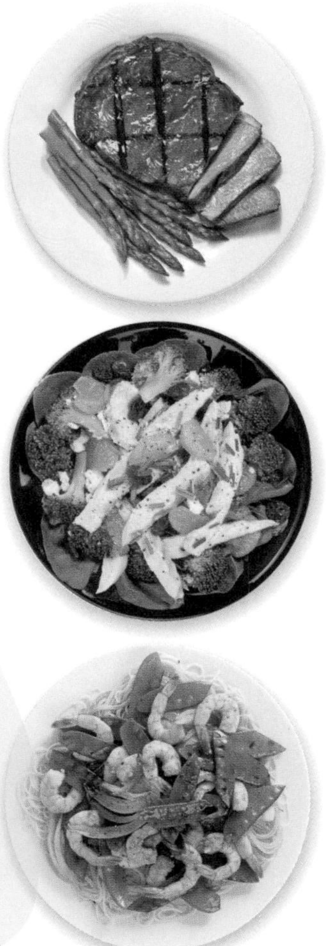

Many of us fill our plates with big pieces of meat or chicken. But for best health, let protein be just one ingredient among many.

2 kg) more than folks in the other group. Dropping visceral fat helps cut "bad" LDL cholesterol. What is especially compelling about these findings is that people who have the highest levels of triglycerides and cholesterol tend to reap the most benefit.

Lower blood pressure. The OmniHeart Study showed that replacing some carbohydrates with either protein or monounsaturated fat nudged blood pressure down by 1 to 3 points.

Lower blood-sugar spikes. When people eat fewer refined carbs and more protein, blood sugar stabilizes. That makes sense, since refined carbs cause dramatic peaks in blood sugar, while protein barely budges blood sugar.

Compared to simple carbohydrates, protein takes far longer to digest. Sugar and other simple carbohydrates have molecules so small and so similar to the glucose molecules that fuel your body's cells that they can be absorbed into the blood with very little fanfare. But protein has huge molecules by comparison. First, your stomach must release enzymes to begin breaking down these large molecules; then, the small intestine generates another batch of enzymes that separate protein into smaller molecules called amino acids. Only then are the protein pieces small enough to pass through the walls of the small intestine and able reach the bloodstream. That involved process means protein foods keep your digestive system occupied for much longer than carbohydrates.

One of the benefits of eating more protein is that, by default, you'll be eating fewer simple carbohydrates, which can inflame arteries and spur overeating.

Weight loss. Protein keeps you full longer than carbs do. It's a proven fact: Of the three macronutrients (carbohydrates, protein, and fat), protein has the greatest power to suppress the "hunger" hormone ghrelin. It's no wonder, then, that it helps people lose weight.

A year-long study from researchers at the University of Illinois and Penn State University divided 130 overweight adults into two groups. One ate a typical low-fat diet in which 55 percent of calories came from carbohydrates and just 15 percent from protein. The other group got only 40 percent of their calories from carbohydrates and 25 to 30 percent from protein. After 12 months, the high-protein group had lost 23 percent more weight, on average and, even more important, 38 percent more body fat. The protein group was also more likely to stay on the plan: Two-thirds followed their diets until the year was up, but less than half of the low-fat group made it that far.

The ease of maintaining a diet that includes more protein is a common theme in research, and it's one reason the Healthy Heart Miracle Diet calls for plenty of protein. People on higher protein diets are more likely to report being satisfied after their meals and less likely to overeat the rest of the day. A review of 50 studies in the *Journal of the American College of Nutrition* found solid evidence that high-protein diets burn more calories (thanks to the extra work your digestive system must do to process the protein) and make you feel more satisfied—so you don't overeat—than low-protein diets.

How Much Is Enough?

In developed parts of the world, the average protein intake is about 15 percent of total calories. For a diet of 2,000 daily calories, that adds up to about 75 grams of protein a day. But according the Harvard School of Public Health, the evidence strongly indicates that increasing protein to 20 to 25 percent of total calories, or around 125 grams a day, will dramatically improve your heart risk profile—especially if the extra protein calories replace simple carbohydrates like white bread and rice.

Of the three macronutrients (carbohydrates, protein, and fat), protein has the greatest power to suppress hunger.

Make no mistake: This isn't a clarion call to go on a beef, bacon, and eggs diet. While research shows that high protein plans like Atkins or the Zone don't always drive up cholesterol or inflame arteries the way most heart experts once thought they would, they can be dangerous to your heart in other ways. Almost no expert believes that you could eat this way for years and not ultimately harm your health. For one thing, getting a group of people to eat such an extreme diet and then following them is something researchers can only do for a limited amount of time; the longest prospective studies on extremely high-meat-protein diets have only lasted about a year-and-a-half.

But populations that traditionally eat a fair amount of protein with most meals along with complex carbohydrates and healthy oils have been tracked for decades, and they tend to have the lowest rates of heart disease in the world. Many of the countries that border the Mediterranean Sea have followed such a diet, and they're among the healthiest in the world.

Eating More Protein: Is It Safe?

When you digest protein, waste products are created that tax the kidneys and liver more than do those from fat or carbohydrates. So doctors worry about extremely high-protein diets, especially in patients with kidney or liver disease. The moderate-protein content of this diet—20 to 25 percent of calories—should be perfectly safe. Even on all-meat-all-the-time plans, healthy adults seem to tolerate the extra protein with no trouble. That said, if you do have kidney or liver disease, ask your doctor how much protein you should eat.

Likewise, the risk to bones posed, in theory, by extremely high-protein diets doesn't apply here. When you eat protein, which is made of amino acids, the body must use more neutral or "base" substances—usually calcium—to balance out the increased acidity. The concern is that when you eat more protein, your body must take calcium reserves from the bones. But even when it comes to Atkins-type diets, the research is conflicting and doesn't clearly show an increase in fracture risk.

Miracle Protein Foods

You'll like this part because you get to enjoy some truly delicious, family-pleasing foods. Strip steak? There's room for that. Pork tenderloin? No problem. Lamb chops? They're okay. The secret lies in choosing lean protein sources that don't contain a lot of saturated fat. (Notice we didn't mention that prime rib or greasy hamburgers or fried chicken was fair game.) You know by now that saturated fat can raise cholesterol levels. But fat also packs 9 calories per gram, versus 4 calories per gram for protein. So, for the most part, the leaner your protein sources, the better. (Fatty fish, loaded with heart-healthy fats, is the major exception. See page 124.) The following is a roundup of excellent protein sources and what you should know about them.

Beans

When our early ancestors first began to gather in small societies to till the earth, it was to grow beans. Archaeologists have found

Complete Proteins: Getting Your Fill

Protein is made up of building blocks called amino acids, which your body needs for making everything from cells to hormones. There are 20 different amino acids in all, including 9 that the body can't make on its own, known as essential amino acids. Foods that supply all 9 essential amino acids in usable amounts are considered complete protein foods. Vegetable proteins such as beans tend to be short of 1 or 2 and therefore are considered incomplete proteins. But not to worry—as long as you get all 9 essential amino acids within a 24-hour period, you'll have what you need. If you decide to eat a primarily vegetarian diet, here are some combinations of plant proteins that add up to complete proteins.

Grains + Legumes

- Beans and rice
- Corn tortillas with beans
- Peanut butter on whole-wheat bread
- Bean soup and whole-grain crackers
- Tofu-vegetable stir-fry over rice or pasta
- Vegetarian chili with bread

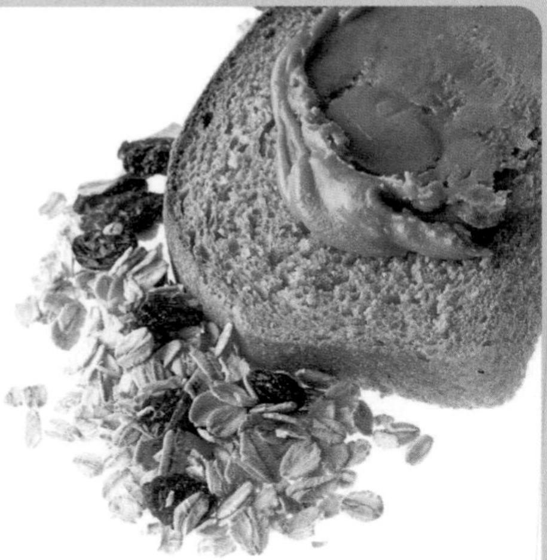

Grains + Nuts or Seeds

- Whole-wheat bun with sesame seeds
- Breadsticks rolled with sesame seeds
- Whole-wheat bread or crackers with peanut butter

Legumes + Nuts or Seeds

- Hummus (chickpeas and sesame paste)
- Trail mix (peanuts and sunflower seeds)
- Salad with chickpeas and corn bread

evidence that beans were a primary part of the diet as far back as 10,000 BC. They've been sustaining us ever since, though they don't play nearly as large a role in the modern diet as they should. Among the richest sources of protein in the plant world, they also deliver a good dose of fiber. Not many foods can boast that kind of double health bonus. In addition to the fiber (much of which is soluble fiber—the kind that lowers blood sugar and cholesterol), they have plenty of complex carbohydrates—in fact, they could just as easily be classified as a carb—which makes them a truly all-purpose food.

For a small number of calories, you get a whopping amount of an important vitamin and minerals. Most beans are rich in heart-protective B vitamins including folate. They also have iron, and if you're eating less meat than you're accustomed to, the beans will fill the iron gap handsomely. They also happen to be a great source of the amino acid arginine, which the body uses to make nitric oxide, the gas that helps keep the walls of arteries relaxed and blood pressure low.

Almost any type of bean you enjoy can be trusted to boost your intake of heart-healthy nutrition, from black, kidney, and pinto beans to lentils and chickpeas. The only bean to limit is black-eyed peas, since they have a higher glycemic load than other beans.

For the best bean experience in terms of flavor and nutrition—not to mention price—you can't go wrong with dried beans. They can be half or less the cost of canned beans, and they're really not that much trouble to prepare. Getting them ready for recipes only requires a moment's planning ahead. Cover them with water and let them soak overnight in the refrigerator; they'll be ready the next morning to toss in the slow-cooker for use in soups or stews. Or just heat them in stock and serve the beans as a side dish. If you need to hurry them along, cover them with water in a pot and bring to a boil, and then let them simmer until they're soft, usually about an hour or two. Split peas and lentils don't even require a presoak; just throw them in the pot when you start your soup or stew, and they'll be done by the time the other ingredients are.

Canned beans also have a place in every kitchen. Keep a variety in your cupboard because you can always use them as a last-minute addition to a dish. Look for lower sodium varieties.

MIRACLE **ADVICE:**

- Rely most often on dried beans.
- Rinse canned beans before using to remove some of the salt.
- Avoid canned baked beans, which can contain shocking amounts of sugar, and certain brands of refried beans, which have amazing amounts of saturated fat.

REMEMBER THIS

What Not to Eat

That basket of Buffalo wings? That tub of fried chicken? Their protein is no excuse for all the saturated fat (and calories) they contain. And those frozen fish sticks and prepackaged breaded fillets aren't what experts mean when they say to get more fish in your diet. Refried beans cooked in lard? Another no-no. As you work to include more protein in your diet, use common sense—if it's breaded, fried, or otherwise filled with fat (what do you think is oozing from that mega-burger?), it's not a lean source of protein, and it doesn't belong on the Healthy Heart Miracle Diet.

Nuts and Seeds

After beans, nuts and seeds are your best plant sources of protein. Green vegetables have enough protein to make an impact on your daily total, but you won't get enough from a head of lettuce to gain all the benefits protein has to offer. Nuts also come into play because they contain a generous amount of "good" heart-healthy fats. They're loaded with minerals that can help lower blood pressure, control blood sugar, and protect against cancer as a bonus. Like beans, nuts tend to have high amounts of the amino acid arginine, and that's good news for your endothelium, the sensitive inner wall of your arteries that is so prone to inflammation.

A caution: Go easy on those standard mixes that contain macadamia and Brazil nuts. Their saturated fat and total fat content are higher than most nuts (including cashews) and macadamias don't offer as much protein. (Chestnuts are also very low in protein.)

Seeds are no slouches either when it comes to your heart. Compared to nuts, they contain more of the plant compounds, called sterols, that act like nature's own cholesterol-beaters. In numerous studies over the past decade, researchers have found that people with high levels of "bad" LDL cholesterol who regularly eat about 1.5 ounces of nuts and seeds a day can expect their LDL to drop by anywhere from 6 to 15 percent. Sesame seeds are the highest in sterols, but sunflower seeds also contain plenty.

Flaxseed deserves special attention for its prowess in protecting against heart disease and diabetes. The research findings are impressive: Adding a couple of tablespoons a day of this tiny seed has been shown to help people with diabetes control blood sugar

Plant Sources of Protein

Meat, poultry, and fish provide the most protein per serving (20 to 30 grams per 3.5 ounces). The next highest is cottage cheese at 14 grams per 1/2 cup. But plant foods also provide a significant amount. Some offer as much or more than a cup of milk (8 grams), an ounce of cheese (7 grams), or an egg (6 grams).

Protein Source	Protein per Serving (g)	Protein Source	Protein per Serving (g)
Oats (1 cup/250 mL cooked)	15	Cashews, hazelnuts, walnuts (1 ounce/30 g)	4
Tofu, firm (3 ounces/ 90 g)	13	Quinoa (1/2 cup/125 mL)	4
Pumpkin seeds (1 ounce/30 g)	9	Pecans (1 ounce/30 g)	3
Spaghetti (1 cup/250 mL cooked)	8	Pine nuts (1 ounce/30 g)	3
Beans and lentils (1/2 cup/125 mL)	7-8	Vegetables (1/2 cup/125 mL cooked or 1 cup/250 mL raw)	3
Peanuts, peanut butter (1 ounce/30 g)	7		
Almonds, pistachios (1 ounce/30 g)	6	Bulgur (1/2 cup/250 mL cooked)	2.5
Flaxseed (1 ounce/30 g)	6	White rice (1/2 cup/250 mL cooked)	2
Sesame & sunflower seeds (1 ounce/30 g)	5	Chestnuts (1 ounce/30 g)	1

it's a myth. YOU NEED TO EAT MORE SOY

For a while, experts thought soy had an almost-magical power to protect health and lower the risk of heart disease. Some studies suggested that the bean could lower cholesterol by as much as 10 percent. But more recently, better studies indicate that the number is only about 3 percent, and that you would have to eat about 50 grams of soy a day—the equivalent of about 1.5 pounds (680 grams) of tofu or 8 glasses of soy milk—to get there. What's more, soy contains hormonelike substances called phytoestrogens, and there's some evidence that, in large amounts, these plant hormones could lower libido in men, spur the growth of some types of breast tumors in women, and possibly increase the risk of certain autoimmune disorders like lupus. Moderate amounts of soy are fine, however. If you enjoy soy, two to four servings a week should be perfectly safe for most people.

and drop LDL cholesterol levels (particularly in women). The seed contains a type of omega-3 fatty acid similar to the fats found in fish—and they're loaded with fiber.

MIRACLE **ADVICE:**

- Use nuts and seeds as a protein source in salads, on cereal, in baked goods, and in vegetable stir-fries.
- Add seeds, especially sesame seeds, to salads, breads, and other baked goods, or eat them as snacks.
- Keep whole flaxseeds on hand in the fridge. Grind them in a spice or coffee grinder when you're ready to add to cereal, yogurt, smoothies, and dough.
- Be wary of the mixed nuts in a can. They're usually oversalted and soaked in trans fats or oils rich in saturated fat.
- Avoid macadamias. Their saturated fat content is extremely high, and the nuts are relatively low in protein.

Peanut Butter

Peanut butter is a great source of easy protein, and a simple way to lower the glycemic load of your breakfast or lunch. But there are good peanut butters and bad ones; read the label to make sure you have the right one. Peanut butter really should have one ingredient: Peanuts. A little added salt is acceptable, but peanut butter too often has added oils like palm, which is very high in saturated fat. And many brands load up on sugar in its many forms; remember to check for syrups and words ending in "-ose", such as fructose and dextrose, on the ingredient list. If yours has sugar, too much salt, food coloring, or additives, buy another brand.

MIRACLE **ADVICE:**

- Keep peanut butter on hand as an easy protein source.
- Avoid brands with added sugar or oils.

Eggs

There's a lot to be said for the humble egg, one of nature's "complete protein" foods (see Complete Proteins: Getting Your Fill on page 94). Long shunned for its cholesterol content, it's only in the last couple of decades that researchers finally tested to see whether eating eggs actually raises blood levels of cholesterol. First, they discovered that eating an egg a day had no impact on heart risk. Further research showed that up to three eggs a day can be eaten without raising cholesterol or otherwise adversely affecting heart risk markers.

An egg contains a modest 2 grams of saturated fat, all in the yolk. If you want to cut back further on saturated fat, eat only the egg white, which contains none of the egg's fat and all of its protein. Eggs are also one of nature's few food sources of vitamin D, which may help guard against high blood pressure and inflammation of the arteries, among its many other benefits. Choline, another beneficial substance of which eggs happen to be a primary source, is vital to nerve, brain, and heart health.

MIRACLE **ADVICE:**

- Unless your doctor tells you otherwise, feel free to eat an average of one egg a day.
- Use eggs as an inexpensive source of complete protein at breakfast, lunch, and even dinner.

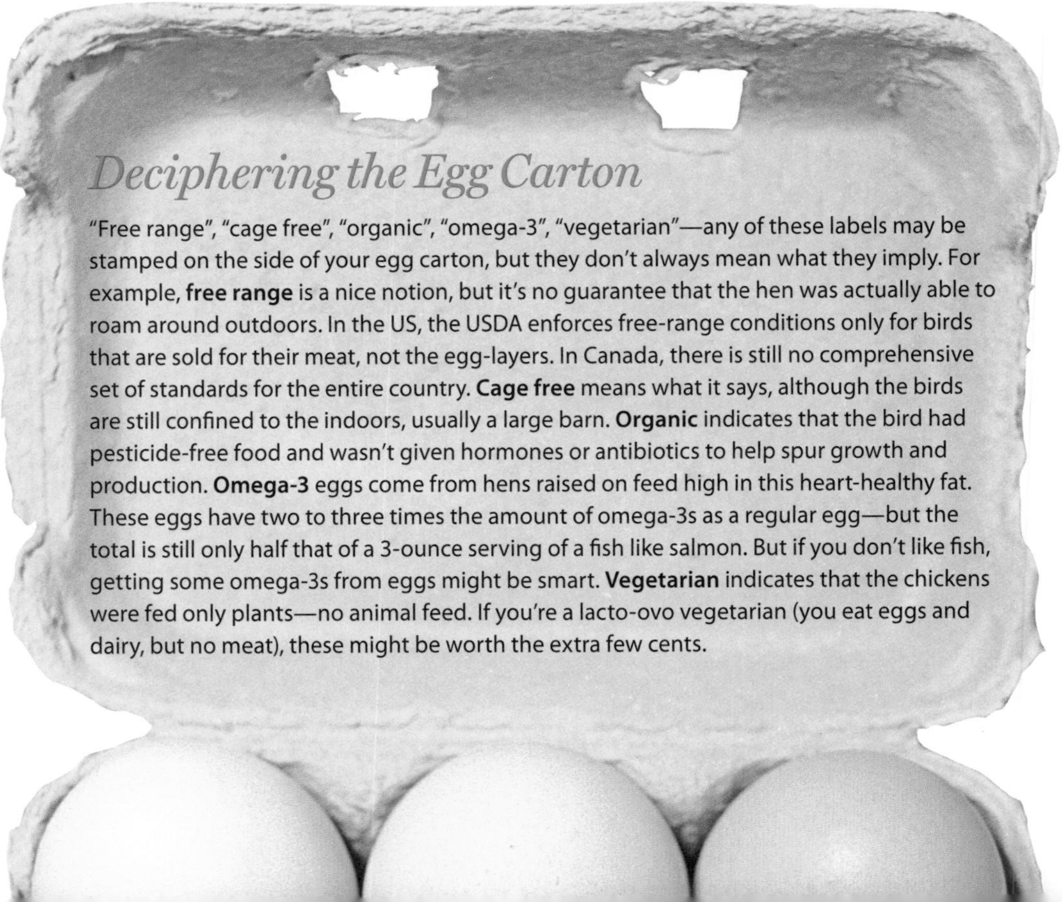

Deciphering the Egg Carton

"Free range", "cage free", "organic", "omega-3", "vegetarian"—any of these labels may be stamped on the side of your egg carton, but they don't always mean what they imply. For example, **free range** is a nice notion, but it's no guarantee that the hen was actually able to roam around outdoors. In the US, the USDA enforces free-range conditions only for birds that are sold for their meat, not the egg-layers. In Canada, there is still no comprehensive set of standards for the entire country. **Cage free** means what it says, although the birds are still confined to the indoors, usually a large barn. **Organic** indicates that the bird had pesticide-free food and wasn't given hormones or antibiotics to help spur growth and production. **Omega-3** eggs come from hens raised on feed high in this heart-healthy fat. These eggs have two to three times the amount of omega-3s as a regular egg—but the total is still only half that of a 3-ounce serving of a fish like salmon. But if you don't like fish, getting some omega-3s from eggs might be smart. **Vegetarian** indicates that the chickens were fed only plants—no animal feed. If you're a lacto-ovo vegetarian (you eat eggs and dairy, but no meat), these might be worth the extra few cents.

Fish

Fish is a terrific, healthy source of protein. Providing an average of 20 grams of protein for a small 3-ounce serving, fish deserves to be a regular player in your meals. White fish like cod, halibut, flounder, and haddock are low in fat while still high in protein. Oily fish like salmon, sardines, mackerel, trout, and tuna are loaded with both protein and "good" fats.

MIRACLE **ADVICE:**

- Eat fish at least twice a week.
- Add canned tuna or salmon to salads to boost the protein content.
- Keep frozen shrimp on hand as an easy protein source (moderate consumption won't raise your cholesterol).

Beef and Lamb

You may think that all-but-eliminating red meat is critical on any heart-healthy diet, but that couldn't be further from the truth. Some recent research suggests that the general alarm over beef's supposed danger to the heart may be in part due to clerical error. Typically, heart researchers lump bacon, hot dogs, and processed deli meats together with unprocessed cuts like steak, London broil, and tenderloin when looking at meat's effect on the heart. So researchers at the Harvard School of Public Health took a fresh look at 20 different diet studies involving more than 1.2 million people to see if they could tease apart the impact of cured, smoked, or salted red meat on heart health versus that of regular red meat.

The results, released in 2010, might surprise you: The researchers found that the risk of heart disease was elevated for people who regularly ate processed meats, *but not* for those who ate fresh cuts of unprocessed meat. One explanation for the lack of trouble with regular beef is its high content of stearic acid, a saturated fat that is converted into healthy monounsaturated fat when it's digested. Beef fat also contains conjugated linoleic acid (CLA), which seems to help control blood sugar. There's even evidence that it can help the body preserve muscle mass and reduce body fat.

As heart experts are quick to point out, however, more research is needed to confirm that the fat in beef is as safe as it appears. And even if beef passes the health test, you still don't want a huge steak dominating your plate every night of the week. The calories alone would crowd out other heart-healthy foods like vegetables, fish, and grains. But there's definitely room for beef in the Healthy Heart Miracle Diet, provided you stick to the leaner cuts. That means avoiding heavily marbled meats including prime rib, filet mignon, T-bone, London broil, and rib steak. All have higher levels of saturated fat and are laced with fat that you can't simply cut away.

Harvard researchers found that the risk of heart disease was elevated for people who regularly ate processed meats, *but not* for those who ate fresh cuts of unprocessed meat.

Skinny Beef

Lean	Extra Lean
Round steak	Eye of round roast
95% lean ground beef	Top round steak
Chuck shoulder roast	Chuck steak
Arm pot roast	Bottom round roast
Shoulder steak	Top sirloin steak
Tenderloin steak	
T-bone steak	

Lamb has one advantage over beef in that there is usually less marbling in the muscle. If you trim away the exposed fat after roasting or grilling, you're getting a protein source that is lower in fat than beef. Lean cuts include leg of lamb, loin chops, and rib chops. Fatty cuts to avoid are the shoulder, blade chops, ribs (as in rack of lamb), and ground lamb.

MIRACLE **ADVICE:**

- If you enjoy meat, go ahead and eat it as a healthy source of protein. Just be sure to choose lean cuts over fatty cuts.
- Leave room on your plate for plenty of vegetables.
- Eat ground beef sparingly (it's fattier than individual cuts), and look for packages labeled 95 percent fat-free.

Pork

The so-called other white meat (it's actually red meat) has made quite a resurgence. A generation or two ago, pork had a different story. Parasites posed a major concern thanks to poor practices in feeding and raising pigs; that meant that people generally cooked chops and tenderloins until they were dry. The cuts were also much fattier because of the type of feed livestock farmers used.

No more: The likelihood that tainted pork will make you ill is low. And pork today contains, on average, 31 percent less fat, 14 percent fewer calories, and 10 percent less cholesterol. In fact, lean cuts such as tenderloin vie with chicken for their low fat content. And you don't have to cook it until it's dry as dust. Even the government health experts say that you can serve pork a little pink in the middle, as long as a meat thermometer reads 160°F (71°C). That means you can serve it with much more juice left in it. You can also cook it with the fat attached and trim it afterward.

The other advantage to pork is in its B vitamins. These can help keep levels of homocysteine in check; high homocysteine levels are linked with increased heart attack risk (see "High Homocysteine" on page 29). One B vitamin in particular, riboflavin, is helpful in metabolizing carbohydrates.

Lean versus Extra Lean

The lean and extra lean designations for meat on these pages hew to this standard: "Lean" means that a 3.5-ounce (100 g) serving of chicken, beef, pork, or any other type of meat has fewer than 10 grams of fat and 4.5 grams of saturated fat. To qualify as "extra lean", a 3.5-ounce (100 g) serving of meat has to deliver less than 5 grams of fat and 2 grams of saturated fat. Both the lean and extra lean cuts also have fewer than 95 mg of cholesterol per serving. That's reassuring to know but, as you may remember, cholesterol in food has little effect on your blood cholesterol levels.

it's a miracle! GRASS-FED LIVESTOCK CONTAINS HEALTHY FATS

If you let cows or sheep graze a field of mixed grass and grains, they'll carefully eat around the grain to get at the grass. That's what they prefer—it's their natural food. Yet today, the majority of livestock are fed grain: It helps fatten them up more quickly and it's less expensive. But all that grain alters the mix of fats in the meat, swapping heart-healthy omega-3 fatty acids for extra saturated fat. Feeding animals grains also increases the overall fat in the animals. One study found that cuts from grass-fed animals have a third of the fat of grain-fed. Grass-fed cuts also contain more conjugated linoleic acid (CLA), a substance that helps the body control blood sugar and may be linked to improved weight-loss success. More and more livestock growers are raising their animals on grass these days, though you'll have to pay extra for these meats. Expect grass-fed cuts to have a slightly stronger and more distinct flavor.

The pork products you need to be wary of are the processed versions: sausage, bacon, cured ham, and hot dogs. However, even sausage and bacon can play a part in your diet if you're careful how you use them. A couple of links of andouille sausage crumbled up and used to flavor a pasta sauce that will end up serving four to six people? There's nothing wrong with that. Four rashers of bacon crumbled over a spinach salad that will feed your entire family? Sure. (But know that bacon contains more fat than protein, so don't think of it as a great protein source.) It's when you serve several links next to eggs at breakfast or have a couple in rolls at a barbecue that you're veering into saturated fat overload. And having three or four pieces of bacon with pancakes or on a BLT will overload your diet not just with saturated fat but also with preservatives and sodium.

Skinny Pork

Lean	Extra Lean
Boneless loin roast	Boneless uncured ham
Boneless loin chops	Pork tenderloin
	Canadian-style bacon

MIRACLE **ADVICE:**

- Enjoy pork tenderloin or pork loin chops as lean sources of protein.
- Use fatty processed products such as bacon and sausage only in very small amounts to flavor a dish.
- Eat deli ham less often. Cured ham has prohibitive levels of salt and contains preservatives like nitrates that are hard on the arteries. Uncured smoked ham may have less salt, but it still contains nitrates. When you want ham, opt, if possible, for uncured, unsmoked ham that you cook yourself.

Poultry

Now that you know you can eat lean cuts of beef and pork, you may find yourself relying less on chicken. But chicken still has its advantages. Aside from having less saturated fat than even lean cuts of beef, skinless chicken breast is very low in calories by comparison. It's also high in selenium. This mineral functions like an antioxidant, and people who have low levels tend to have problems with unstable blood sugar levels. People with diabetes who are low in selenium are more likely to suffer complications from their condition, which has led researchers to speculate that selenium may offer some protection against the damage to cells caused by high blood sugar.

Turkey breast actually has more protein and selenium than chicken, and it's lower in calories to boot, making it one of the leanest, lower calorie sources of protein you can find. One major caveat: If you're buying ground turkey, make sure to look for a package labeled ground turkey *breast*. Other types of ground turkey include some turkey skin and possibly dark meat, making it closer to ground beef in terms of nutritional value.

In general, choosing the leanest cuts of poultry is much more straightforward than it is with other types of meat: Favor white meat. And don't eat the skin. If you want to cook the bird with the skin on to make sure the chicken stays moist and juicy, that's fine; just remove it before you eat.

REMEMBER THIS

One of your main goals on the Healthy Heart Miracle Diet is to eat more fresh foods and fewer processed foods. That extends even to chicken. You're far better off cooking a chicken or turkey breast at home and slicing the meat for sandwiches than buying deli meat. Deli meats often contain added salt and sugar as well as nitrates, preservatives that are known carcinogens.

MIRACLE **ADVICE:**

- Always remove the skin before eating chicken, and if you opt for ground turkey, look for ground turkey ***breast***.
- Use white-meat chicken to add extra protein to salads and pasta dishes.
- Cook turkey breast more often for an even leaner, lower calorie source of protein.

Dairy

You'd probably never guess that a daily glass or two of milk could offer serious heart protection. But if you stopped drinking milk after childhood, it's high time to start again (unless of course you're lactose intolerant).

Most dairy foods, including milk, yogurt, and cheese, are excellent sources of protein and low in carbohydrates. That alone is a reason to eat or drink more, as long as you choose low-fat or fat-free (skim) versions to avoid the extra saturated fat and calories. But dairy can also help lower your blood pressure and protect your arteries in other ways, too.

Chalk up the blood pressure benefits in part to the calcium, magnesium, and potassium in dairy. In the landmark DASH (Dietary Approaches to Stop Hypertension) study, people who ate diets rich in fruits and vegetables and had three daily servings of low-fat dairy products dropped their blood pressures by 11.4/5.5 mmHg, on average. Meanwhile, people following the same diet but without the dairy lowered their blood pressures by only 7.2/2.8 mmHg, on average. Some researchers believe that the whey protein in dairy foods acts like widely prescribed blood pressure drugs called ACE inhibitors.

it's a miracle! COTTAGE CHEESE IS SMART FOR YOUR HEART

Ounce for ounce, cottage cheese contains the most protein of any dairy product. A half-cup serving has 15 grams of protein and only 3 grams of carbohydrates. Go with the low-sodium, low-fat version. (If it's too bland, add a little salt on your own.) Avoid nonfat cottage cheese, which often has added sugar and extra salt. A half-cup of low-fat cottage cheese has about 100 calories, which is just right for a Healthy Heart Miracle Diet snack.

What's more, the milk you pour on your breakfast cereal and the cheese you add (sparingly) to your green salad also help fight insulin resistance, an early sign of diabetes that's also linked to heart disease. Researchers have found that people who get at least a couple of servings of dairy on a daily basis are 21 percent less likely to develop insulin resistance than people whose diets are similar minus the dairy.

Milk is generously kind to your arteries, too, suppressing artery inflammation, which contributes to heart attacks. One study showed that a combination of dieting and consuming low-fat dairy foods cut a key measure of inflammation by 29 percent. And its vitamin D helps keep blood vessels flexible. Many Westerners are woefully low in the sunshine vitamin, making a daily glass of milk especially important during the long winter months.

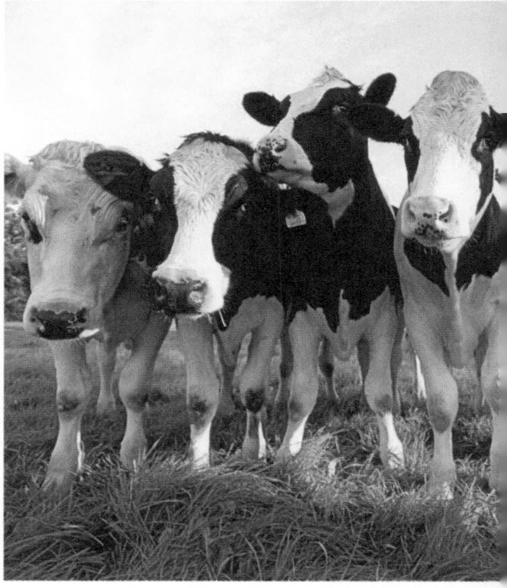

Finally, people who eat and drink lots of high-calcium foods and beverages tend to weigh less than those who don't. Why? When you're low on calcium, certain hormones that make the body store fat rise. In one 6-month study, people who cut calories and ate diets low in dairy and calcium lost 14.5 pounds (7.25 kg). A similar group that cut calories but included three servings of low-fat dairy foods a day shed about twice as much weight.

Cheese is rich in protein, but it's a bit trickier since it also contains a lot of saturated fat. It's a part of this plan because dairy in all its various forms seems to help protect against insulin resistance. Because of the saturated fat factor, enjoy cheese in sensible amounts. Invest in an adjustable wire cheese slicer and set it as thin as possible when you're cutting slices for a sandwich. When you want shredded cheese for a salad, use a fine grater and don't work with the entire block. Instead, cut off the amount you plan to use and grate that to control your serving size.

MIRACLE **ADVICE**

- Drink more milk, but make it 1% or fat-free (skim) milk to cut back on saturated fat and calories.
- Look to plain low-fat yogurt for the perfect breakfast or snack. Add your own fruit and other flavorings, such as wheat germ or ground flaxseed.
- Eat full-fat cheese in moderation. Buy the sharpest cheese and treat it as a flavoring, not a main ingredient.

Stocking a High-Protein Kitchen

Keeping plenty of protein-rich foods on hand will help ensure that you reach the suggested 20 to 25 percent of calories from protein on the Healthy Heart Miracle Diet.

food item	helpful hints	simple uses
Anchovies	You'd be surprised how many experienced chefs sneak anchovies into a variety of foods—with no one the wiser. They add a distinct savory flavor known as umami, and when your audience doesn't know what's providing the flavor, they'll rave about the depth and richness of your dishes.	Chop and add to salad dressings, pasta sauces, marinades, stews, and soups.
Canned tuna	Choose tuna packed in water, not oil. You'll save some calories, but you'll also protect the healthy fat content of the tuna; the oil tuna is packed in can leach out some of the heart-healthy omega-3 fatty acids in the fish.	Pile on whole-grain crackers with a drizzle of lemon juice to add protein to snacks.
Frozen chicken tenders	Keep a bag of frozen chicken tenders in the freezer to ensure you're always ready to put together a quick healthy protein meal.	Skip the ketchup, which is loaded with sweetener, and use mustard, marinara, or salsa as a dip.
Canned salmon	Canned salmon is a wonderful option because all salmon used for canning is wild, not farmed, therefore it's less likely to contain contaminants. And it tends to be less expensive than fresh or frozen.	Drain a can and stuff a tomato with the salmon mixed with lemon juice and minced red onion. Or mix salmon in a small bowl with 2 egg whites and 1/4 cup (50 mL) bread crumbs. Form into patties, sear in a nonstick skillet until lightly golden, and serve on greens or a whole-grain roll.
Eggs	Store them skinny end down, in the carton, on the lowest rack of the fridge, not in the door, where they'll lose nutrients to the cool dry air.	Have a hard-boiled egg for a mid-morning snack. Beat an egg and drizzle into a serving of chicken soup on the stove for a quick eggdrop soup.

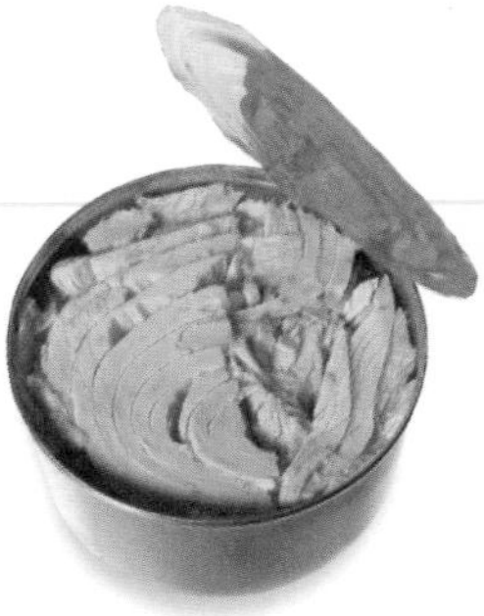

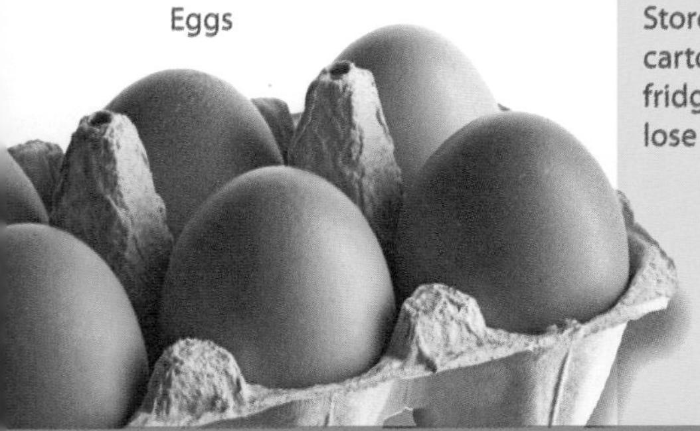

food item	helpful hints	simple uses
Frozen meat	Most meats freeze nicely, and you can keep roasts, steaks, and chops for at least 6 months without an appreciable loss of nutrients or flavor. Write the date on the package when you place meat in the freezer. To thaw, place on the top shelf in the fridge (wrap well to avoid dripping) overnight.	Save a few slices from your steak to add to a lunch salad tomorrow.
Hummus	Plain hummus is delicious, but you can also find it flavored with a variety of ingredients, such as garlic, peppers, and sun-dried tomatoes.	Make fresh vegetable and hummus sandwiches. Offer as a dip with baked nacho chips, whole-grain crackers, or triangles of fresh bread.
Frozen edamame	Buy these green soybeans in the freezer section, either in or out of the pod.	Add shelled edamame to soups and salads. Steam edamame in their pods and enjoy with a little salt as a snack.
Sardines	Canned sardines are great sources of protein and "good" fat for people who like them. Buy them stored in water or their own juices.	Top crusty bread with drained skinless, boneless sardines mashed with minced shallot and a drop of balsamic vinegar. Broil for 2 minutes. Drizzle with lemon.
Yogurt	Buy plain low-fat yogurt and add your own flavorings. Choose Greek-style yogurt for its higher protein content.	Use yogurt in baking in place of some of the oil, or mix with mayonnaise to lower fat and calories. Also use in place of sour cream as a topping on baked potatoes or Mexican-style dishes.
Seeds	Keep unsalted pumpkin or sunflower seeds on hand as snacks.	Add to salads and baked goods.
Nuts	Favor almonds and walnuts above all.	Add to salads. Throw into stir fries. Even add to vegetable dishes like green beans or spinach.

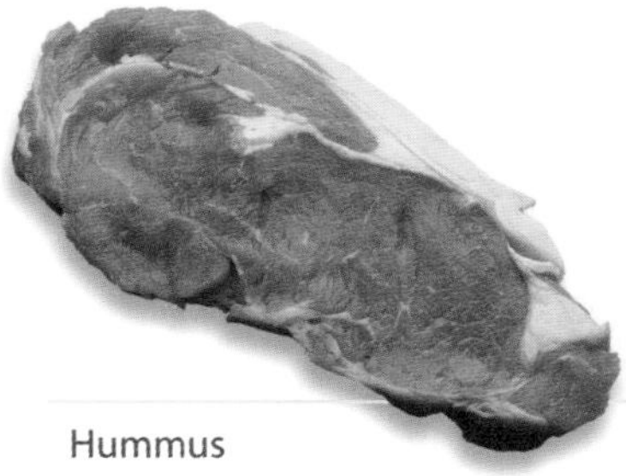

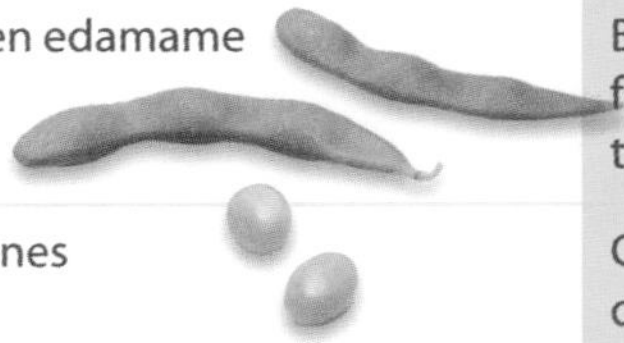

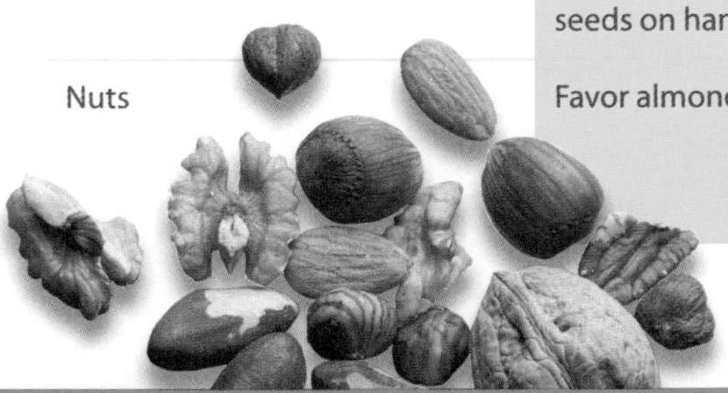

POWER UP YOUR PROTEIN: Your Meal-by-Meal Plan

Enjoying more protein at every meal will help keep you full and satisfied, and also stave off cravings for sugary foods and simple carbs. This is one of those instances in which something that sounds too good to be true actually *is* true, if you take care to choose sources of protein that are low in saturated fat.

Are you ready to put the protein plan into action? It's easiest to start with breakfast: Adding more protein to your morning meal is one of the most important steps you'll take on the Healthy Heart Miracle Diet because it will influence how you eat for the rest of the day. When you're ready, move on to another meal, or change your snacks. Getting more protein at snack time can be a challenge, but wait until you see what a difference it makes.

In chapter 9, you'll find a 14-day meal plan that shows you in detail exactly how to eat on the Healthy Heart Miracle Diet, including what the right amount of protein actually looks like across three meals. The meals there feature some of the recipes you'll find in part 4, but you should feel free to pick out some of those recipes now to help you incorporate more high-protein dishes into your day.

YOUR PROTEIN PLAN at Breakfast

1	Have eggs for breakfast several times a week.
2	Look for cereals with at least 3 grams of protein, and add nuts or seeds for extra protein.
3	If you have fruit, serve it over 1 cup (250 mL) of nonfat yogurt.
4	Oatmeal is surprisingly rich in protein, another reason to favor it for breakfast. Make it with milk instead of water for even more protein.
5	If you have toast, stick with 1 large slice or 2 small slices and add peanut butter or low-fat cream cheese.

Breakfast

Eating breakfast every day is one of the must-dos on the Healthy Heart Miracle Diet. If you eat breakfast *and* you make sure it contains protein (one reason that fruit by itself is not a great way to start the day), you'll be amazed at how easy it is to control your eating throughout the rest of the day.

It's this simple: When you eat more protein and fewer carbs, the fullness lasts longer. In a study published in 2010, University of Connecticut researchers fed men a breakfast of 1 1/2 pieces of toast and three scrambled eggs on one day. On another day, they ate a large plain bagel with just a smear of cream cheese and a small cup of yogurt. The breakfasts had the same number of calories, yet when the men ate eggs for breakfast, they ate 400 fewer calories over the next 24 hours compared to when they ate the bagel and cream cheese. What was the difference? Remember ghrelin, the hunger hormone? The researchers found that the men had much higher levels of the hunger hormone following the high-carb breakfast.

Most people naturally reach for carbs at breakfast, but adding more protein isn't difficult.

Make eggs for breakfast. One of the easiest ways to get enough protein for breakfast is to have an egg. Poached is a great way to go, or choose hard-cooked for convenience; you can hard-cook several eggs on Sunday to take with you on weekday mornings if you're in a rush. Obviously, you can also scramble or cook your eggs over easy—just use nonstick cooking spray instead of butter to keep down the calories and saturated fat. If you're looking for a breakfast the whole family can sit down and appreciate, how about French toast? You can dip whole-grain bread in an egg mixture and cook it up on a griddle sprayed with a monounsaturated vegetable oil. The eggs will help balance out the carbs in the bread.

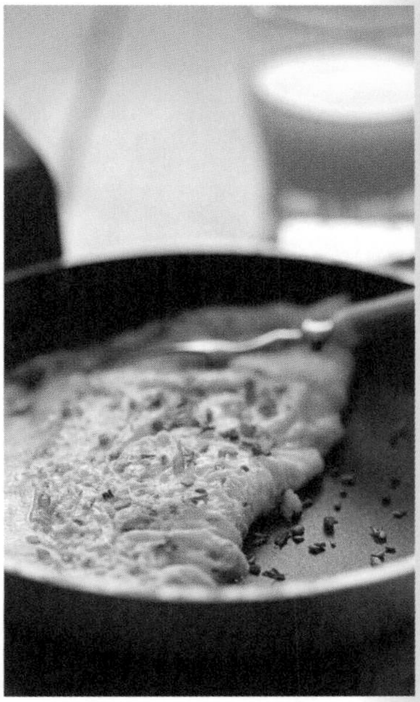

Remember dairy. Dairy is another good protein choice; just remember to stick to low-fat or skim options. Low-fat or fat-free (skim) milk over a whole-grain cereal (many of which will deliver a decent amount of protein on their own) will get your day off to a great start. And don't limit yourself to milk: Yogurt offers another source of protein. Some brands contain as many as 15 grams of protein per 6 ounces (175 g)—that's as much as two eggs. Greek-style yogurt tends to contain significantly more protein because the straining process makes it thicker. If you buy yogurt that contains live, active cultures, you'll also get beneficial bacteria that help you digest food, power up your immune system, and reduce your risk of colon cancer.

Add cut-up pineapple, banana, apple, and low-fat yogurt into a blender for a delicious smoothie that you can take with you, and that will stay with you until lunch. Or make a yogurt parfait by layering cereal, yogurt, and chopped fruit for a filling, relatively low-carb breakfast.

Get nutty. On the Healthy Heart Miracle Diet, you'll want to make nuts and seeds a regular part of your daily diet. If you love toast for breakfast, spread some peanut butter on it. You can also add toasted nuts to your cereal, and sprinkle ground flaxseed (also a source of "good" fats) to hot or cold cereal or to yogurt or smoothies.

Breakfast Suggestions

1 or 2 eggs with 1 to 2 slices of whole-grain toast

Yogurt parfait with fresh fruit, granola, and 1 cup (250 mL) plain low-fat yogurt

1 to 2 slices of whole-grain toast or 1 English muffin with 1 tablespoon (15 mL) peanut butter

Yogurt-and-fruit smoothie

Lunch

Having enough protein at lunch is the key to staying awake between the sleep-inducing hours of 2:00 and 4:00 in the afternoon. And if you do, you'll find yourself less ravenous when you walk in the door in the evening and less likely to reach for carb-heavy before-dinner snacks.

Look to vegetable proteins at lunch. Because you'll often have meat with your evening meal, lunch provides the chance to squeeze in some protein from vegetarian sources. Bean soups such as chili, split-pea, or lentil will set you up nicely for your afternoon. Three-bean salad is another healthy choice, and most delis carry it. Chickpeas can be mashed with olive oil and lemon juice to make hummus, a Middle-Eastern spread. Use it as a sandwich or pita-bread filling along with vegetables like tomatoes, cucumbers, and bean sprouts. Toss any kind of rinsed canned beans, such as black beans or red kidney beans, over a salad. If you're looking for other nonmeat sandwich options, consider peanut butter or soy nut butter.

YOUR PROTEIN PLAN at Lunch

1	Favor vegetable proteins from sources like beans.
2	Avoid cured deli meats and use home-cooked turkey or chicken, when possible.
3	Add protein to salads in the form of meat, chicken, or beans.

Choose your lunch meats carefully. Home-cooked chicken or turkey that you slice yourself is the best "lunch meat" of all because it's free of additives, preservatives, and extra sodium, and you know what you're eating. If you want sandwich meat from the deli, look for meats that haven't been cured (it's not always obvious—even some turkey meat is cured—so read the label if you can or ask at the counter). Turkey and chicken are the best choices. Choose roast beef less often; it contains about twice the calories per ounce than turkey and more saturated fat. Remember to choose whole-grain bread, or skip the bread altogether and have a chef's salad with rolled or shredded deli meats and plenty of greens and vegetables such as red onions, carrots, tomatoes, and whatever else sounds appealing.

Consider eggs again. If you didn't have eggs for breakfast, consider them at lunch. It's easy enough to add a sliced hard-cooked egg to a green salad, or chop it and mix it with low-fat yogurt and low-fat mayo for a sandwich filling (along with veggies such as lettuce and red onions).

Don't forget fish. Lunch is where canned tuna and salmon really come in handy—in sandwiches, on salads, or even wrapped in lettuce leaves.

Lunch Suggestions

Split-pea or lentil soup

Vegetarian chili

Three-bean salad

Half a deli sandwich made with turkey or ham, Swiss or cheddar cheese, lettuce, tomatoes, pickles, and onions

Chef's salad with deli cuts, cheese, and vegetables

Green salad with tuna or salmon and beans

Dinner

Most of us get most of our protein at dinner (though on the Healthy Heart Miracle Diet, you'll be aiming to include more of it at breakfast and lunch, too). That's because meat, poultry, and fish—typical Western dinner fare—are all rich in it. So the problem at dinner isn't necessarily getting enough protein, it's getting the right protein, which mainly comes down to keeping saturated fat in check. It's also about keeping portion sizes in check. If a piece of meat or chicken takes up most of your plate, it's way too big.

Think beans again. Legume dishes, bean and barley soups, split-pea soup, and pasta e fagioli (cannellini beans with noodles), are all excellent vegetable protein main courses.

Feel free to have meat several times a week. But choose lean cuts—which, incidentally, don't include most ground beef. And instead of a giant steak, serve yourself a portion that takes up only one-quarter to one-third of your plate. In fact, think about using meat as a flavoring and protein-booster for other dishes, such as a vegetable stir-fry or a pasta dish. By cutting it into strips and then using it in a stir-fry, with kebabs, in a stew, or with onions and colorful bell peppers in fajitas, you will satisfy your carnivorous desires and get the protein you need, but limit the calories and saturated fat.

If you apply the meat-as-flavoring approach, you can even enjoy sausage. You can find flavorful versions of andouille, brats, chorizo, and other sausages made with turkey or chicken. While you'll still want to break up these sausages and use them for flavor rather than as the focus of a meal, by switching to poultry links, you further limit the saturated fat in your dinner.

Many lean cuts of meat such as sirloin and top round can come out tough if you're not careful. If you'd like to avoid a workout for your jaw muscles, make a marinade that uses wine or citrus juice; the acids in the liquid will soften the tough fibers. You can also pound meat to make it thinner and loosen up the cut before cooking. Cook lean cuts either very quickly (over high heat) or very slowly (over low heat). By searing meat over high heat, you'll preserve the beef flavor. Letting it roast slowly while basting will allow the meat to take on the flavors of the sauce and conversely flavor the sauce with that distinctive beef taste.

Pork works in stir-fries and in rice and vegetable dishes and stews. But a pork tenderloin is not only a perfect source of lean protein, it's a delicious cut that deserves to stand on its own. Brown it on the stove top, let it cool, and then rub it with spices, mustard, or the sauce of your choice and roast it slowly in the oven. Be sure to take it out before it's overdone (an internal temperature of 160°F (71°C) will mean the pork is done and still pink in the center), slice it in 1/4-inch (0.5-cm) medallions, and serve it on a platter with its own juices or a quick sauce made by deglazing the roasting pan with white wine or vermouth.

Get creative with chicken. To keep a relationship interesting, you need to try new things together. To keep chicken interesting, you need to try new recipes. When possible, cook chicken with the skin on and then remove it before you eat the dish. That way, the meat stays moist. When you're working with skinless, boneless chicken breasts, pounding the cuts will keep the meat tender and allow it to retain more of the juices in which it's been prepared. Preparing the

YOUR PROTEIN PLAN at Dinner

1	Make sure a protein-rich food such as fish or chicken fills at least one-quarter to one-third of your plate.
2	At least two times a week, choose vegetable protein, such as beans, for your main course.
3	Plan a fish main course at least once a week.

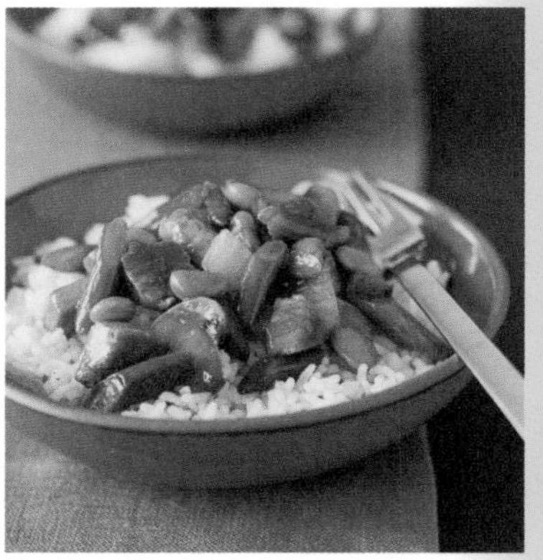

breasts in, say, a lemon-caper sauce and cooling them in the refrigerator will allow you to quickly turn salads into a main event at dinner or, with some quick heating, add extra protein to pasta dishes.

For a fast dinner, serve fish. Want fast food? Ready in as little as 10 minutes, fish is it. Salmon is one of the easiest, most versatile fish to work with, and it's rich in heart-healthy fats. But any other type of fish will do, too, as long as it's not fried or drowned in butter.

Power up your pasta. On nights that you're having a carb-focused meal, add chicken strips, beans, or another source of protein to your dish along with vegetables. Pasta and beans are a classic combination.

Dinner Suggestions

Bean and barley vegetable stew

Pork or chicken and vegetable stir-fry

Salmon with lemon-caper sauce

Sirloin steak salad

Pasta primavera

Steak fajitas with onions and bell peppers

Snacks

The difficult truth discovered by anyone trying to add more protein to their diets is that most easy-to-grab snack foods consist mainly of carbohydrates. That holds true whether you're reaching for fruit, pretzels, granola bars, or candy. (Fruit is still a healthy snack of course—but if you add a smear of peanut butter to that apple, it will keep you full longer.) The trick is planning ahead so you'll have a protein-filled snack handy when your hunger hits.

YOUR PROTEIN PLAN at Snack Time

1	Instead of grabbing chips or pretzels, plan ahead for protein-rich snacks.
2	If you have fruit as a snack, add a small amount of peanut butter or a piece of cheese for protein.

Keep hard-cooked eggs in the fridge and edamame in the freezer. Both make for excellent high-protein snacks.

Carry nuts or seeds with you for anytime snacks. Nuts are one of the great joys of following the Healthy Heart Miracle Diet in that they're satisfying, flavorful, and good for you. Moderation is key, of course: These little flavor bombs are loaded with calories. Since you aren't eating too many of the nuts, getting the salted version is fine. (Check with your doctor—if you have high blood pressure that is very sensitive to salt, you may need to choose unsalted nuts.) A bag of almonds or sunflower seeds in the car can help you resist the temptation to stop at fast-food outlets or other roadside lures.

Keep nuts in their shell in a bowl at home. Next to that bowl of fresh fruit you keep on the counter, put a bowl of mixed nuts in the shell. Cracking a few walnuts, almonds, or hazelnuts when you feel peckish will quell your need for something to chew on and give you something to occupy your hands. Pistachios, sunflower seeds, walnuts, hazelnuts, almonds, and most other types of popular nuts can be found in the shell.

Keep a jar of peanut butter handy. Whether you're snacking on apple slices, baby carrots, celery sticks, or whole-wheat crackers, peanut butter (remember: no added sugar or fats) is an excellent and tasty way to add protein and balance out the carbs.

Snack Suggestions

- 1 hard-cooked egg white filled with hummus
- 1 ounce (30 g) low-fat mozzarella cheese stick with veggie slices
- Fresh turkey slices with veggie sticks
- 1 cup (250 mL) steamed edamame
- Peanut butter on fruit or whole-grain crackers
- Canned tuna on crackers
- 1.5 ounces (45 g) roasted soy nuts

RECIPE

Easy "Roasted" Nuts

When commercial roasters roast nuts and seeds, some nutrients are inevitably lost. For a roasted taste with the most healthy oils, vitamins, and minerals preserved, the University of Nebraska recommends this easy microwave method. It works well for amounts ranging from a tablespoon to 1/2 cup (125 mL). (With larger amounts, some nuts or seeds are likely to turn dark quicker than others.) The time will vary depending on the size, type, and temperature of the nuts or seeds and also may be influenced by the type of microwave you have.

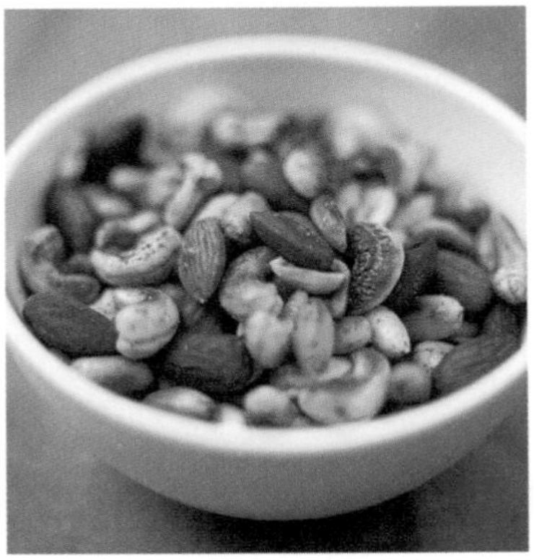

1. Spread up to 1/2 cup (125 mL) nuts or seeds evenly in a single layer on a flat, microwavable dish, such as a 9-inch glass pie plate.
2. Add a small amount of oil. Use about 1/2 teaspoon (2 mL) oil per 1/2 cup (125 mL) nuts or seeds. Stir to thinly coat. This small amount of oil helps with browning, speeds up the toasting process, and adds only about 20 calories per 1/2 cup nuts (125 mL) or seeds.
3. Microwave on high for 1 minute.
4. Stir, then microwave for another minute.
5. Check to see how the toasting is proceeding. Add more cooking time 1 minute at a time, stirring after each minute. Thin nuts (for example, sliced almonds or pine nuts) may be finished at 2 minutes. Larger nuts, such as whole almonds, walnuts, or pecans, will take an additional minute or two to become lightly browned and smell fragrant. Store any extra toasted nuts in an airtight container in the refrigerator for 1 to 2 weeks or freeze them for 1 to 3 months.

8

Fix Your Fats

"Fat" used to be a dirty word. Today, if you're still trying to cut most of the fat out of your diet, you're doing yourself a disservice. Eating more of the right fats can cut your risk of a heart attack and even help you to shed some weight.

Have you swapped the rice cakes that used to be your midday snack for a handful of nuts? Does sliced avocado sound like a healthy addition to your sandwich or salad? Do you have a favorite olive oil? If so, then obviously you got the memo: Fat is good.

Doctors used to think that certain types of fat in foods were, at best, neutral in terms of their effect on health. But years of research now show that so-called good fats are critical to heart health. Stacks of

YOUR FAT PLAN at a Glance

1	Eat more "good" fat foods like fish, nuts, seeds, and avocados.
2	Eliminate man-made trans fats, which clog arteries and contribute to heart disease.
3	Reduce sources of saturated fat, such as butter and marbled meats—but do eat dairy.
4	Don't stint on healthy cooking oils such as olive and canola oil.

compelling studies indicate that if your diet is missing or running low on good fats, you aren't the getting the full and potent health protection that food can provide.

You'll learn about some common fat myths in this chapter, but here's the biggest one of all: Most people consume too much fat. It's simply not true. In the United States, for instance, about one third of the calories consumed by the average person come from fat. Believe it or not, that's just fine. In fact, if you've been eating a lot of low-fat foods because you believe they reduce your risk for heart attacks, you're in for a pleasant surprise: You'll be increasing your fat intake on the Healthy Heart Miracle Diet.

The problem is that most people scarf down too much of the wrong kind of fat. That means the solution couldn't be more straightforward: Ramp up your intake of the right fats and curb your appetite for others. One of the major goals of the Healthy Heart Miracle Diet is to bring your fat intake back into balance. And that's not as hard to do as you might think. Consider: A Harvard study found that a woman who swaps just 5 percent of the unhealthy fat in her diet for good fats could cut her risk for suffering a heart attack by 42 percent. Other studies suggest that making simple additions to your diet, such as eating a few weekly servings of seafood (some of which are rich in good fats), can lead to dramatic reductions in the threat of cardiovascular disease, too.

What's more, new research suggests that you can fight fat—the kind that creates belly rolls and flabby thighs—with the fat you eat. That's more than just good news for your figure: Excess body fat, especially the kind that accumulates about the waistline, is closely linked to metabolic syndrome, a cluster of conditions (including high blood pressure, elevated blood sugar, and unhealthy levels of blood fats) that increase the risk not only for heart disease but also for strokes, type 2 diabetes, and other diseases. Eating more good fats could be an important key to reversing it. University of Washington researchers found that people with metabolic syndrome who took up diets filled with good fats fared much better than patients who ate typical low-fat diets. In particular, their LDL ("bad") cholesterol dropped nearly 3 times more and their triglycerides, another dangerous blood fat, dipped about 2.5 times more.

Research suggests that you can fight fat—the kind that creates belly rolls and flabby thighs—with the fat you eat.

Just to be clear: The Healthy Heart Miracle Diet is not a fat free-for-all. There are still fats that you should limit or avoid altogether. However, as you'll see, depriving yourself of favorite foods with that familiar luscious texture and gooey "mouth feel" that only fat can provide just isn't necessary.

Why Fat Is Fundamental

Do yourself a favor: If there's a fat-free cookbook gathering dust on your kitchen shelf, toss it in the recycling bin. Remember that when most people cut fat from their diets, they replace it with carbohydrates—often the refined kind—which is one of the main reasons that low-fat diets often fail to reduce the risk of heart disease.

Drastically cutting all fat from your diet was never a good idea, and many nutrition scientists say that overemphasis on reducing this vital nutrient may have backfired, making some people more vulnerable to heart disease and other health problems. Here's why fat is fundamental to your diet:

- Fat travels slowly through your gastrointestinal system. Because it takes a while to digest, it slows the rate at which food leaves your stomach, keeping your belly busy and your appetite satisfied. Even better, having fat with a meal slows down the digestion of carbohydrates, which helps to prevent blood sugar spikes and crashes that can lead to cravings for high-calorie snacks, not to mention increase the risk for insulin resistance, a precursor to diabetes.
- Fat is essential for your body's daily upkeep. Among other things, fat is a critical component of cell membranes, so you'd literally fall apart without it. You also need it to absorb so-called fat-soluble vitamins, including vitamins A, D, E, and K.

Do yourself a favor: If there's a fat-free cookbook gathering dust on your kitchen shelf, toss it in the recycling bin.

The Healthy Heart Miracle Diet emphasizes two kind of "good" fats: monounsaturated fatty acids, or MUFAs, and polyunsaturated fatty acids, or PUFAs. Aim to make these the source of 25 percent to 30 percent of the calories you consume. The 14-Day Meal Plan in the next chapter will show you exactly how. If you have been eating a typical Western-style diet, chances are good that you're not getting enough MUFAs and too little of an important variety of PUFA known as omega-3 fatty acids. Here's a closer look at why these good fats are so important for heart health.

MUFAs: The Mediterranean Diet's Must-Have Fat

Remember when olive oil was just something you kept in a little cruet and mixed with vinegar to make salad dressing? Once a bit player in most kitchens, olive oil is now heralded as a nutritional knight in shining armor. Avocados and nuts—formerly deemed guilty pleasures due to their high fat content—have undergone image makeovers, too. The reason: Research shows that people who eat plenty of these foods and others rich in MUFAs have low rates of heart disease.

This phenomenon was first discovered in the early 1970s, when researchers noted that people on the Greek islands of Crete and Corfu had shockingly few heart attacks. The observation eventually helped to popularize the so-called Mediterranean diet. There is no single Mediterranean diet, of course; the cuisine of southern France has little in common with the culinary tastes of Egypt, for example. What's more, people who eat traditional diets in this region tend to consume plenty of fish, whole grains, fruit, vegetables, and other heart-friendly foods. Yet MUFA-rich olive oil is the common food that unites the region.

Is there a bottle of olive oil in your pantry? If not, then you probably aren't getting enough MUFAs. Major studies suggest that cooking with olive oil or canola oil, and eating other foods high in MUFAs, can dramatically boost your defense against heart disease.

Is there a bottle of olive oil in your pantry? If not, then you probably aren't getting enough MUFAs.

Lower risk of a second heart attack. In a French study, people who had suffered a heart attack—and were therefore at risk for another—went on a MUFA-rich diet featuring olive oil. Four years later, they were 50 to 70 percent less likely to suffer a second heart attack or stroke than a group who ate other types of fat.

it's a miracle! FAT THAT BURNS FAT

It seems completely counterintuitive: Fat contains twice as many calories as carbohydrates and protein. Yet new research suggests that MUFAs (monounsaturated fatty acids) not only don't make you fat but they may help defend your body against the worst kind of flab: visceral fat deep in your abdomen. For example, some studies suggest that the body burns MUFAs—especially the kind in olive oil—faster than saturated fat. Whether that means eating more MUFAs will help you lose weight remains controversial. However, in a small 2007 study by Australian researchers, overweight people given a high-carb diet were more likely to pack on belly flab than others who ate a diet with the same calorie content but that was high in MUFAs.

Reversal of metabolic syndrome. Italian researchers put a group of patients on a typical low-fat diet, which included about 30 percent of total calories from fat, while a second group followed a diet with the same amount of fat, but primarily from olive oil, nuts, and other sources of MUFAs. Two years later, half of the dieters in the MUFA group no longer had metabolic syndrome—they lost weight, their blood fats improved, they processed sugar more efficiently, and their arteries were healthier. Just 12 of the original 90 patients who ate the old-fashioned low-fat diet had overcome metabolic syndrome.

A healthier heart-risk profile. A trial called the OmniHeart (Optimal Macronutrient Intake Trial for Heart Health) Study compared several different weight-loss diets and found that people who got much of their fat from MUFAs slashed their level of high triglycerides (an artery-clogging fat) and "bad" LDL cholesterol while lowering blood pressure dramatically—their systolic (top number) blood pressure dropped almost 16 points, while their diastolic (bottom number) readings fell by 8 points. And, as you'll see, making MUFAs a mainstay in your diet may even help with girth control.

Olive Oil

If you asked a chef to select a cooking oil to bring to a desert island, chances are he would choose olive oil. And with all the good news about olive oil and health, you may be tempted to use this golden nectar in recipes as often as possible. Olive oil is not only a top source of MUFAs but it's also rich in antioxidants called phenols, which block the destructive effects of free radicals—the unstable molecules that promote heart disease, cancer, and other diseases. But you'll enjoy olive oil's unique flavor and gain more of its potent protection against heart disease and other conditions if you use it wisely—and know when to opt for another oil.

Extra-virgin olive oil. This finest quality olive oil, sometimes abbreviated EVOO, comes from the first batch of oil that's "cold-pressed" from ground-up olives. It's not only the most flavorful olive oil but it also contains the most antioxidants.

it's a myth. FAT-FREE SALAD DRESSING IS A SMART CHOICE

Never mind that fat-free salad dressing can leave your taste buds disappointed; some nutritionists think they're a terrible idea. The reason: Oil-based dressings are an excellent source of good fats. One huge study by Harvard researchers found that women who had a simple oil-and-vinegar salad dressing five or six times a week cut their risk for heart attacks in half. The authors of the study felt that the results were so convincing they considered the use of fat-free salad dressings to be a public health concern.

Best for: Making salad dressings, drizzling over cooked vegetables or fish, and as a dip for crusty bread. This is not the oil to use when you sauté or fry foods. It will begin to smoke at a lower temperature than most other oils, producing harsh odors and flavors. (The precise smoke point depends on the brand, but some brands may begin to smolder at as low as 320°F (160°C), though others remain stable at up to 400°F (205°C). What's more, heat robs the oil of antioxidants. One recent study found that olive oil in a skillet heated to 350°F (177°C) lost 60 percent of its phenol content after 30 minutes.

Keep Oil Fresh

Here's another rule of thumb for making sure that you're cooking with healthy fats: Don't let the oil spoil. Olive oil, canola oil, and other oils may offer a potent defense against heart disease, but they are nonetheless vulnerable to the damaging effects of air, light, and heat. Rancid cooking oil not only tastes lousy but the spoilage may create disease-causing free radicals. Check your cooking oil IQ with this quiz.

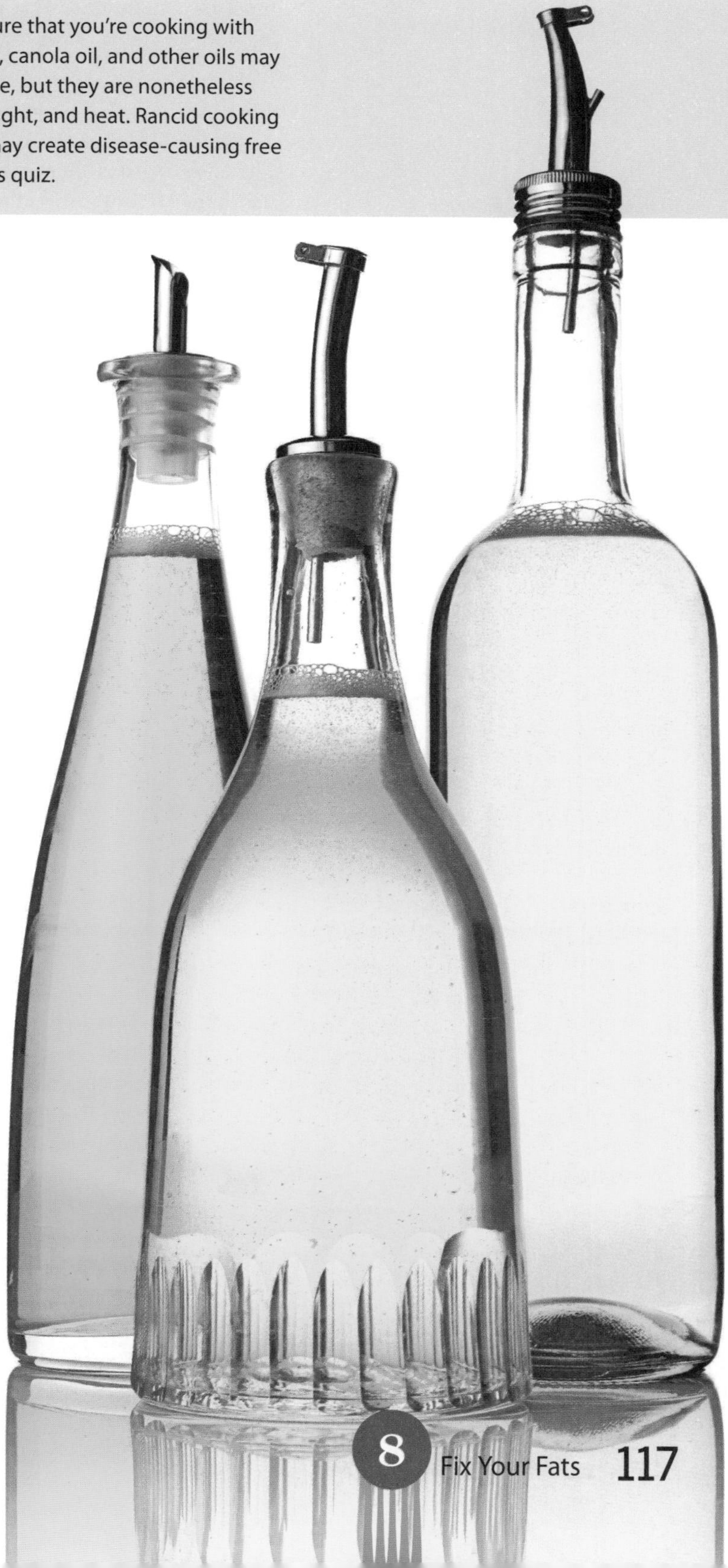

Do you store it near the stove? ...or another hot spot? If so, the heat could be draining the oil's antioxidants and speeding up the spoilage process. Move it to a cooler spot in the kitchen.

Do you leave it on the counter? Another mistake: Light damages cooking oil. Store it in a dark cupboard in an opaque container.

Did you buy it ages ago? As a rule, vegetable oils stay fresh for about 6 months or so, while olive oil keeps for about a year. Now and then, give a bottle of cooking oil the sniff test. If it has an off-odor, it's probably turned bad, so toss it out. If you buy a large container of cooking oil, pour a pint or so into a smaller bottle for everyday use. Avoid opening the original container too often.

Do you keep your oil in the refrigerator? No problem. Some cooking oils must be kept cool to stave off spoilage, such as walnut oil and almond oil. However, storing any oil in the fridge will keep it fresh longer. The oil may turn solid, but take it out of the refrigerator shortly before cooking and it will reliquefy.

Do you pour old cooking oil down the drain? If so, do you know a good plumber? You'll have a clogged sink before long. Put old or used cooking oil in a leak-proof container and throw it out with the trash.

Olive oil. Sometimes labeled "pure" or "virgin" olive oil, this oil lacks EVOO's big flavor, but it has other important advantages that make it a must for any kitchen. Regular olive oil is not only cheaper than EVOO, but its higher smoke point and milder taste make it more versatile.

Best for: Making salad dressings or preparing any other recipe where you don't want the flavor of olive oil to dominate. You can fry with regular olive oil, too, but other oils (such as peanut oil) are cheaper and less likely to burn at very high temperatures.

"Light" or "extra light" olive oil. Sold in the United States and some other countries, this refined olive oil has a neutral flavor and very high smoke point. However, it also has a lower concentration of antioxidants.

Best for: People who don't like the taste of olive oil, but still want at least some of its benefits. Light olive oil's higher smoke point makes it acceptable for frying.

Canola Oil

It may lack olive oil's mystique (and rich flavor, though that can be an advantage), but canola oil deserves a place in the kitchen of any health-conscious cook. Canola oil was developed by Canadian researchers and introduced in 1974. There are several reasons it quickly gained a reputation as one of the healthiest of all cooking fats. Among its peers, it has the lowest amount of saturated fat, with a scant 6 percent of calories. (For comparison, olive oil contains 14 percent saturated fat; butter checks in at 62 percent.) While olive oil is the champ in terms of MUFAs—74 percent of its fat takes this heart-healthy form—canola oil is a close second, at 62 percent.

The Best of the Rest: Choose the Right Oil for the Job

You can think of olive oil and canola oil as the foundation fats for the Healthy Heart Miracle Diet, but that doesn't mean you can't or shouldn't stock other cooking oils as well. This chart will help you choose the right oil for your dish. What about good old corn oil? Corn, sunflower, and safflower oils may be heart healthier choices compared to butter and stick margarine because they have less saturated fat and trans fat, but they also contain less monounsaturated fat than other oils. If you do choose sunflower oil, look for "high-oleic" sunflower oil, which is processed to contain mostly MUFAs.

Type of oil	Description	Good Source of	Used for
Grapeseed	Mild flavor; contains a small amount of vitamin E	PUFAs	Sautéing and frying; can tolerate high heat
Peanut	Nutty flavor; often used in Asian cuisine	MUFAs	Stir-frying
Sesame	Strong flavor; essential for Asian cuisine	MUFAs and PUFAs	Marinades, salad dressings, sauces
Walnut	Strong flavor; contains a small amount of ALA, an omega-3 fatty acid	PUFAs	Salad dressings, sautéing

What's more, canola oil carries a potential bonus: It contains a small amount of alpha-linolenic acid (ALA), which is a type of omega-3 fatty acid. (Other sources of ALA include walnuts and flaxseed oil.) Although the evidence is far from conclusive, some studies suggest that ALA may have important heart benefits. With its neutral flavor and friendly price, canola oil is a versatile cooking fat and a great choice if you're not a fan of olive oil's rich taste or you want other flavors in a recipe to stand out.

When you shop: Choosing canola oil is usually pretty straightforward—buy whatever is inexpensive, since flavor isn't an issue (though some specialty retailers carry extra-virgin canola oil; it's said to have a subtle, nutty flavor). Avoid higher-priced canola oils that claim to be supplemented with fish oil or other healthy-sounding ingredients; they probably contain too little to make a difference in your health. You may also come across unrefined canola oil, which you should avoid since it burns at very low temperatures.

Best for: Just about any type of cooking, including sautéing, stir-frying, and baking. Although other oils (such as peanut or safflower oil) have higher smoke points, many restaurant chefs use canola oil for deep-frying.

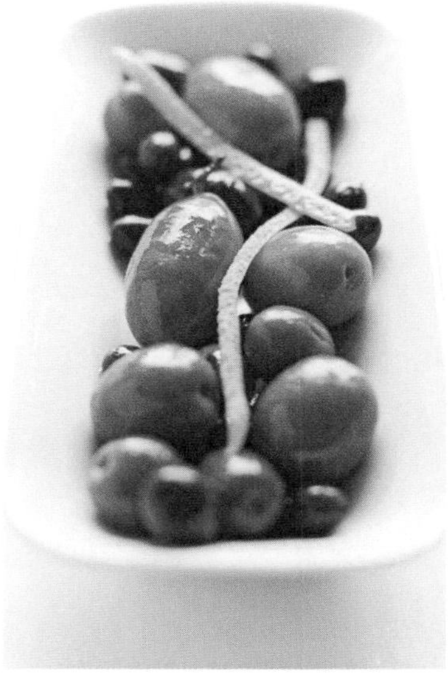

Olives

You already know about olive oil and its important role in protecting the heart. So why not go straight to the source? If that jar of Spanish olives in the back of your refrigerator only surfaces when you mix an occasional martini, bring it to the fore and put these nutritional powerhouses to work as part of the Healthy Heart Miracle Diet. Better yet, discover other varieties of olives, such as briny black Kalamatas or the tiny niçoise, perfect for the French salad of the same name. There are gaetas, ligurias, luganos, and others, too—many supermarkets now feature gourmet olive bars, which will allow you to sample the various fruits that grow on the *Olea europaea* tree.

For true olive taste, buy fresh ones from the deli section, not canned olives. And remember that the goal is to replace other fat sources (such as cheese) with good fats sources, not to add more calories to your diet.

Nuts and Peanut Butter

If you have yet to be convinced to eat peanut butter, you have some explaining to do. As you know, it's rich in protein. And taste can't be the issue: Whether you prefer crunchy or smooth, few foods can top peanut butter's big flavor and palate-pleasing texture. If you think peanut butter is for kids, think again: Research shows that its high content of MUFAs and PUFAs make it an extremely healthy food. In fact, in a major study published in the *Journal of the American*

Medical Association, researchers found that women who ate peanut butter five times a week cut their risk for type 2 diabetes by 21 percent. No one is sure why, though some studies suggest that diets rich in good fats make the hormone insulin more effective, which helps keep blood sugar under control—and thereby also reduces heart disease risk.

Eating peanut butter regularly makes sense if you already have diabetes, too. A 2009 study found that women with the condition cut their risk for heart attacks and strokes nearly in half by eating just a tablespoon of peanut butter (or an ounce of nuts) on most days of the week.

The best peanut butter has the shortest ingredients list: Roasted peanuts and salt (though you can certainly shrink the list even further by choosing unsalted). Most conventional brands contain added sugar; once you get used to all-natural peanut butter, you'll never turn back. (But beware of "no-stir" varieties; see page 132 to find out why.)

More Reasons to Nibble on Nuts, Seek Out Seeds

You already know that nuts and seeds are a great source of protein. Well, if we all munched on almonds, nibbled on pistachios, and savored some luscious cashews more often, the number of heart

What's in a Nut?

Adding nuts to your dishes is a great way to hit the Healthy Heart Miracle Diet target of about 30 grams of MUFAs every day. Don't forget calories, though; most nuts contain between 160 and 200 calories per ounce (30 g), so overeating nuts can offset the benefits. And some nuts contain more saturated fat than others (one reason to go easy on macadamias and Brazil nuts). Your best bet? Eat all types of nuts. And don't skip walnuts just because they're low in MUFAs; they contain other valuable nutrients, including a form of omega-3 fatty acid called ALA.

Type of Nut	MUFAs per oz/ 30 g	Saturated fat per oz/30 g
Macadamia	16.8	3.4
Hazelnut	13	1.3
Pecan	11.6	1.8
Almond	8.7	1
Cashew	7.7	2.6
Brazil nut	7	4.3
Peanut	7	2
Pistachio	6.9	1.6
Walnut	2.5	1.7

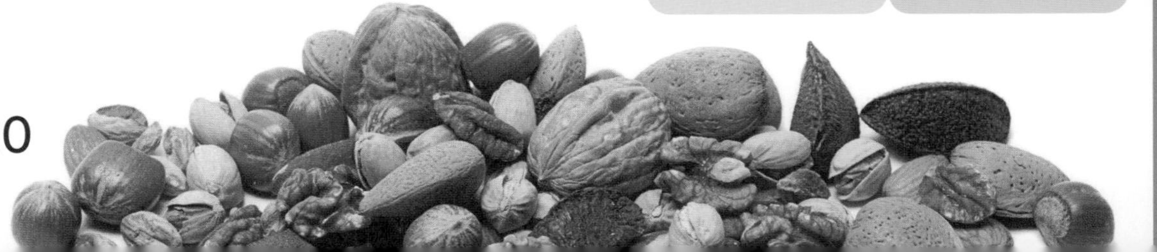

attacks that strike each year would drop dramatically. That was the conclusion of a team of nutrition scientists from Harvard, Penn State, and other leading universities who examined the impressive and consistent evidence in favor of eating nuts for a healthy heart. In study after study, the results are the same: Eating nuts helps prevent cardiovascular disease. In fact, the combined results of four huge studies, including more than 170,000 men and women, show that munching on nuts on all or most days of the week cuts the risk of heart attack by an incredible 35 percent.

What is it about walnuts? How do peanuts protect the heart? This much is clear: Eating nuts in place of less healthy foods can lower total and LDL ("bad") cholesterol by an average of 12 percent and 18 percent, respectively. Nuts are one of nature's best sources of MUFAs, with a healthy dose of PUFAs, too, and a lesser amount of saturated fat. That's good news for your blood fats, but better cholesterol doesn't tell the whole story, scientists say. Nut-lovers have such good heart health that there has to be something else about these crunchy snacks that guards against cardiovascular disease. To be sure, nuts are brimming with nutrients that appear to promote strong hearts. To name just a few: vitamin E, a potent antioxidant; arginine, an amino acid that helps blood vessels relax; and an array of micronutrients, especially one headline-grabber called resveratrol.

Munching on nuts on all or most days of the week cuts the risk of heart attack by an incredible 35%.

The latter has gained a reputation as an antiaging compound in recent years, and while that may sound like hype, the science behind resveratrol is hard to ignore. Lab mice fed resveratrol live about 15 percent longer than other mice, even when they become obese from eating high-calorie, junk-food diets. While it seems to take high doses of resveratrol to bring about health benefits, it's worth noting that peanuts (which are technically legumes, not nuts) are a top source of this substance. (Red wine contains the most.)

Go Green: Eat Avocados

If the only time you have avocados is when you order the guacamole in a Mexican restaurant, then you're missing out on a delectable treat that should be a regular feature in any heart-healthy diet. It's a rare fruit in that it contains huge quantities of fat—up to 30 grams in one avocado, which is more than you'd get from a fast-food double cheeseburger. Fortunately, most of that fat is in the form of good-for-you MUFAs.

Although it's a bit extreme, one study gives some idea why adding avocados to your diet could benefit your heart. In the study, 37 people with high cholesterol ate lots of avocados—enough to provide nearly 50 grams of MUFAs a day, which is considerably more than you'll be consuming on the Healthy Heart Miracle Diet. In just a week, their blood fats experienced some rather remarkable changes: On average, their total cholesterol dropped 17 percent, while their unhealthy LDL cholesterol and triglycerides fell even more—22 percent.

There's more than MUFAs to avocados, by the way. They're also good sources of vitamin C, vitamin E, folate, magnesium, potassium, and zinc. Fiber, too: Half an avocado provides 6 to 7 grams, much of it the soluble kind that lowers cholesterol. (For comparison, an apple has about 5 grams of fiber.) Of course, avocados are high in calories, too, so beware of portion control.

How to tell if an avocado is ripe: The skin should be firm yet yield to gentle pressure. Press down with a finger. If it gives just a little, it's ripe and ready to eat. If pressing leaves a permanent dent, it may be too ripe.

How to make an avocado ripen faster: Put it in a paper bag with a banana. Fruit gives off a gas called ethylene that causes ripening; the closed quarters will cause the avocado to absorb more ethylene.

it's a miracle! EATING AVOCADO ADDS MULTIPLE HEALTH BENEFITS

Adding sliced avocado to salad greens and vegetables makes their nutrients easier to absorb. In one study, Ohio State University researchers asked healthy volunteers to eat salsa with and without mashed avocado. In another part of the experiment, they fed the men and women a simple green salad with and without avocado. Blood samples showed that when avocado was included, the volunteers absorbed nearly 4.5 more times lycopene, a compound that may guard against some cancers; 5 times more lutein, which combats macular degeneration, a leading cause of blindness; and up to 7 times more alpha-carotene and 15 times more beta-carotene, which together protect against heart disease and cancer.

Dark Chocolate

In the past, anyone concerned about cardiovascular health would have been advised to keep right on strolling past the candy aisle. Yet there's now solid evidence that the quintessential splurge food—chocolate—helps keep a heart healthy. One recent study in Germany found that people who snacked on a small piece of chocolate every day cut their risk for heart attacks and strokes by 39 percent when compared to others who rarely or never ate chocolate.

The fat in chocolate, which comes from cocoa butter, is made up of equal parts MUFAs and saturated fat (including one form of saturated fat, called stearic acid, that's thought to be less harmful to health than other types of this fat).

Of course, there is a catch—two, really. For starters, most scientists agree that dark chocolate is the only real choice for promoting heart health. Compared to milk chocolate, the dark variety is a much richer source of antioxidants called flavonoids that appear to have several critical cardiovascular benefits. And it's much lower in saturated fat and sugar.

A number of studies have shown that eating dark chocolate induces a modest drop in blood pressure, and you might be surprised what a difference a few points makes. In a 2007 study published in *Journal of the American Medical Association*, a group of men and women with mildly elevated blood pressures started eating small amounts of dark chocolate every day. Four months later, the typical chocolate-eater's blood pressure had dropped a few points—but that was enough to mean that 20 percent of them no longer had high blood pressure. (Eating white chocolate had no effect on blood pressure.) Other studies have shown that eating dark chocolate helps the arteries relax and dilate, promoting better blood flow. This bitter, sweet candy may also turn down chronic, low-grade inflammation, another potential heart threat.

The other catch? Less is definitely more when it comes to eating dark chocolate for your heart's sake. Chocolate is chock-full of calories, of course, so chomping too much will backfire in the form of climbing numbers on the bathroom scale. The good news is that it takes just a small piece of dark chocolate to get big heart benefits—a portion slightly larger than a Hershey's Kiss every day.

When you buy chocolate: Read labels and look for bars that contains at least 60 percent cocoa to be sure that you're getting a full dose of heart-friendly flavonoids.

Miracle MUFAs

If you'd like to keep score, here are the benefits you get by eating more MUFAs:

- Lowers triglycerides and "bad" LDL cholesterol
- Lower blood pressure
- Improved insulin sensitivity
- Less visceral fat

PUFAs: A *Miracle* Fat from the Land and Sea

While MUFAs are important for heart health, PUFAs may be even more critical. Vegetable oils are packed with PUFAs and represent one of the most common sources of these good fats in most people's diets. But it's important to get your fill from other foods, too. Key among them: fish, nature's best source of a type of PUFAs known as omega-3 fatty acids. Overwhelming research now suggests that omega-3s may be the best fats of all for your cardiovascular system and all-around health.

The Healthy Heart Miracle Diet includes at least two servings of fish per week, which could lower your risk of heart attack by 36 percent, according to a review of more than 30 large studies by researchers at the Harvard School of Public Health. Fish-lovers suffer fewer strokes, too. Seafood is a great source of protein, vitamin D, selenium, and other important nutrients, which alone makes it a nutritional standout. However, it's fish oil that's the true heart medicine. In particular, it prevents sudden cardiac death, which is death caused when the heart suddenly stops beating (usually due to underlying heart disease). The omega-3 fatty acids in fish oil also reduce levels of dangerous blood fats called triglycerides, lower blood pressure, and chill out inflammation in the arteries, which can trigger heart attacks. Eating fish also seems to help lower insulin resistance, the metabolic problem that leads to type 2 diabetes.

Meanwhile, omega-6 fatty acids, which are by far the most common type of PUFA in most diets, offer another key heart benefit: They reduce "bad" LDL cholesterol when used to replace less-healthy saturated and trans fats (from foods like butter and stick margarine). Vegetable oils are good sources of PUFAs, as are walnuts, flaxseeds, and soy nuts. A 2009 study led by Danish researchers found that swapping just 5 percent of the saturated fat in your daily diet with an equal amount of PUFAs could cut the risk of fatal heart attack by 26 percent.

Take the Plunge: Eat More Fish

How much fish do you eat? If you're like most people, the simple answer is: not enough. In many countries, only about one person in five eats seafood twice a week, the amount the Healthy Heart Miracle Diet recommends. Even that figure is misleading, however, since lots of folks like seafood breaded and deep-fried, which offsets the cardiovascular protection you get from the omega-3 fatty acids. (A serving of breaded fried shrimp has nearly as much saturated fat as two glazed doughnuts.)

Furthermore, many people eat only white-fleshed fish, like cod and tilapia. There's nothing wrong with these fish, which are lean sources of protein. But other fish in the sea offer your heart a much bigger dose of omega-3s per mouthful. Fatty fish is rich in two types of omega-3 fatty acids, known as EPA and DHA. Experts recommend consuming between 1,500 and 2,000 milligrams of DHA and EPA, combined, each week. The best way to do that is to eat a few servings of dark-fleshed, oily fish, which are nature's richest

it's a miracle! FISH OIL FIGHTS FLAB

How's this for a bonus from the sea? The good fats in fish could help you lose weight. Although most of the research has involved laboratory animals, studies suggest that consuming the omega-3 fatty acids in seafood can block the effects of eating less-healthy fats. Obese lab rats fed diets rich in omega-3s lose body fat. Why? No one's certain, but evidence suggests that omega-3s suppress appetite. One Spanish study found that people who eat fish as part of a low-calorie diet are less likely to complain about feeling hungry. Other lab research suggests that fish oil switches on genes that tell the body to burn fat instead of storing it as flab.

How Does Your Favorite Fish Rate?

If you're already hooked on fish, scan this chart for your favorite varieties and use the legend below to determine whether you're getting enough omega-3s.

♡♡♡
Best choices. If you eat these fish at least twice a week, you're getting the full protection of the omega-3 fatty acids DHA and EPA.

♡♡
These fish are fine choices, though they contain somewhat lower levels of omega-3s. When you choose one of these varieties, be sure to have fish that's very high in omega-3s in the same week.

♡
These varieties are all good sources of lean protein, but they're relatively low in omega-3s. They make an excellent alternative to red meat on weeks when you want to have an extra seafood dinner.

Note: If you don't see your favorite fish here, it could be that it's too high in mercury; see page 126 to find out why you should avoid four types of fish.

Fish (3.5 oz/100 g serving, unless noted)	**Omega-3 Content**
Atlantic herring	♡♡♡
Atlantic mackerel	♡♡♡
Mussels	♡♡♡
Sablefish (also called black cod)	♡♡♡
Salmon (farmed)	♡♡♡
Salmon (wild)	♡♡♡
Trout	♡♡♡
Tuna (albacore)	♡♡♡
Alaskan pollock	♡♡
Anchovy (serving of 5)	♡♡
Arctic char	♡♡
Crab	♡♡
Halibut	♡♡
Oysters	♡♡
Scallops	♡♡
Shrimp	♡♡
Snapper	♡♡
Sole	♡♡
Squid	♡♡
Atlantic cod	♡
Catfish	♡
Clams	♡
Haddock	♡
Lobster	♡
Mahimahi	♡
Sardines (serving of 2)	♡
Tilapia	♡
Tuna (light)	♡

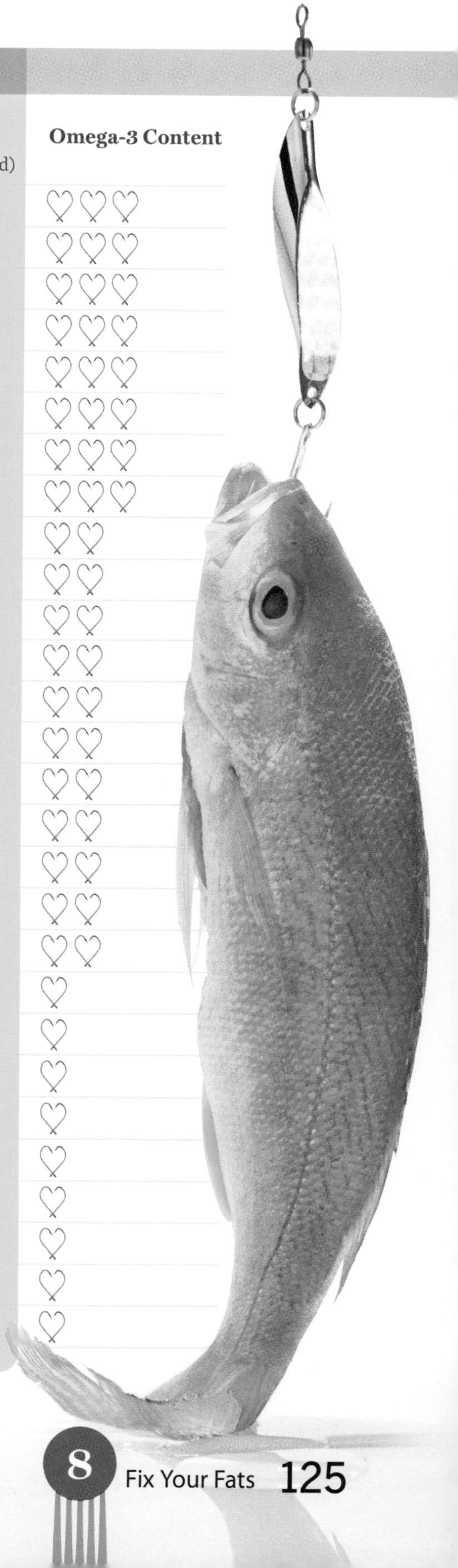

source of nourishing omega-3s. That doesn't mean other fish are off the menu, but knowing how to mix up your selections can help ensure that you're getting your weekly ration of omega-3s. Use the chart "How Does Your Favorite Fish Rate?" on page 125 to guide your choices. (This list isn't exhaustive. Depending on where you live, your local fishmonger may offer delicious varieties that also fit the bill.)

What about Mercury?

Mercury is a justifiable concern—who wants a heavy metal with their halibut? But knowing the facts about mercury will help you realize that there are fish you can choose without worry.

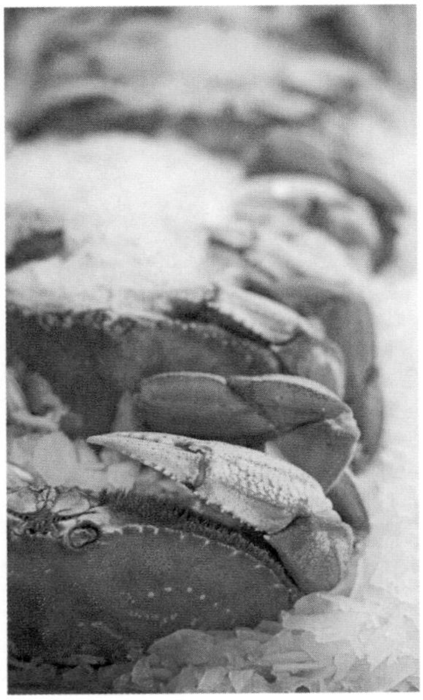

First, the hard reality: All fish contains mercury. This common element occurs naturally in the environment, but much of the mercury that ends up in fresh and saltwater comes from industrial pollution. Another inescapable truth: Seafood is the number one source of mercury in the human diet. Finally, the scary part: Mercury is a known toxin that can cause brain damage in developing fetuses and very young children exposed to high levels.

But here's the all-important counterpoint: Most fish and shellfish species contain only tiny traces of mercury. A relatively small number of fish have high levels, all of them large predators that live for many years and spend their days gobbling up smaller fish. The U.S. Food and Drug Administration and Environmental Protection Agency have determined that women of childbearing age and children under 12 should follow these rules:

- Eat no more than 12 ounces (360 g) of fish per week.
- Eat no more than 6 ounces (180 g) of albacore tuna per week.
- Don't eat the following large predators: swordfish, shark, king mackerel, and tilefish.

For everyone else, there's not enough evidence to suggest that eating any amount of fish will make you sick, though if you want to be on the safe side—sorry, swordfish-lovers—it's probably wise to follow that last rule.

Current Health Canada guidelines for eating fresh or frozen tuna, shark, swordfish, marlin, orange roughy and escolar recommend limiting consumption as follows: Women who are pregnant, may become pregnant or are breastfeeding, 150 g/month; children 5 to 11 years old, 125 g/month; children 1 to 4 years old, 75 g/month; general population, 150 g/week. Guidelines for canned albacore (white) tuna—not light tuna—are as follows: Women who are pregnant, may become pregnant or are breastfeeding, 300 g/week; children 5 to 11 years old, 150 g/week; children 1 to 4 years old, 75 g/week.

The Bad Fats: Saturated Fat and Trans Fat

Think of them as bad and badder: These fats increase the risk for heart disease, and that's only the beginning. The Healthy Heart Miracle Diet will help you cut back on these fats to less than 10 percent of your calories for saturated fat, and as close as possible to zero for trans fat. That doesn't mean that you should worry about feeling deprived because there is room on the plan for your favorite foods. In fact, some foods you may think of as prime sources of saturated fat, like dairy products and chocolate, can have surprising benefits for your heart and waistline, while protecting against other conditions, such as diabetes.

Saturated Fat = Belly Fat, Bad Cholesterol, and Worse

You have been hearing the message for years: For a healthy heart, you must cut back on butter, whole milk, juicy meats, and other foods laden with saturated fat. Eating saturated fat increases "bad" LDL cholesterol and leads to cardiovascular disease. That's why it may surprise you to learn that, in recent years, a few researchers have pointed out an inconvenient truth: Some scientific studies have failed to show that curbing our intake of saturated fat prevents heart attacks.

Spared: A Day's Worth of Saturated Fat—In One Meal

You can easily pack more than a day's worth of saturated fat into a single meal if you're not careful. Here's how making some simple changes to a traditional steak-and-potatoes dinner can help you stay within your budget for saturated fat, which for most people should be no more than about 20 grams per day.

Bad Fats Meal	Saturated Fat (g)	Good Fats Alternative Meal	Saturated Fat (g)
Rib-eye steak (3.5 oz/100 g)	5.7	Beef tenderloin (3.5 oz/100g)	3.8
Butter for frying (1 Tbs/15 mL)	7.3	Olive oil for frying (1 Tbs/15 mL)	3.8
Sour cream for potato (2 Tbs/25 mL)	2.7	Herbed nonfat yogurt for potato (2 Tbs/25 mL)	0
Whole milk (1 cup/250 mL)	4.6	1% milk (1 cup/250 mL)	1.6
Chocolate ice cream (1 cup/250 mL)	9	Fresh strawberries (1 cup/250 mL)	0
TOTAL	**29.3**	**TOTAL**	**9.2**

But don't start making that bacon-and-cheese sandwich just yet, because this doesn't mean saturated fat is off the hook. As researchers looked closer at these studies, they discovered that simply eating less saturated fat isn't the whole solution; how you replace those calories matters. In other words, cutting back on excessive amounts of saturated fat could be a waste of time if you replace it with foods that are equally punishing to the heart. And, as you know now, many people do just that by filling up on white bread, white rice, and other high-glycemic carbohydrates, which raise triglycerides, lower "good" HDL cholesterol, and create other problems in the cardiovascular system.

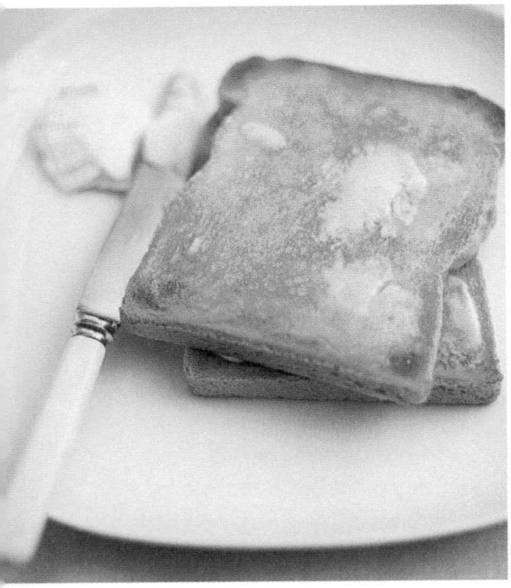

There are other very good reasons to cut back on saturated fat. For one, studies suggest that your body prefers using the saturated variety to fill out your abdomen. Belly flab is closely linked to high blood pressure, elevated triglycerides, and other scary features of metabolic syndrome. Meanwhile, there is good evidence that replacing some saturated fat with unsaturated varieties (MUFAs and PUFAs) will slash your risk for heart attacks, strokes, and other cardiovascular problems.

What About Butter?

Butter isn't banished from the Healthy Heart Miracle Diet, but let's face it: At more than 7 grams of saturated fat per tablespoon, you won't always have room in your daily fat budget for it, if you're trying to stay under 20 grams of saturated fat a day. When you really need butter (some dishes aren't the same without it), go for just a small pat, which contains 2 to 3 grams of saturated fat. If you like to bake cookies, cakes, and pies, you probably consider butter a must. If so, try mixing it with a trans-fat-free margarine to keep down the saturated fat content of your baked goods.

If you mostly use butter for spreading on bread or toast, consider using whipped butter. It won't work in baking or most other recipes (heat causes it to melt too fast), but for cold uses, it's the healthier choice. Trade a tablespoon of regular butter for the whipped variety and you'll spare yourself 35 calories and 2.5 grams of saturated fat.

	Saturated Fat (g)	Calories
Butter (1 Tbs/15 mL)	7.3	102
Whipped butter (1 Tbs/15 mL)	4.7	67

Trans Fats: Heart-Stoppers and Belly-Busters

Doctors may debate which form of fat—MUFAs or PUFAs—is best for your heart, but there's no disagreement over which one is worst. Trans fats are by far the most dangerous form of fat for the cardiovascular system. Some experts estimate that if these bad fats suddenly disappeared, the number of heart attacks worldwide would drop by 20 percent almost overnight.

Furthermore, disturbing new research suggests that trans fats may even be a major hidden cause of obesity. That's why the Healthy Heart Miracle Diet is designed to bring your intake of trans fats way down—as close to zero as possible. Fortunately, that's getting easier to do every day.

A tiny amount of trans fat—representing 0.5 percent of calories or less in most diets—occurs naturally in dairy foods, beef, lamb, and some other meats. (And at least one study found that naturally occurring trans fats don't increase the risk for heart disease.) But the overwhelming source in most diets is partially hydrogenated vegetable oil, which is vegetable oil that has been treated to give it a semisolid texture. Partially hydrogenated vegetable oil offers foods a longer shelf life, which is one reason processed food manufacturers like it. Your heart, however, doesn't. Here's a short list of problems you may be experiencing if you consume too many foods packed with these fats.

- High levels of "bad" LDL cholesterol, especially small, dense LDL particles that appear to be especially damaging
- Low levels of "good" HDL cholesterol
- Elevated triglycerides, a dangerous type of blood fat
- High levels of Lp(a) lipoprotein, a molecule in the blood that may increase the risk for heart attacks

And that's not all. Some studies suggest that trans fats spark chronic inflammation in the body and cause damage to the lining of blood vessels. (As mentioned in chapter 2, endothelial dysfunction is a major contributor to heart attacks.) It's no wonder that researchers estimate that widespread cutbacks on trans fat could prevent about one in five heart attacks.

Some experts estimate that if trans fats suddenly disappeared, the number of heart attacks worldwide would drop by 20 percent.

Fat That Makes You Fat

Scientists have long argued that a calorie is a calorie when it comes to weight gain. There's no difference whether it comes from fat, carbohydrates, or protein—all calories pack on fat the same way. Or so the thinking went. But new research offers powerful evidence that trans fats don't follow the rules. Wake Forest University researchers fed one group of lab monkeys diets high in trans fat. They fed a second group a diet with the same number of daily calories that was high in MUFAs. After 6 years, the monkeys that ate trans fats gained *three times* more weight than the other monkeys. Even worse, much of the extra weight took the form of belly fat, which is a key factor in metabolic syndrome.

Tossing back a handful of cheese crackers could actually make you fatter than eating a hot dog.

This research is still preliminary, but the implications are mind-boggling: Tossing back a handful of cheese crackers could actually make you fatter than eating a hot dog. Trans fats are increasingly linked to other diseases, too. For instance, a 2008 study found that people who consume the most trans fats may be up to 86 percent more likely to develop colon cancer.

There is good news about these bad fats, however: A growing number of food processors have quit using them. That means that you're probably consuming fewer trans fats today than you were a few years ago. For instance, Canadians used to be among the world's most voracious consumers of trans fats, putting away about 8.4 grams per person every day back in the mid 1990s. But in 2005, the Canadian government asked manufacturers to lower levels of trans fats in processed foods. By 2008, average consumption in Canada had dropped to 3.4 grams daily.

While that's encouraging, experts say it's not low enough. The World Health Organization recommends keeping your intake of trans fats to less than 1 percent of your daily calories. That's just 2 grams a day if you're following a 2,000-calorie diet. See "Trans Fat Disaster Foods" below to find out if you're exposing your body to the worst sources of this bad fat.

Trans Fat Disaster Foods

Many restaurants and food processors have cut back on or stopped using partially hydrogenated oils, the main source of deadly trans fats, but many others have yet to make the switch. The following foods are the worst potential culprits. The only way to know if a food contains trans fat is to ask restaurant servers (assuming they have a clue) and read food labels closely.

Danger Food	Trans Fat Threat		
Fast-food French fries	💣💣💣💣	Frozen French fries	💣💣
Breaded fish sandwich	💣💣💣💣	Doughnuts	💣💣
Chicken nuggets	💣💣💣💣	Stick margarine	💣💣
Pie	💣💣💣	Enchilada	💣💣
Danish	💣💣💣	Crackers	💣💣

SOURCE: Adapted from *The New England Journal of Medicine, CITETK*

it's a myth. "0 GRAMS OF TRANS FAT!"

Okay, it's not quite a myth, but it's often not true. Due to legal loopholes in the United States, Canada, and some other countries, manufacturers are permitted to claim that a product contains no trans fats even if it has small amounts, which can add up if you eat too many processed foods. In the United States, the threshold is 0.5 gram per serving, while Canada permits a maximum of 0.2 gram. How can you tell which products contain invisible trans fat? Check the ingredients lists. If you see any oil listed that's prefaced by the phrase "partially hydrogenated," the product is not completely free of trans fat.

Out with the bad fats:

A Kitchen Purge

You've already cleaned out the bad carbs in your kitchen; now it's time to get rid of the unhealthy fats. This may take a bit of detective work, in the form of scrutinizing package labels for certain key words that are tip-offs that a food needs to be exiled. The following categories represent the bad fats foods on which you should focus.

Old-Fashioned Shortening

If you like to bake, you may keep a tub of vegetable shortening in the cupboard. Vegetable shortening is a solid fat that's usually made from a mix of oils, such as soybean and cottonseed oils. It's cheap, flavorless, and some bakers feel it's a better choice than butter for making light, airy cakes and getting just the right flakiness in a pie crust. Unfortunately, the only form of vegetable shortening available for many years was made with hydrogenated oils—in other words, trans fats. But now, major food processors sell reformulated versions that are largely free of trans fats. If you must buy shortening, look for one of these brands.

That doesn't mean that these products are good for you. They usually contain palm oil, which is high in saturated fat, as well as tiny amounts of trans fat (though by law, in the United States, Canada, and some other countries, it can be advertised as "trans-fat free"). But they're better than old-fashioned shortening, which contains up to 2 grams—your maximum daily amount—of trans fats per tablespoon.

Foods That Contain Tropical Oils

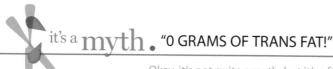

Coconut oil, palm oil, palm kernel oil—they come from plants so they must be good for you, right? Wrong. All vegetable oils contain at least a small amount of saturated fat, but tropical oils are mostly saturated fat. Coconut oil is 87 percent saturated fat—significantly worse than butter, which contains 62 percent saturated fat. Palm kernel oil has slightly less than coconut oil, and palm oil is about half saturated.

You may be reading this section and thinking: Why worry? I don't have any bottles of palm or coconut oil in my cupboard. Maybe not, but you probably have some snacks, breakfast foods, and other packaged goods that contain these awful oils. Manufacturers add these fats to foods to improve the taste, texture, and shelf life of a wide range of products. (To make matters worse, these oils are often partially hydrogenated, which make them even more unhealthy.) Start eyeballing the labels of packaged goods and you may be shocked to learn that many brands of the following foods—including some unlikely suspects—contain small amounts of saturated fat from tropical oils.

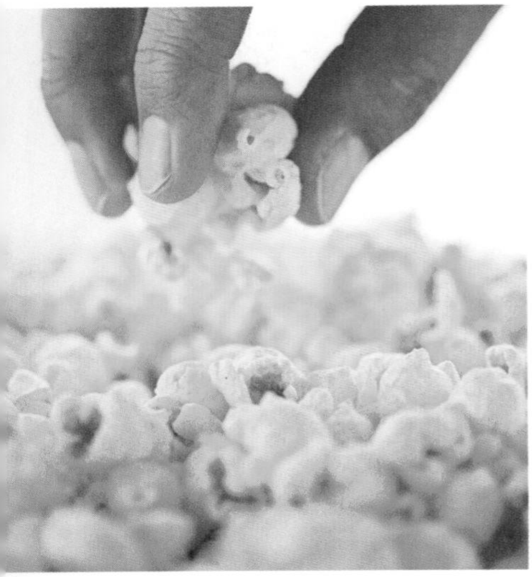

No-stir "all-natural" peanut butter. Peanut butter is a fantastic food. And buying all-natural varieties helps you avoid high-fructose corn syrup and other unwanted ingredients. Yet not all all-natural peanut butters are created equal. If the label reads "no-stir," be very suspicious—and turn the jar around to inspect the fine print. Chances are, the ingredients list includes palm oil, which some manufacturers add to prevent the peanut oil from separating from the peanut butter.

Breakfast cereal and breakfast bars. Choosing the wrong breakfast cereal can start your day off with a major dose of bad carbs. But even if you've switched to granola or a whole-grain brand of cereal, beware: Some healthy-seeming varieties contain added tropical oils. For instance, one popular oat cereal serves up a surprising—and completely avoidable—3 grams of saturated fat per bowl. The same is often true of breakfast bars, including some varieties that are marketed as healthy choices for people on the go. There are plenty of good breakfast cereals and energy bars to choose from that contain zero grams of saturated fat; make sure yours is one of them.

Candy, cookies, and cakes. Here's a little-known fact: Some candy bars are worse for you than others. That's because some contain tropical oils that ratchet up the saturated fat content. Consider: Some candy bars have more saturated fat (up to 11 grams) than a cheeseburger (9 grams), due in large measure to added palm oil and palm kernel oil. It's not as though you should never eat candy again; in fact, a little dark chocolate now and then is good for your heart. But don't buy sweets of any kind with added tropical oils.

Chips, crackers, and other salty snacks. Palm oil stands up well to heat, so manufacturers often use it to fry potato chips and bake crackers. Bagel crisps may be cooked with palm oil, too, as are those addictive wasabi peas that have become so popular recently—toss back a few handfuls and you could tack a few grams of saturated fat onto your daily total. Chips, crackers, and other salty snacks are high-calorie treats, so you'll want to choose healthier foods for between-meal munching. But when you do indulge a taste for salty snacks, look for varieties cooked in a healthier fat, such as canola oil.

Instant noodles. They're a budget-friendly meal you can whip up in a minute, but do you realize that a single cup of instant noodles can pack more saturated fat than a medium-size order of French fries? There's little else to recommend about quick noodles, nutrition-wise—they're usually high in sodium and brimming with unpronounceable chemicals, too. Bottom line: Don't buy instant noodles. If you can boil water, you can make regular noodles instead.

Microwave popcorn. Popcorn is an ideal healthy snack—unless it's popped with palm oil. Microwave popcorn may be convenient, but many brands contain saturated fat from this ubiquitous tropical oil. Buy real popping corn and pop it in an air-popper to keep it light, airy, and low-fat.

Pancake mix. What are tropical oils doing in your pancake mix? Adding 2 grams of saturated fat per serving, even before you've topped the stack with a pat of butter. Don't buy pancake mix. If you like flapjacks, make them from scratch with flour (mix in some whole-wheat with the white), baking powder, eggs, sugar, milk, and salt.

Powdered coffee creamer. Nondairy doesn't mean nonfat. This stuff often contains coconut oil. True, it's only 0.5 gram of saturated fat per cup (250 mL). But if you have a few cups a day, seven days a week—you get the idea. Fat-free milk is a much better choice if you like your coffee a lighter shade.

Foods That Contain Trans Fats

Look for the words "partially hydrogenated" before any type of oil on ingredients lists. Pay particularly close attention to packaged foods such as the ones listed below. The good news: Just about any food you toss out that contains partially hydrogenated oil can be replaced by a trans-fat-free alternative.

- Stick margarine
- Baked goods such as cookies, cakes, doughnuts, and muffins
- Breaded chicken nuggets
- Breakfast bars
- Candy
- Chips and crackers
- Frozen French fries
- Tortillas, burritos, and enchiladas

FIX YOUR FATS: Your Meal-by-Meal Plan

Now that you've fixed the carbs and the proteins in your meals, it's time to tackle the last—but not least important—macronutrient: fat. The goal is not to achieve a low-fat diet but to replace saturated fat and trans fat with "good" fat. Remember, you're looking to get 25 to 30 percent of the calories you consume from good fats. So subtracting isn't the name of the game; swapping is. Within a week, you'll find that your breakfasts will be more filling, your lunches more satisfying, and your dinners a miracle mix of flavor and health.

Breakfast

For many people the morning meal means one of two things, fat-wise, and neither is positive. At one extreme, maybe you grab a carb-heavy bagel and eat it plain, skipping the cream cheese to avoid the extra calories. That's bad news for your blood sugar and can trigger hunger spikes later in the day, not to mention foster insulin resistance. As you learned in the last chapter, it's better to incorporate some protein to keep you full. If you add some good fat to the equation, your carbs will digest more slowly, balancing out any blood-sugar swings.

At the other extreme, you can easily devour a day's worth of saturated fat at breakfast if you eat at a fast-food joint (think sausage patties with cheese) or serve yourself a plateful of bacon.

The truth is, many of the foods we associate with good fats—olive oil, fish, avocados—are more commonly included as part of lunch and dinner. But it is possible to add good fats to breakfast.

Think nuts. If your cereal doesn't contain nuts, add some chopped almonds, walnuts, or pecans yourself. If you're enjoying a piece of toast or a whole-wheat English muffin, peanut butter is the perfect spread. You can also add chopped nuts to waffle, pancake, and muffin batter.

Use a smart margarine. Vegetable oils contain PUFAs, one of the good types of fat. And margarine is made from vegetable oil. So if you're careful to choose a brand that doesn't contain any trans fats (remember, don't trust the front of the label on this issue; scan the ingredients list looking for the words "partially hydrogenated"), margarine is a fine addition to your morning meal. Look for a brand that contains 2 grams or less of saturated fat per tablespoon. (All fatty foods include some of each major type of fat, and vegetable oils are no exception: All contain some saturated fat, but some use oils

YOUR FAT PLAN at Breakfast

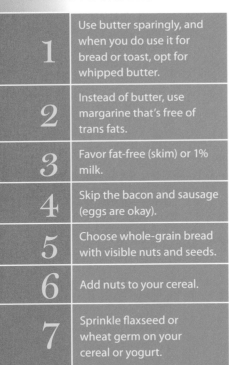

1	Use butter sparingly, and when you do use it for bread or toast, opt for whipped butter.
2	Instead of butter, use margarine that's free of trans fats.
3	Favor fat-free (skim) or 1% milk.
4	Skip the bacon and sausage (eggs are okay).
5	Choose whole-grain bread with visible nuts and seeds.
6	Add nuts to your cereal.
7	Sprinkle flaxseed or wheat germ on your cereal or yogurt.

with more than others). Don't bother with high-priced products that contain added omega-3 fatty acids. A tablespoon of one such margarine has only traces of DHA and EPA, the healthful omega-3s in fish oil—which is 20 times less than you'd get from a 3-ounce serving of salmon.

Get the flax. Flaxseeds are loaded with ALA, a form of PUFA that resembles omega-3 fatty acids. And they have a pleasant, slightly nutty taste. Buy whole flaxseeds, store them in the fridge, and grind them as needed. Don't eat whole flaxseeds or they'll come out the way they went in.

Don't forget eggs. They're nature's best source of protein, and here's a little-known fact: One large egg contains 2 grams of MUFAs, the good fats also found in nuts and olive oil.

Breakfast Suggestions

Whole-grain cereal sprinkled with chopped nuts

Granola topped with chopped pumpkin seeds or sunflower seeds

1 whole-wheat English muffin with 1 tablespoon (15 mL) peanut butter

Scrambled eggs with smoked salmon

Lunch

If you've quit getting takeout burgers and mayonnaise-smothered deli sandwiches for lunch, then pat yourself on the back. But if you switched to green salads and find your stomach groaning by 2:00 p.m., then your midday meal needs some help, especially if you're raiding the pantry or vending machine for high-calorie, tide-you-over snacks. Adding good fats to your lunch—either on the side or right on top of that salad—will give your midday meal a first-class upgrade.

Give yourself an A for avocados. Replace the cheese in your sandwich or salad with avocado slices. Or mash some avocado and use it as a spread in place of mayonnaise. Avocado slices are also great additions to black bean soup.

Fall in love with peanut butter again. Talk about an easy lunch: Start with a slice of whole-grain bread (and, here again, choosing a brand with lots of visible nuts and seeds boosts your intake of good fats even further), slather on a few tablespoons of peanut butter, and you've got a belly-filling companion for that lonely green salad.

Other ideas for peanut butter and nuts at lunch:

- Slather peanut butter on a banana or some apple slices.
- Top whole-wheat noodles with spicy Asian peanut sauce (which you can whip up fast with peanut butter, soy sauce, ginger, lime juice, and a few other ingredients).
- For a change of pace, try almond butter. (But skip Nutella; it contains more sugar than nuts.)

Give tahini a try. Like nuts, seeds are full of good fats. Try seed spreads, such as tahini, an essential food in Middle-Eastern cuisine that's made from sesame paste. Tahini is delicious on its own—you

YOUR FAT PLAN at Lunch

1	Use avocado slices or cubes to add good fat to just about anything.
2	Rediscover the wonder of peanut butter.
3	Sprinkle nuts over your salad.
4	Look to include canned tuna and salmon as one of your twice-weekly fish meals.

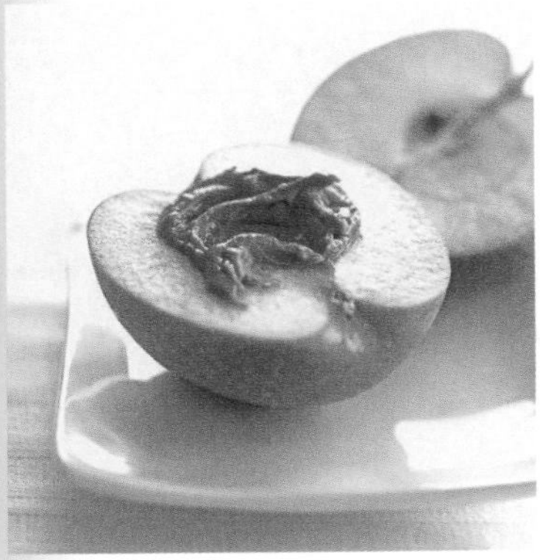

Lunch Suggestions

Tomato stuffed with tuna salad made with low-fat mayonnaise or plain yogurt, hard-cooked egg, chopped apples, celery, and onions

Tuna or salmon sandwich with lettuce and onions on whole-grain bread

Green salad topped with dried cranberries, chopped nuts, and an olive-oil-based dressing

Mixed-greens salad with peanut-butter-smeared apple slices on the side

can spread it on bread like peanut butter—but it's also the key ingredient in easy-to-make healthy dishes such as hummus (prepared with mashed chickpeas, lemon juice, and garlic) and baba ghanoush (made with pureed eggplant, lemon juice, garlic, and oil).

Soup up your salad. There are two ways to go wrong with a lunch salad. If your ingredients list starts with lettuce, cucumbers, and tomatoes—and pretty much ends there—then it's no wonder your stomach starts sounding the hunger alarm long before dinner. While these salad favorites all have nutritional merits, satisfying appetite isn't one of them. On the other hand, piling grated cheese or fatty deli meats on a salad may make it a rib-sticking meal, but also heaps on many grams of saturated fat. Adding good fats instead will make a salad more satisfying and heart healthy. Choosing an oil-based (preferably olive, canola, or flaxseed) salad dressing is a good start. But don't stop there. Try these nutritious, heart-friendly additions.

- ¼ avocado
- A palmful of chopped walnuts or pecans
- 8 chopped olives

Dinner

For most people with busy schedules, dinner is the meal where you are most likely to strap on the apron and do some real cooking. That makes the evening meal a prime window of opportunity for fitting in more good fats, since some of the best sources are cooking oils (tops for MUFAs) and seafood (unparalleled for omega-3 fatty acids). If you don't think of yourself as much of a cook, don't worry: The Healthy Heart Miracle Diet includes simple, easy-prep meals that provide all the good fats you need.

Don't fear olive oil. In fact, feel free to drizzle it over cooked vegetables to make them more appealing. And if you're serving a crusty whole-grain or sourdough bread with dinner, put out a small bowl of olive oil for dipping. Other cooking oils are good for you, too, in moderation. Choose one from the chart on page 118 to complement your meal.

Cook fish—it's easy. One of the main reasons people offer for avoiding fish is the cooking difficulty factor: It's just too hard to make a great-tasting fish dinner, they claim. Count that as another myth. Try these simple ideas.

- **Steam it.** For an easy, healthy fish dinner, try steaming just about any fish. Using hot, moist air to prepare fish is practically foolproof, since it's almost impossible to overcook the fish this way. If you don't own a steamer, you can pick up a bamboo steamer basket at an Asian market or online for about $10. Use stock or broth instead of water for more flavor and top the steamed fish with fresh herbs, a spritz of lemon, and dash or two of salt.

- **Bake it in foil.** Baking fish in foil packets makes a perfect fish meal surprisingly easy to pull off. Just coat a couple of fish fillets with olive oil, lemon juice, salt and pepper, a fresh herb of your choice, and bake in a 400°F (200°C) oven for 15 to 20 minutes. For a complete meal, throw cut-up vegetables, such as zucchini, red peppers, and scallions, into the foil packet, too.
- **Turn to the tins.** For many people, preparing a fish dinner begins with digging through the kitchen drawers for a can opener. Great idea, since canned tuna and sardines are both good sources of heart-healthy omega-3 fatty acids. For a quick dinner, try albacore tuna with cannellini beans, sliced red peppers, cucumbers, and onions, tossed with an olive-oil-based dressing.
- **Give it a grilling.** Thick, firm-textured varieties of fish such as salmon or fresh tuna are perfect for an outdoor barbecue. Just be sure to brush the grill with oil (or use cooking spray) to prevent sticking. White-fleshed filets such as sole or tilapia are too tender and will break up, though you can grill them using a wire fish basket.

Use nuts in place of meat. Nuts, especially peanuts and cashews, are tasty, filling stand-ins for meat in veggie-heavy stir-fry dishes. (Remember to serve the stir-fry over brown rice and use low-sodium soy sauce.)

Add some sesame seeds. They liven up broccoli, and they're another great addition to Asian-inspired stir-fries and beef and chicken dishes.

Odor-Free Fish

Does the family complain that your famous salmon specialty stinks up the house? The best defense against fishy odors is to buy the freshest seafood available. But since you can't always get seafood right off the boat, try these tips to fight fishy fragrance.

- Cook with acidic ingredients, such as lemon juice and vinegar, which can neutralize the fish smell.
- Cook in a stainless steel pan.
- Leave a small cup of white vinegar in the kitchen to help absorb odor overnight.
- Simmer cloves in a small pot of water while you tidy up after dinner.

YOUR FAT PLAN at Dinner

1	Sauté meat, poultry, and other proteins in good fats such as olive, canola, or peanut oil.
2	Use extra-virgin olive oil to top salads and cooked vegetables.
3	Eat fish for dinner at least once a week (twice a week, if you're not having it for lunch).
4	Add nuts to stir-fries.
5	Add seeds to steamed or sautéed vegetables.
6	If you eat meat, choose a lean cut of grass-fed beef, which contains more omega-3s and less saturated fat.

Dinner Suggestions

4 ounces (125 mL) of fish that's baked, steamed, grilled, or cooked in foil

Pasta tossed with olive oil, basil, pine nuts, and sun-dried tomatoes

Sardines canned in tomato sauce heated along with sautéed garlic and onions and served on top of whole-wheat pasta

Shrimp and vegetable stir-fry

Grilled skewers of fish, shrimp, and/or scallops and vegetables such as onions and cherry tomatoes

Fish tacos with heated (not fried) corn tortillas

it's a miracle! YOU *CAN* HAVE CHIPS

Corn and tortilla chips may not sound heart-friendly, but a University of Alabama study found that they can be a better choice than some other healthy-sounding foods. Researchers asked 45 men and women to snack on corn and tortilla chips fried in PUFA-rich corn oil for 25 days, then switched the group to low-fat snacks such as fat-free cookies and cereal bars for a similar period. The men and women lowered their "bad" LDL cholesterol on both diets, but their triglycerides dropped while they were snacking on chips. (Note: the corn oil was *not* the partially hydrogenated variety commonly used in processed foods.) If you're watching your salt intake, choose low-salt chips.

Snacks

Aside from giving you a moment to pause and relax in the middle of a busy day, having a snack serves an important purpose: It staves off hunger between meals and helps keep your blood sugar from spiraling downward—but only if you choose the right snacks. Choosing a snack with protein is job one. But snack time is also an opportunity to fit in some good fats.

One snack fits both bills nicely: nuts. In fact, if you plan to snack on a handful of nuts every day, your snack decision making is done. Almonds are a particularly good choice. If you prefer peanuts, buy them in the shell to keep your hands busy. And don't forget about peanut butter; enjoy it on whole-wheat crackers or smeared on apple slices or celery sticks.

If you need a hit of sugar at snack time, enjoy nuts paired with a *small* amount of raisins or other dried fruit, such as dried apricots. Seeds are also a good choice, so think unsalted pumpkin or sunflower seeds.

They're not as portable, but avocado slices are another healthy option. And remember that if you choose a hard-cooked egg as your snack, you'll get a healthy dose of protein along with about 2 grams of good fat.

YOUR FAT PLAN at Snack Time

1	Avoid candy bars and granola bars that contain tropical oils.
2	Check all your favorite snacks, including crackers for trans fats/hydrogenated oils—that's where these fats like to hide.
3	Make nuts your new favorite snack food.

Snack Suggestions

- Tapenade (olive spread) on toasted whole-wheat pita triangles
- Spiced almonds (1 ounce/30 g)
- ¼ of an avocado drizzled with lemon juice or avocado slices on whole-wheat crackers
- A handful of pumpkin or sunflower seeds
- 1 tablespoon all-natural peanut butter on whole-wheat crackers
- 1 ounce/30 g of soy nuts (roasted soybeans)

Dessert

The Healthy Heart Miracle Diet dessert philosophy is simple: Don't eat it every day, and keep portion sizes small. Frankly, if you follow this advice, you can indulge in just about any dessert you want. But, of course, some desserts are far healthier than others—and in some cases, the healthier desserts taste just as good or even better.

Dessert is the time to indulge in some antioxidant-rich dark chocolate. If you're having fruit for dessert, top it off with shavings of dark chocolate to make it more indulgent. Or enjoy a homemade chocolate pudding for very little saturated fat. You can make it in 5 minutes with just 5 ingredients: cocoa, sugar, 1% milk, cornstarch, and vanilla.

Nuts make a wonderful addition to many desserts, especially when they're chopped and baked or toasted. If you're having ice cream (yes, it can fit into the Healthy Heart Miracle Diet), splurge on the good stuff but stick to 2 small scoops the size of golf balls (this can be one of your dairy servings for the day), and add some crushed nuts on top. Or you can experiment with low-fat versions of ice cream to see if you can find one that satisfies your need for sweet. Nuts also pair well with baked fruits, as the Greeks and other Mediterraneans have discovered.

YOUR FAT PLAN at Dessert

1. Avoid store-bought cakes and cookies that contain tropical oils.
2. If you have ice cream, limit yourself to two scoops the size of golf balls.
3. Think nuts again, which are terrific in a variety of desserts.
4. Make dark chocolate a regular choice.

Dessert Suggestions

- Greek yogurt with honey and crushed hazelnuts
- Dark-chocolate-covered almonds
- 1 small slice of flourless chocolate cake
- 1/2 apple baked with cinnamon, walnuts, and maple syrup
- 1/2 fresh peach basted with honey and cardamom, and topped with toasted ground almonds

Putting the Healthy Heart Miracle Diet into Action

Now you know exactly how to correct your carbs, power up your protein, and fix your fats. But what does the Healthy Heart Miracle Diet actually look like? How do all the pieces fit together? See for yourself in the 14-Day Diet Plan, coming up next. Every meal and snack you'll eat is spelled out, in the proper portion sizes. Stick to the plan for the full 2 weeks, and you'll find yourself with an intuitive understanding of how to put the Healthy Heart Miracle Diet into action to last a lifetime. Are you ready to begin?

9

The Healthy Heart Miracle Diet
14-Day Meal Plan

Knowing the rules of healthy eating is a great first step. But more important is knowing how to *apply* the rules. These daily meal plans make it easy. Model your eating after these menus, and the "miracle" of great health is sure to follow.

Reading about how to do something well and *wanting* to do something well doesn't mean that you can just snap your fingers and automatically *do* it well. That's true whether you're learning a new language, improving your dance technique, or changing how you eat...*especially* changing how you eat.

You can be certain, though, that eating the Healthy Heart Miracle Diet way is satisfying, filling, and easy. Once it becomes routine, you'll never look back (unless it's to admire your improved figure!). But getting from here to there is unquestionably challenging. With this in mind, you'll want to take advantage of the powerful and useful tool found in the menus that follow.

On the pages ahead are 14 days of morning-to-night menus that adhere perfectly to the Healthy Heart Miracle Diet. If you follow them to the letter, you will reap all the health benefits you've read about in the program, and more. But, realistically—and understandably—few of us like to be told exactly what to eat. Even if that's the case, these meal plans are still extremely useful, because they also reveal what a day of eating generally looks like.

For example, you'll see that you can have some big snacks and make up for it at dinner by emphasizing vegetables. You'll see, too, that dessert is definitely on the menu, but in light and refreshing forms, rather than in behemoth slices of frosted cake. Breakfasts are small but yummy. There's plenty of meat, but in limited portion sizes.

Study these menus closely and observe the patterns to help you master the concept of the plan easily. Even if you don't follow the daily choices to the letter, emulate them in terms of portion sizes, nutrient combinations, and even the pacing of eating throughout the day. They truly represent the Healthy Heart Miracle Diet in action.

About the Menus

The daily menus were built to deliver the calories just as described in the past several chapters. Each day provides the following:

Total calories: 1,800
From protein: 25%
From carbohydrates: 40%
From unsaturated fat: 25%
From saturated fat: 10%

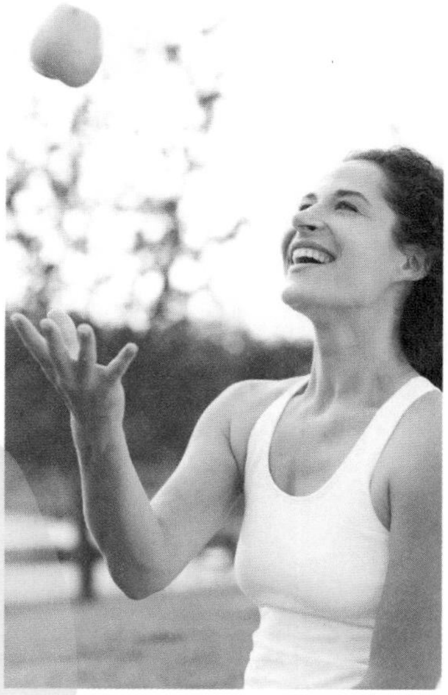

Each menu also explains how to add 200 calories, if that is what your body requires, or how to trim 200 calories, if you are seeking to lose weight or only require 1,600 calories.

Since most food packages give nutrients in weights, not percentages, each day's total provides nutrient tallies in grams. In general, you should be striving for roughly these amounts of each macronutrient:

Protein: 110 grams
Carbohydrates: 200 grams
Unsaturated fat: 50 grams
Saturated fat: 20 grams or less

That's powerful information, because it gives context to the packaged foods around you. For example, a McDonald's Quarter Pounder with Cheese has 12 grams of saturated fat and 26 grams of total fat. Eat one, and you've consumed well over half your total fat needs for the day.

You'll also find fiber information for each day's meals. The meals deliver 35 to 45 grams of fiber per day, a substantial amount that will contribute in many ways to great health, lower weight, and a well-protected heart.

Finally, to make things even more simple, the menus are peppered with portions from the guilt-free recipes that appear later in the book (see page 213). These dishes were carefully crafted to be easy, tasty, inexpensive, and 100 percent consistent with our healthy-heart guidelines. Give them a try!

Day 1

TODAY'S TALLY

fiber	35 g
saturated fat	14 g
unsaturated fat	55 g
protein	112 g
carbs	201 g

LUNCH: Add 1/2 cup (125 mL) chickpeas to the salad.

SNACK: Eat 2 teaspoons (10 mL) all-natural peanut butter with the apple.

200 CALORIES

LUNCH: Have 1/2 whole-grain roll (1 ounce/30 g) instead of a whole roll; use 1 1/2 teaspoons (7 mL) olive oil instead of 1 tablespoon (15 mL).

DINNER: Eliminate the salad.

Breakfast
1 serving Whole-Grain French Toast with Sautéed Apples (page 216)
1 cup (250 mL) fat-free milk (cold or steamed)

Lunch
Grilled chicken salad made with:
1/2 grilled chicken breast, 3 cups (750 mL) torn romaine lettuce, 1/2 cup (125 mL) chopped tomato, 7 walnut halves
2-ounce (60 g) hearty whole-grain roll
1 tablespoon (15 mL) olive oil

Snack
1 medium apple

Dinner
1 serving Broiled Fish Steaks with Tomato, Peach, and Orange Salsa (page 281)
2 servings Roasted Asparagus with Orange Gremolata (page 300)
1 serving Wild Rice with Two-Mushroom Sauté and Toasted Hazelnuts (page 324)
2 cups (500 mL) mixed greens with 1 tablespoon (15 mL) olive oil and balsamic vinegar

Dessert
1 cup (250 mL) plain low-fat yogurt
1 1/4 cups (300 mL) sliced fresh strawberries
Dark chocolate shavings (about 4 grams, the size of a Hershey's Kiss)

Day 2

TODAY'S TALLY

fiber	42 g
saturated fat	19 g
unsaturated fat	50 g
protein	109 g
carbs	207 g

BREAKFAST: Add tomato slices.

LUNCH: Eat 2 servings of soup.

200 CALORIES

LUNCH: Have 2 crisp breads instead of 4; have 1 ounce (30 g) of goat cheese instead of 2 ounces (60 g).

SNACK: Use 1/2 medium banana in the smoothie instead of a whole banana.

Breakfast
1 whole-grain English muffin
2 ounces (60 g) smoked salmon
1 tablespoon (15 mL) vegetable-oil-based spread (0 trans fats)
2 onion slices
1 cup (250 mL) melon cubes

Lunch
1 serving Creamy Curried Carrot Soup (page 256)
4 multi-grain crisp breads
2 ounces (60 g) goat cheese

Snack
Raspberry smoothie made with:
1 medium banana, 1 cup (250 mL) raspberries, 1 cup (250 mL) low-fat (1%) milk, 4 ice cubes

Dinner
1 serving Hazelnut-Crusted Turkey Cutlets with Parmesan and Rosemary (page 266)
2 servings Velvet Spinach with Sesame (page 314)
Pasta made with:
1 ounce (30 g) whole-grain penne, 2 teaspoons (10 mL) olive oil, Minced garlic, to taste

Day 3

Breakfast	1 serving Individual Breakfast Tortilla (page 220) 1 cup (250 mL) sliced mango 1/2 medium banana
Lunch	Seasonal fruit parfait made with: 1/4 cup (50 mL) blueberries, 1 cup (250 mL) raspberries, 2 cups (500 mL) low-fat Greek yogurt, 1/4 cup (50 mL) chopped walnuts
Snack	2 slices low-sodium turkey breast 1 cup (250 mL) raw carrot strips 1/4 cup (50 mL) hummus
Dinner	1 serving Curried Chicken Breasts with Butternut Squash, Green Beans, and Tomatoes (page 262) 2 servings Green Beans with Ground Toasted Almonds (page 301) 1 serving Bulgur Pilaf with Dried Cranberries and Pistachios (page 326)

TODAY'S TALLY

fiber	47 g
saturated fat	16 g
unsaturated fat	48 g
protein	113 g
carbs	212 g

SNACK: Add 3 more slices of turkey.

DINNER: Eat 2 servings of bulgur pilaf.

200 CALORIES

BREAKFAST: Eliminate the mango.

SNACK: Eliminate the turkey.

Day 4

Breakfast	1 1/2 cups (375 mL) fat-free milk 1 1/2 cups (375 mL) high-fiber, low-sugar, whole-grain cereal 1 1/4 cups (300 mL) sliced fresh strawberries
Lunch	Veggie pita pizzas made with: 2 small whole-grain pita breads, 2 ounces (60 g) low-fat mozzarella cheese, 1/4 cup (50 mL) tomato sauce, 1/2 cup (125 mL) seeded and chopped green bell pepper, 1/2 cup (125 mL) chopped mushrooms Salad made with: 2 cups (500 mL) shredded romaine lettuce, 1 tablespoon (15 mL) Italian dressing, 16 large ripe olives
Snack	1 large Granny Smith apple, sliced 1 tablespoon almond butter
Dinner	1 serving Zinfandel Beef Stew with Roasted Vegetables (page 276) Sautéed green beans made with: 1/2 pound (250 g) green beans, 1 tablespoon (15 mL) olive oil, 1 clove pressed garlic

TODAY'S TALLY

fiber	43 g
saturated fat	15 g
unsaturated fat	54 g
protein	91 g
carbs	218 g

ADD: Parfait made with 1/2 cup (125 mL) fresh pitted cherries, 1/3 cup (75 mL) part-skim ricotta cheese, 1 tablespoon (15 mL) slivered almonds

200 CALORIES

BREAKFAST: Eat 1 cup (250 mL) cereal instead of 1 1/2 cups (375 mL); use 1 cup (250 mL) milk instead of 1 1/2 cups (375 mL).

LUNCH: Have 7 olives instead of 16.

SNACK: Use 2 teaspoons (10 mL) almond butter instead of 1 tablespoon (15 mL).

Day 5

TODAY'S TALLY

fiber	35 g
saturated fat	12 g
unsaturated fat	59 g
protein	113 g
carbs	187 g

BREAKFAST: Add 1 cup (250 mL) fat-free milk.

SNACK: Add 1 3/4 ounces (52 g) mixed dried fruit.

200 CALORIES

LUNCH: Eat 1 1/2 servings of the salad instead of 2.

DINNER: Eat 1 1/2 servings of the salad instead of 2.

Breakfast
Veggie egg-white omelet made with:
3 large egg whites, 1/4 cup (50 mL) chopped broccoli florets, 1/4 cup (50 mL) chopped onion, 1 teaspoon (5 mL) canola oil

2 slices whole-grain toast, 1 1/2 teaspoons (7 mL) vegetable-oil-based spread (0 trans fats)

1 navel orange

Lunch
2 servings Chicken, Arugula, Avocado, and Tomato Salad with Lemon-Garlic Dressing and Black Olives (page 238)

2 bread sticks

Snack
1 cup (250 mL) plain nonfat yogurt sprinkled with cinnamon (if desired)

16 pistachios

Dinner
1 serving Three-Bean Vegetarian Chili with Tomato, Avocado, and Corn Topping (page 299)

1/2 cup (125 mL) cooked brown rice

2 servings Cantaloupe and Watercress Salad with Feta cheese (page 251)

Day 6

TODAY'S TALLY

fiber	44 g
saturated fat	10 g
unsaturated fat	59 g
protein	111 g
carbs	203 g

BREAKFAST: Eat 2 servings of cereal bars.

LUNCH: Add 1 1/2 teaspoons (7 mL) of peanut butter; use a whole banana.

200 CALORIES

LUNCH: Eliminate 1 slice of bread; use 1 teaspoon (5 mL) of peanut butter instead of 1 tablespoon (15 mL).

DINNER: Eat 1 1/2 servings of the lentils instead of 2.

Breakfast
1 serving Strawberry, Pineapple, and Almond Smoothies (page 215)

1 serving Cranberry-Peanut Cereal Bars (page 228)

Lunch
Open-faced peanut butter and banana sandwich made with:
2 slices whole multi-grain bread, 1 tablespoon (15 mL) peanut butter, 1/2 medium banana, sliced

Greek yogurt delight made with:
1 cup (250 mL) nonfat Greek yogurt, 1 teaspoon (5 mL) honey, 5 walnut halves, 1 cup (250 mL) blackberries

Snack
Fresh avocado and tomato salad made with:
1/4 avocado, peeled, pitted, and cubed, 1 large tomato, cubed, 1 medium cucumber, peeled and cubed, 1/2 teaspoon (2 mL) olive oil, Pinch of dried basil, Salt, to taste

Dinner
1 1/2 servings Orange-Glazed Roasted Salmon with Tricolor Bell Peppers (page 280)

2 servings Lentils with Dill and Sun-Dried Tomatoes (page 322)

Sautéed asparagus made with:
1/2 pound (250 g) asparagus, cut into pieces, 1 teaspoon (5 mL) olive oil, Salt, to taste, Freshly ground black pepper, to taste, Minced garlic, to taste

Day 7

Breakfast 1 serving Smoked Salmon and Asparagus Frittata (page 223)

Warm breakfast salad sauté made with:
2 cups (500 mL) torn spinach, 1/2 cup (125 mL) chopped mushrooms, 1/2 cup (125 mL) seeded and chopped red bell pepper, 1 teaspoon (5 mL) canola oil, Fresh crushed pepper, to taste

1 cup (250 mL) low-fat (1%) milk

Lunch French tuna plate made with:
3 ounces (90 g) water-packed canned tuna, drained, 1 ounce (30 g) anchovies, 1 cup (250 mL) cut green beans, 1/2 cup (125 mL) chopped tomato, 1 small boiled potato, 1 teaspoon (5 mL) olive oil, 2 teaspoons (10 mL) balsamic vinegar, 4 whole-grain crackers/crisps

Snack Cottage cheese parfait made with:
1/2 cup (125 mL) low-fat cottage cheese, 5 pecan halves, 2 fresh apricots, pitted and sliced

Dinner 2 servings Barley Risotto with Mushrooms and Spinach (page 295)

2 servings Carrots and Sugar Snaps with Tarragon and Orange (page 309)

Dessert 1 ounce (30 g) blue cheese with 5 almonds

TODAY'S TALLY

fiber	42 g
saturated fat	19 g
unsaturated fat	48 g
protein	110 g
carbs	202 g

BREAKFAST: Add 1 medium peach.

SNACK: Add 5 additional pecan halves.

DESSERT: Add 6 dried apple rings.

200 CALORIES

LUNCH: Eliminate the anchovies.

DINNER: Have 1 serving of carrots and sugar snaps instead of 2.

DESSERT: Eliminate the almonds.

Day 8

Breakfast Toasted breakfast protein wrap made with:
1 slice low-sodium turkey breast, 2 slices low-fat Swiss cheese, 1 tablespoon (5 mL) salsa, 1/4 avocado, peeled, pitted, and sliced, 1 medium whole-grain tortilla

1/2 cup (125 mL) raspberries

1 cup (250 mL) plain low-fat yogurt

Lunch 1 serving Black Bean Soup with Chipotle Chiles (page 260)

1 serving Sweet Potato, Green Apple, and Peanut Salad with Apple-Cider-Vinegar Dressing (page 242)

Snack Banana–almond butter smoothie made with:
1 sliced frozen medium banana, 1 tablespoon (15 mL) unsalted almond butter, 1 cup (250 mL) low-fat (1%) milk

Dinner 1 serving Pork Tenderloin Medallions with Lemon and Honey Mustard Sauce (page 273)

1 serving Orzo Pilaf with Spinach and Walnuts (page 321)

Dessert 1 serving Fresh Fruit and Cheese Tartlets (page 330)

TODAY'S TALLY

fiber	33 g
saturated fat	15 g
unsaturated fat	45 g
protein	111 g
carbs	217 g

LUNCH: Eat 2 servings of the salad.

200 CALORIES

SNACK: Use 3/4 of a banana instead of a whole banana.

DESSERT: Eliminate dessert.

Day 9

TODAY'S TALLY

fiber	42 g
saturated fat	13 g
unsaturated fat	48 g
protein	115 g
carbs	209 g

DINNER: Add 1 medium baked potato (with skin) topped with 1 tablespoon (15 mL) vegetable-oil-based spread (zero trans fats).

200 CALORIES

LUNCH: Use 2 ounces (60 g) of tuna instead of 3 ounces (90 g); use 1 slice of multi-grain bread instead of 2 slices.

SNACK: Eliminate the baby carrots.

Breakfast 2 servings Cooked Oatmeal-and-Bulgur Cereal with Apples and Dates (page 218)

1/4 cup (50 mL) walnuts

Lunch Tuna melt made with:

3 ounces (90 g) water-packed tuna, drained, 1/2 small tomato, chopped, 2 teaspoons (10 mL) chopped red onion, 1 black olive, chopped, 1 marinated artichoke heart, chopped, Fresh lemon juice, 1 tablespoon (15 mL) feta cheese, 2 slices multi-grain bread, 1/2 teaspoon canola oil (to brown bread)

17 red seedless grapes

Snack Yogurt dip made with:

1 cup (250 mL) nonfat Greek yogurt, 1/4 cup (50 mL) chopped red bell pepper, 2 teaspoons (10 mL) chopped onion, 1 teaspoon (5 mL) dried dill, Pinch of minced garlic, Salt and red pepper flakes, to taste

15 baby carrots and 1 medium green bell pepper, sliced

10 whole-grain crackers

Dinner 1 serving Grilled Flank Steak and Sweet Potatoes with Dried Tomato, Caper, and Parsley Sauce (page 274)

2 servings Oven-Roasted Cauliflower with Madras Curry Powder (page 312)

Day 10

TODAY'S TALLY

fiber	30 g
saturated fat	16 g
unsaturated fat	50 g
protein	96 g
carbs	218 g

LUNCH: Add an extra 1/2 tomato to the salad.

DINNER: Eat 1 1/2 servings of the fish.

200 CALORIES

BREAKFAST: Have 1 waffle instead of 2; use 1 teaspoon (5 mL) of the spread instead of 2 teaspoons (10 mL).

LUNCH: Eat 3/4 of a serving of the pasta instead of a whole serving.

Breakfast 1 cup (250 mL) low-fat cottage cheese

1/2 large grapefruit

2 small whole-grain waffles

2 teaspoons (10 mL) vegetable-oil-based spread (0 trans fats)

1 tablespoon (15 mL) fruit preserves

Lunch 1 serving Fusilli with Pinto Beans, Kalamata Olives, Tomatoes, and Broccolini (page 294)

Mediterranean cucumber and tomato salad made with:

1 large tomato and 1 cucumber, chopped, 1/2 red bell pepper, chopped, 1 scallion, chopped, 1 teaspoon (5 mL) olive oil, Fresh lemon juice, Salt and pepper, to taste

Snack 1 cup (250 mL) cubed melon

1/2 ounce (15 g) dark chocolate (at least 70% cocoa)

1 cup (250 mL) nonfat café latte (regular or decaf)

Dinner 1 serving Oven-Roasted Mackerel with Cherry Tomatoes, Potatoes, and Smoked Paprika (page 288)

2 servings Summer Squash, Edamame, and Leek Sauté with Lemon and Thyme (page 319)

Side salad made with:

2 cups shredded romaine lettuce, 4 cherry tomatoes, 1 teaspoon (5 mL) olive oil

Day 11

Breakfast	1 serving One-Egg Omelets with Chopped Broccoli, Tomatoes, and Cheddar (page 222) 1 cup (250 mL) low-fat (1%) milk 1 cup (250 mL) pineapple chunks
Lunch	Pita pocket made with: 1 large whole-wheat pita, 1/2 grilled skinless chicken breast, sliced, 1/2 cup (125 mL) shredded lettuce, 2 tomato slices, 2 tablespoons (25 mL) low-sodium grated Parmesan cheese, 1 tablespoon (15 mL) reduced-calorie Caesar dressing 3 medium carrots, peeled
Snack	1 medium apple, sliced 1 ounce (30 g) mixed nuts
Dinner	1 serving Orange-and-Soy-Glazed Beef Stir-Fry with Green Beans, Mini Bell Peppers, and Peanuts (page 277) 2 servings Braised Mixed Greens with Slow-Cooked Garlic and Dried Currants (page 313) 1 serving Quinoa Pilaf with Dried Apples and Sliced Almonds (page 323)
Dessert	1 serving Three-Berry Oatmeal and Almond Crisp (page 334)

TODAY'S TALLY

fiber	41 g
saturated fat	16 g
unsaturated fat	48 g
protein	102 g
carbs	219 g

↑ DINNER: Eat 2 servings of the quinoa pilaf.

200 CALORIES

↓ DINNER: Eliminate the quinoa pilaf.

Day 12

Breakfast	1 serving Blueberry-Orange Yogurt Smoothies (page 215) 1/4 cup (50 mL) pistachios
Lunch	Spinach salad made with: 3 ounces (90 g) canned salmon, 4 cups (1 L) chopped spinach, 1/2 cup (125 mL) sliced mushrooms, 1/2 cup (125 mL) peas, 2 tablespoons (25 mL) of a 1-part-olive oil-to-2-parts-balsamic-vinegar dressing, 1 tablespoon (15 mL) sesame seeds 2 crisp breads
Snack	1/4 cup (50 mL) fruit-and-nut whole-grain granola
Dinner	1 serving Braised Chicken Breasts with Garlic, Lentils, and Asparagus (page 264) 1 serving Rough-Mashed Olive Oil and Garlic Potatoes (page 318)
Dessert	6 ounces (175 g) plain low-fat yogurt 1 cup (250 mL) raspberries 1/2 cup (125 mL) sliced banana A cherry on top

TODAY'S TALLY

fiber	42 g
saturated fat	13 g
unsaturated fat	50 g
protein	113 g
carbs	202 g

↑ LUNCH: Add 1 cup sliced pears.

SNACK: Eat 1/2 cup (125 mL) of the granola.

200 CALORIES

↓ DINNER: Eat 1/2 serving of the chicken instead of a whole serving.

Day 13

TODAY'S TALLY

fiber	36 g
saturated fat	17 g
unsaturated fat	51 g
protein	99 g
carbs	211 g

SNACK: Have 2 turkey roll-ups.

200 CALORIES

SNACK: Make the turkey roll-up without the tortilla.

DINNER: Use 1 1/2 ounces (45 mL) linguine instead of 2 ounces (60 g).

Breakfast

2 whole-grain crisp breads

2 tablespoons (25 mL) cashew butter

1/2 cup (125 mL) sliced strawberries

1 cup (250 mL) nonfat Greek yogurt

1 teaspoon (5 mL) honey

Lunch

Pita pizza made with:
2 small whole-wheat pitas (4-inch/10-cm), 1/2 cup (125 mL) shredded mozzarella, 2 tablespoons (25 mL) tomato sauce, 2 tablespoons (25 mL) sliced olives, Basil, to taste, Oregano, to taste

Red pepper flakes, to taste

1 medium green pepper, seeded and sliced

1 Clementine

Snack

Easy turkey roll-up made with:
1 whole-grain tortilla, 2 slices turkey breast, 1/4 cup (50 mL) shredded lettuce, 1 teaspoon (5 mL) mayonnaise

Dinner

1 serving Lamb Stew with Artichoke Hearts and New Potatoes (page 269)

Pasta made with:
2 ounces (60 g) whole-grain linguine, cooked, 2 teaspoons (10 mL) olive oil

2 servings Broccoli Rabe with Sautéed Cremini Mushrooms (page 306)

Day 14

Breakfast	Scrambled tofu made with: 1/2 block firm tofu, water removed and crumbled, 1 1/2 teaspoons (7 mL) olive oil, 1/2 red bell pepper, seeded and chopped, 1/2 red onion, chopped, 1/2 teaspoon (2 mL) soy sauce, Dash of turmeric, Dash of paprika, Dash of black pepper 1 cup (250 mL) plain low-fat yogurt 1 kiwifruit, sliced
Lunch	1 serving Butternut Squash and Apple Soup (page 257) 1 serving White Bean, Fennel, and Onion Salad with Red-Wine Vinaigrette (page 245)
Snack	10 assorted olives 1 ounce (30 g) Parmesan cheese
Dinner	2 servings Whole-Grain Pasta Primavera with Ricotta (page 289)
Dessert	1 cup (250 mL) sliced strawberries 1/4 cup (50 mL) whipped cream

TODAY'S TALLY

fiber	45 g
saturated fat	19 g
unsaturated fat	44 g
protein	112 g
carbs	198 g

SNACK: Add 1 ounce (30 g) more Parmesan and 25 red seedless grapes.

200 CALORIES

SNACK: Eat 2/3 ounce (20 g) of Parmesan instead of 1 ounce (30 g).

DINNER: Eat 1 1/2 servings of pasta instead of 2.

10

Maintaining the Miracle

The Healthy Heart Miracle Diet isn't a plan you follow until your health improves; it's a new way of living that will make you feel so good that you won't ever want to go back.

It really *is* a miracle: Unlike hard-to-maintain low-fat diets that often leave you hungry and wanting something more, the Healthy Heart Miracle Diet is, by nature, satisfying and easy to follow (not to mention incredibly effective at slashing the risk of heart attack and stroke).

Research proves that eating fewer simple carbs and getting more "good" fat and lean protein—the three main tenets of eating on this plan—are the secrets to feeling full and avoiding the types of cravings that can ruin your efforts to eat well. You may have already discovered that this approach boosts your willpower between meals, allowing you to cruise through your day full of energy and able to resist temptations in ways you never thought possible.

On the Healthy Heart Miracle Diet, there are no "banned" foods and few hard-and-fast rules. There are just three critical guidelines plus a 14-day eating plan to set you on the right course, along with 100 recipes to help you put the plan into action day by day, week by week, and month by month. This is not a diet but rather an approach to eating that should ultimately help you enjoy food *more*, not less.

Still, change is always hard, at least at first, and changing your relationship with food is no exception. Following the Healthy Heart Miracle Diet means planning ahead a little more and cooking more meals at home. It means paying a little more attention to what, where, and even why you're eating. You're willing to do that, or you wouldn't have read this far. Yet when life throws you curveballs, they can have you ducking back into bad habits. Old cravings will reassert themselves at your weakest moments. And challenges will arise when it comes to staying on track in different settings, like at work or in restaurants.

Behavior specialists are well aware of the pitfalls that can waylay health-conscious eaters, and they've been studying various methods to help people avoid them. Read on to learn the research-proven secrets that will help you stick with the Healthy Heart Miracle Diet until it becomes second nature.

People who keep food diaries start cutting back their calorie intake and begin losing weight even if they aren't trying to.

Simple Tricks to Staying the Course

Eating right is a little like maintaining a good relationship: You can't just expect it to happen on its own—you have to put in a little bit of work. But that effort carries a huge reward, which you'll start reaping right away.

Some of the tips below will help you become more conscious about what you're putting on your plate. Others will allow you to control your portions without having to think about it. At first, try all the tips. After a few weeks, you may find that you don't need to, say, keep a food diary. Other strategies may stay with you for the rest of your life.

Keep a Food Diary

In all the diet research that's been done over the last half-century, one technique has truly proven its worth: keeping a food diary. The simple act of writing down what you consume can, by making you more conscious of what you're putting in your mouth, almost magically changes the way you eat. You don't even have to count up the calories—just put pen to paper, detailing everything that passes your lips, drinks included. The method is so effective that, in studies, people who keep food diaries start cutting back their calorie intake and begin losing weight even if they aren't trying to.

Purchase a small notebook that you can keep with you at all times, preferably in a pocket along with a pen. Whether or not you've begun following the Healthy Heart Miracle Diet, start writing down what you eat morning, noon, and night. Some typical entries for a person who hasn't started the diet might be:

Breakfast

Bagel w/cream cheese

Coffee with milk and sugar

Coffee break

Cruller

Coffee w/milk and sugar

Lunch

1 slice pepperoni pizza

Can of cola

Salad with bleu cheese dressing

Afternoon snack

Bag of potato chips (2 oz/60 g.)

Can of cola

REMEMBER THIS

Taking a photo of your meal before digging in can help you become more conscious of your portion sizes. You can even refer to the photo later when you want to write down what you ate and how much. And if looking at the photo makes you change your mind about indulging, good for you; use the erase button to eliminate the photo—not to mention the extra calories.

And so on. You can learn a lot from this list, even at first glance. For instance, this person consumed no fruit and hardly any vegetables during the day—hard to make up for at dinner alone. His breakfast contained too many carbs and didn't provide enough protein to get him through the morning, leaving him craving a sugary treat before lunch. Do a little detective work and you'll also realize that the snacks in this person's day deliver more calories than either breakfast or lunch.

You don't have to list the calories in what you eat—research shows that a food diary is effective whether you do or not. But when you first start keeping the diary, you may find that tracking calories for a few days or a week reveals some important insights. For instance, maybe you're consuming more total calories than you thought (studies show that people tend to underestimate their calories by as much as 50 percent), or you're getting more calories from your beverages than you ever imagined. Many people discover that they snack much more than they realize (or care to admit). If you do find that snacks dominate your afternoons, or that postdinner noshing is a problem, you may find that tallying the caloric consequences of that behavior to be an excellent deterrent. Use one of the many online calorie counters to help you fill in the calorie blanks.

"Check" Your Way to Success

Everyone likes to check off accomplishments. Why not use the same approach when it comes to your diet? It can be easy to forget how many times you've had fish this week, or to tell whether produce is playing a big enough part in your meals.

A simple solution: Keep a checklist on your refrigerator. The list below could work for you, or you can adapt it to your needs if, say, produce tends to be the part of the Diet that you struggle with.

Protein at breakfast? ☐ **Yes** ☐ **Not much**

☐ **Veggies today :**

☐ **Fruit today:**

☐ **"Good" fats today (fish, nuts, olive oil, etc.)**

☐ **Beans or whole grains today:**

☐ **Dairy today:**

Downsize Your Plates and Glasses

Using smaller-diameter plates (10 in/25 cm instead of 12 in/30 cm) can cut the amount of food you consume by as much as 25 percent, according to Cornell University behavioral psychologist Brian Wansink, PhD. Dr. Wansink has found that, by shrinking your plates, you could drop as much as 18 pounds/9 kg a year (of course, you'll have to hold off on seconds as well). Purchase just the salad plates for you and your family's everyday dining. These plates usually run about 8 in/20 cm to 10 in/25 cm in diameter. Fill the plate to the brim and your eye and your brain will be tricked into thinking you're getting a bigger portion of food than you really are.

REMEMBER THIS

You've heard it before, but it bears repeating: When it's time to eat, make sure that you're not sitting in front of the computer or the television. Multitasking generally means that the several things demanding your attention get short shrift, and that's especially true when you're eating. It's far better to focus on your meal and make it count. Behavioral psychologists say that being more "mindful" of the food you consume can help you cut unnecessary calories.

Apply the same logic to the rest of your dining ware as well. Most dessert bowls are a great size for your cereal in the morning. Try eating your cereal, soup, and ice cream with a teaspoon instead of a tablespoon, and using the dessert fork for your dinners. By eating with smaller utensils, you'll find that it takes about the same amount of time to eat the smaller portions; that can help convince your brain and belly that it's getting the same amount of food. When it comes to beverages, studies show that people consume 34 percent fewer liquid calories when they drink out of a tall skinny glass instead of a short, stubby one.

Choose Foods You Enjoy—And Eat Till You're Full

One of the advantages of the Healthy Heart Miracle Diet is its remarkable flexibility. Don't like avocados? Don't eat them. Choose another source of "good" fats instead, such as walnuts or olives. Not an egg fan at breakfast? Get your protein from cottage cheese (topped with fresh fruit) instead. Do you avoid meat? You can get plenty of protein from eggs, fish, beans, and other sources. Love pasta? No problem; just be sure to add plenty of vegetables to your dish to lower the glycemic load. There are infinite ways to follow the general principles of the diet, so find the ones that work best for you. If that takes some trial and error, that's okay. Remember, you're not looking to change your diet overnight, you're looking to change it gradually and forever.

If you're choosing meals from the plan that contain plenty of fiber, protein, and "good" fat, and you're taking time to savor them, yet you find that they're leaving you hungry, eat more. Seriously. While it's smart to not overstuff yourself, it's just as smart to not let yourself go hungry. Feeling ravenous between meals makes you more likely to overeat later—and probably not the kinds of foods that you should be eating. It's much better to consume a bit more when you have good choices in front of you if it prevents an unhealthy binge later. At dinner, for example, give yourself a half portion more, and savor it as slowly as you did the first time around. Between meals, try adding an extra Healthy Heart Miracle Diet snack like nuts or cut fresh vegetables.

Measure Your Progress

You can't actually see your heart or blood vessels getting healthier from one week to the next. You can't see your arteries become wider, more relaxed, or more flexible, and you can't watch the lining of those vessels—your first and best defense against heart disease—becoming smoother, healthier, and more resistant to attacks by cholesterol particles. You can't witness a decrease in the deep belly fat that encases your internal organs or observe your cells becoming less resistant to insulin. And that's too bad, because each of these things will happen on the Healthy Heart Miracle Diet, and each of them will significantly lessen your risk of a heart attack or stroke.

While you can't look inside your body and watch it change from day to day, there are other ways to measure your successes on the Healthy Heart Miracle Diet. Seeing progress is the best motivator of all, no matter what your goal. Some (but not all) of these ways involve your doctor. He should measure your blood pressure at every visit and tell you the numbers. Write them down so that if your blood pressure drops over time you'll know it. It also pays to buy a blood pressure monitor and take your blood pressure at home between visits.

Your cholesterol levels are another obvious measure of your progress. Officially, you need to check your cholesterol only once a year or less (if you don't have high cholesterol or other signs of heart disease), but if your doctor knows you're serious about making changes to bring down your cholesterol, he may authorize an extra test at 6 months to see how you're doing. Remember that it's your ratios of "good" and "bad" cholesterol that count more than your total cholesterol number (making many home tests all but useless).

While it's smart to not overstuff yourself, it's just as smart to not let yourself go hungry.

Meanwhile, if your efforts to change your diet are paying off by shrinking the amount of dangerous visceral fat deep in your abdomen, your waist should eventually shrink, and that's easy to measure. Use the "Progress Tracker" on page 156 to record the changes that take place. You can also record less tangible changes, such improvements in your energy level and decreases in hunger and cravings for sweet, fatty, or carbohydrate-laden treats. Chances are, you'll be pleasantly surprised at the progress you make.

Do a progress check each month for at least a year. By then, you'll have a new cholesterol test to compare to your original. This record of success can be a powerful source of motivation, especially during times when you're feeling down or discouraged. Hit a plateau in your progress? Take a look at your track record of success, and you'll know that you can push through.

Progress Tracker

Start Date /		1 Month	2 Months	3 Months	4 Months	5 Months	6 Months
Blood Pressure							
Waist							
Weight							
Hunger (scale of 1–5)							
Cravings (scale of 1–5)							
Energy (scale of 1–5)							

Cholesterol

	Start Date /	6 Months	1 Year
Total cholesterol			
HDL cholesterol			
LDL cholesterol			
HDL/LDL Ratio			
Triglycerides			

Keeping Weekends on Track

You might expect weekends to be the perfect time to build on your healthy eating efforts. After all, you have more leisure time to prepare and eat healthy meals. Unfortunately, it's often just the opposite: Many people treat the two-day break from the work week as a break from sensible eating. Researchers at the Washington University School of Medicine tracked the weight, eating habits, and exercise levels of 48 men and women for a year. The intensive study required participants to weigh and record everything they ate, weigh themselves every morning, and wear heart-rate monitors that tracked their physical exertion.

The goal was to have the volunteers follow a diet for a year, but they began recording their food and weight a month before the diet began. Turns out that the participants were already eating enough extra on the weekends to gain an average of 9 pounds (4.5 kg) a year. That behavior didn't change once they began the diet: They continued to overeat on the weekends to the tune of about 300 calories each day, an amount that, over a year, added back at least 9 pounds (4.5 kg) to whatever they managed to lose. As a result, few people lost a significant amount of weight.

Weekends present a lot of challenges, from plenty of free time for random snacking to parties and dining out. Here's how you can soar above these obstacles.

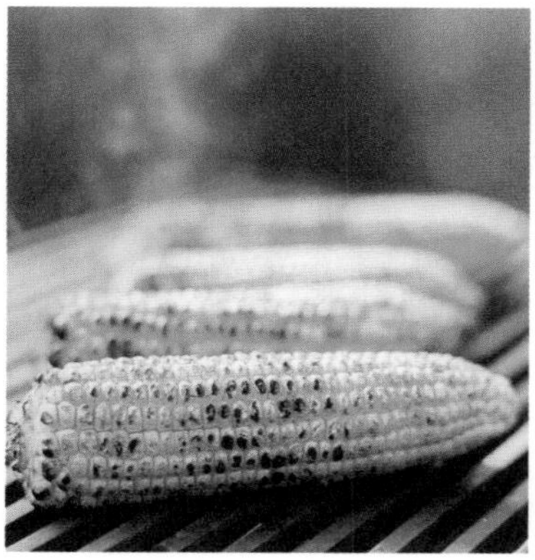

Schedule Your Meals

We love weekends exactly because they're free and easy. Yet too much spontaneity and unstructured eating are the very issues that lead us to overeat and indulge in the wrong foods. So, especially when you're first adjusting to the Healthy Heart Miracle Diet approach to eating, sit down over breakfast on Saturday morning with a list of your activities for the weekend and figure out where and what you'll be eating. If you see some danger spots, you can plan your strategy for ensuring that you don't overdo it, whatever the event.

If you're heading for the mall, bring a portable snack, or plan to shop right after breakfast or lunch, so you won't need to rely on mall food while you're there. Going to a barbecue? Give yourself a healthy snack before you go, and plan to start with a vegetable like salad or corn on the cob, and then sample one each of the BBQ meat (within reason, of course): Have a rib and a chicken breast, for example, or a sausage minus the bun plus some pulled pork.

If you're looking at running from one event to another with no options but fast food, you may want to pack a meal or at least some protein-rich snacks like nuts, trail mix, or dried apricots to tide you over until you get home. (By the way, you *can* make some good fast-food choices—see page 166.)

For stay-at-home weekend dinners, take advantage of your extra time by planning a more ambitious meal than you might cook during the week. Reward your extra effort by doubling the recipe and keeping the leftovers for future lunches and dinners. By thinking ahead about how to approach the dining aspect of your weekend, you can avoid the slide into mindless noshing.

Do a Little Party Planning

As you'll discover in part 3, a happy social life is every bit as good for your heart as a smart diet. So if you've been invited to a party, good for you! Just use a little common sense to keep your eating in line with the Healthy Heart Miracle Diet.

While drinking in moderation reduces the chances of having a heart attack, heavy drinking increases the risk of heart failure and sudden cardiac death.

Unless it's a dinner party, start by having a healthy snack or meal before you leave the house so you don't arrive hungry. Once you arrive, survey the scene. If food is laid out in an inviting spread, settle on a plan of attack so you don't find yourself eating all evening long. Plan only one or two trips to the appetizer table, then avoid it for the rest of the night. Once you've eaten, move away from the food to another area of the room and focus on the social aspects of the evening. If servers are carrying around trays of appetizers, plan to sample only every third item that comes around.

If you're drinking alcohol, keep in mind that the safe amount for your heart is up to one to two drinks for women and up to two drinks for men. While drinking in moderation reduces the chances of having a heart attack, heavy drinking increases the risk of heart failure and sudden cardiac death, among other health problems. It's especially important not to drink too much if you're taking aspirin for your heart; the combination can damage the stomach lining and cause bleeding. In managing your alcohol intake, consider alternating your alcoholic beverage with a glass of seltzer (add a splash of juice for a little color and flavor). That will keep your total calories down, help you avoid becoming too tipsy, and shore up your willpower to resist all those tempting treats.

Let Activity Replace Lunch with Friends

Nurturing your friendships is essential to your emotional *and* physical health. But remember that not every weekend get-together needs to involve food. Maybe you automatically default to meeting your friends for lunch or brunch—but that could easily add hundreds of calories to the meal (a cup of soup, a sandwich) that you'd otherwise eat at home. The combination of restaurant food and good company can lead you to order, and consume, a lot more than you intended. If you're trying to improve your diet, you can't ignore the fact that the more often you eat at home, the better you'll eat.

Instead of meeting at a restaurant, kill two birds with one stone and ask your friends to join you for a stroll at the local park or a ride on the bike path. You'll subtract calories and add exercise to your day. Plus, the enjoyable distraction of catching up with friends will allow you to cover more ground than you might on your own. Walk or cycle for an hour and you'll burn 300 to 600 calories; sit down at a restaurant and you could easily take in 1,200 calories. That's 1,500 to 1,800 calories you've cut from your day. It's easy to see the advantage to pursuing the active alternative.

To help make exercise a regular habit in your life (more on this in part 3), why not sign up for a dance class with another couple, or join a neighborhood tennis league with friends? Once these activities are built into your social life, you won't need to come up with a new activity idea every time you want to get together.

If you're trying to improve your diet, you can't ignore the fact that the more often you eat at home, the better you'll eat.

Conquering Restaurant Eating

Going to a restaurant when you're trying to eat right can be a little like going to a bar when you're trying to quit drinking: Temptation is everywhere. Fortunately, plenty of the most tempting foods fit the guidelines of this plan. Many of the items that were off the menu of a low-fat, high-carb diet—steak, guacamole, shrimp cocktail—are back on. But you'll still want to use a little caution when ordering. Some dishes hide ingredients that can send blood sugar soaring and inflame arteries. And restaurant chefs are notorious for seasoning food with too much salt and sugar. This kind of extreme flavor can put you back on an extreme eating roller coaster: All the salt can push you toward sugary treats, followed by a desire for more sodium-heavy food, and so on. The cuisine-by-cuisine tips below can help keep you on a more even keel.

Some restaurant dishes hide ingredients that can send blood sugar soaring and inflame arteries.

Ask questions. Don't hesitate to pump the waitperson for information like how big the appetizers or entrées are, how dishes are prepared, and whether you can substitute salad for the mashed potatoes. Many restaurants and waitstaff will accommodate your desires if it means repeat business. Also, you aren't the first person to make such requests, and you definitely won't be the last. If the staff doesn't respond well to your queries, they don't deserve your money.

Order creatively. Scan the appetizers for a possible entrée. You may find something on the list there that appeals to you as a main course, and given the portion sizes at most restaurants, an appetizer or salad may be enough for a full meal. Mussels in marinara sauce, chicken Caesar salad, clams or oysters on the half shell, shrimp cocktail, California roll, seviche, the soup of the day—all make nice Healthy Heart Miracle Diet main courses.

Take control of portion sizes. There's no law that says you need to stare at a plate overloaded with an excessive amount of food when you eat out. Remember, you're the customer, which means you're in charge. Since many restaurants tend to pile on portions that are double or triple the size of a healthy serving, splitting entrées is a wise idea. Another way to go is to ask for half the meal to be placed in a take-home container even before you are served (out of sight, out of mind). Any dessert concocted at a restaurant was definitely meant to be split by two or more; most are large enough to satisfy four people. Take a look at other tables to see if you can scope out the size of the desserts. If the slice of molten chocolate cake is generous, order one and ask for extra forks. Order a coffee or espresso drink on the side. Have a sip for every bite you take, and savor how the rich sweet and bitter flavors mix. Being able to "ooh" and "aah" over the dessert with your dining companion makes the whole experience more pleasurable. And after three or four bites, you'll be satisfied.

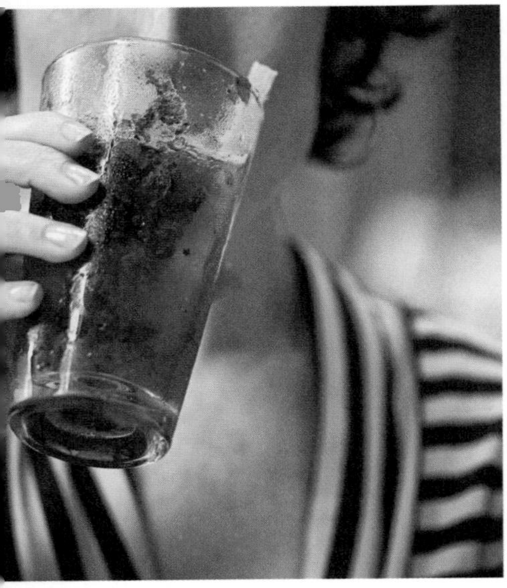

Keep sauces on the side. Most chefs are only too happy to drown their creations in buttery, salty sauces, with no regard for health or calories. Don't stand for it: Ask for sauces and dressings on the side.

Send back the bread. Always ask the server to hold the bread. The butter and bread can add up to 500 or so calories before you've even begun to eat, and the bread is typically made with white flour.

Drink alcohol during dinner, not before. Alcohol can lower inhibitions, quieting the voice in your head that tells you to avoid the chips or stop after half the steak. When the waiter takes your drink order, ask to have the drink arrive with the meal. You'll also end up drinking fewer calories from alcohol this way. (Women should try to limit themselves to one drink with dinner; men can have two. Besides staying sober enough to drive home safely, this is the amount of alcohol researchers have found is heart healthy.) Before your meal arrives, fill up on water or seltzer instead of wine or beer. Remember that it's easy to confuse feeling thirsty with being hungry, so this strategy may help you eat less.

Splurge when it's time to splurge. If it's your birthday or anniversary, feel free to toss caution to the wind. Every once in awhile, you can and should order without worrying about portion sizes, glycemic load, or the health of your arteries. *Carpe diem.*

Chinese

The watchword with this cuisine is "fried." Chinese can be a great choice as long as you avoid the fried rice and noodles, fried wontons, fried potstickers, fried egg rolls—you get the idea. (You may have to ask how the item is cooked: Not all fried dishes have the word "fried"

The Safe Way to Negotiate a Buffet

All-you-can-eat buffets are a good deal, economically speaking, only if you overeat. You may as well spend money at a restaurant where the food wasn't prepared hours earlier and hasn't been slowly losing its flavor and nutrients in a steam tray. But sometimes you can't avoid buffet-style eating. Weddings, banquets, and benefit dinners all can feature this type of meal. When you do find yourself tempted by the myriad offerings, try these research-tested tricks developed by Brian Wansink, PhD, at Cornell University.

1. Don't pick up a plate until you've perused the entire buffet and thought about what items you want. That way, you won't load up on a dish early in the line and then end up overloading your plate with the stuff you really want toward the end of the line. A bonus: Sometimes restaurants place the more expensive items, such as peel-and-eat shrimp, at the end so you won't have room for it on the plate—but if you follow this strategy, you will.

2. Sit on the far side of the room from the food tables, and don't sit facing the food.

3. If you think you'll have a tough time not going back for more, limit yourself to only two items per visit. Say you start with the Caesar salad and the chicken piccata. When you go back, you can get the mixed vegetables and sliced beef tenderloin. At that point, you'll probably be full and, although you'll most likely have eaten more calories than is wise, at least you won't have overstuffed yourself.

in the name.) It should go without saying that you need to be doubly wary of twice-fried dishes like General Tso's chicken and crispy beef or chicken. "Crispy" usually indicates frying twice, though anything that comes heavily breaded has typically been dipped in oil and fried more than once, too. Sweet-and-sour dishes are usually breaded and fried as well, so ask your waitperson before ordering those items. And while nuts get the green light on the Healthy Heart Miracle Diet, the walnuts in Chinese dishes are often caramelized and fried, which cancels out their health benefits. (The peanuts in Szechuan dishes are usually fine, however.) Here are some more strategies to help ensure that your meal meets Healthy Heart Miracle Diet standards.

MIRACLE **ADVICE:**

- Choose brown rice over white. Or if you really can't do without white rice, get only a small bowl or container (about a cup's worth) for two people and mix it with vegetables and/or meat to lower the simple carbohydrate shock to your system.
- Order soup for an appetizer: Wonton, egg drop, and hot-and-sour soups are all good choices. The broth is very salty, however, so don't add any soy sauce (which is very high in sodium). That broth will help take the edge off your hunger, making it easy for you to eat less of the main course.
- Steamed dumplings and potstickers are also good choices if you want more than soup for an appetizer. Although the dough is made with

white flour, it's thin and the vegetable and meat filling helps balance out the effects of the simple carbohydrates.

- Good main courses that are steamed, braised, roasted, and—the exception to the frying rule—stir-fried. For stir-fries, ask the waiter if you can have yours made with less oil than usual. And be wary of the sauces that come with any dish since these can be loaded with fat. Leave it on the plate or in the bottom of the takeout container.
- Use those chopsticks! Talk about an easy way to slow down your eating. You can pick up only a limited amount of food, so you'll have to slow down.

Italian

Along the Mediterranean shores of Italy, you can find some of the healthiest food and eating habits in the world. Unfortunately, many Italian restaurants forgo their cultural heritage and instead serve up capacious plates of overcooked noodles drowned in butter, cheese, and cream sauces. Huge slices of pizza groan under the weight of a one inch- (2-cm) thick coating of mozzarella.

The first hurdle is the overflowing basket of bread the server brings to the table. As you're being seated, ask that the bread not be brought to your table. Don't be fooled by the "salad" designation on the antipasto, which is primarily cured meats and fatty cheeses. And although many Italian restaurants treat pasta as a preliminary course to the main dish, you'll be better off thinking of it as a main course.

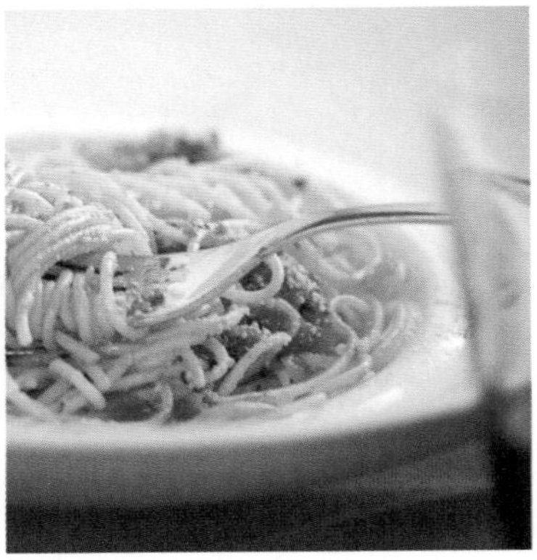

MIRACLE **ADVICE:**

- Consider Italian soups such as pasta fagioli or minestrone. Full of beans and vegetables, a small bowl of these soups will take the edge off your hunger in a hurry.
- A Caesar salad is a nice way to start your meal. The anchovies used in the dressing (authentic restaurants will also lay whole fillets on the salad) are one of the best sources of healthy omega-3 fats. That said, you'll still want to ask for the dressing on the side if only to limit the amount of calories: Some restaurants will drown the romaine.
- Choose red pasta sauces like the red clam, marinara, and vegetable sauces over white cream sauces. White wine–and garlic-based sauces are also fine if they're not made with too much butter. Ask how the pasta primavera is made before you order; many restaurants load it up with cream.
- Look for piccata, cacciatore, and marsala fish, chicken, or beef dishes.
- Choose seafood that's been cooked in olive oil or wine broths, not the breaded and fried types.

Mexican

The chips on the table; the margaritas; the mounds of refried beans and rice. This is one cuisine where overdoing it seems unavoidable. But you can also find pinto and black beans that haven't been refried, fajitas with grilled bell peppers and onions, and fish steamed and slathered in fresh tomatilla sauce. The trick is all in the ordering.

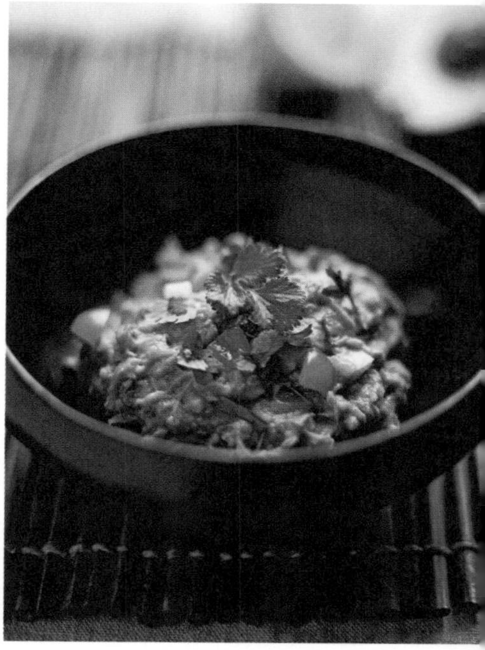

Avoid anything with flour tortillas. These carb bombs can deliver nearly a meal's worth of calories on their own, and they're made of refined white flour. The refried beans are often loaded with lard and, as the name implies, they're fried. Cheese is another area where most restaurants go crazy: You can get a 1/2-pound (250 g) of it shredded over most dishes or stuffed into enchiladas and rellenos. Chimichangas—deep-fried burritos—are obviously a bad choice. And watch out for salads that come in deep-fried tortilla bowls, which can contain about 400 calories in the bowl alone. (If you can limit yourself to the greens inside, fine.)

The biggest trap at Mexican restaurants is the portion sizes. Try ordering à la carte, (minus the rice—usually fried—and beans—refried or cooked with loads of salt and fat) and definitely plan to split the meal, either with your dining companion or to take home for another meal.

MIRACLE **ADVICE:**

- Ask that the chips not be brought to the table. But keep the salsa—it's loaded with antioxidants and the vinegar and tomatoes can offer help in controlling blood sugar. Use it as a healthy way to spice up anything on your plate.
- For appetizers, consider seviche—chopped up raw fish marinated in lime, cilantro, and other spices—or gazpacho—spicy vegetable soup served cool.
- Guacamole is full of healthy fats, but also calories. Lighten the load by eating it with soft corn tortillas—these are loaded with fiber and are a good substitute for deep-fried tortilla chips and flour tortillas.
- Favor fish entrées as long as they're not breaded and deep-fried or smothered in cheese. Fish tacos are fine when they're made with corn tortillas and fresh fish.
- Scan the menu for grilled items such as fajitas, which you can get made with beef, chicken, or fish. (Go easy on the tortillas, and focus on the filling instead.) The dishes will have that smoky grilled taste and you can use salsa to add even more flavor.

Indian

Indian buffets can be an exception to the rule about avoiding all-you-can-eat restaurants, as long as you use some caution. Most of the offerings are high in quality protein. The tandoori chicken is skinless and baked in a clay oven with very little oil. The curries use a lot of spices such as turmeric, cumin, and coriander that are rich in antioxidants that have anti-inflammatory properties. And many dishes are full of beans like lentils and chickpeas.

But there are still traps like samosas and kachori (deep-fried pockets of dough filled with potatoes, meat, and occasionally vegetables), and many of the curries will be loaded with cream or ghee, a clarified butter used in many Indian dishes. Do a little investigating at the restaurant before you dig in. Find out which soups and curries are broth-based and stick with those to avoid loading up on saturated fat.

MIRACLE **ADVICE:**

- Order the roti bread. It's typically made with whole-wheat flour or a whole-wheat blend. Skip the naan, a white-flour bread brushed with clarified butter.
- Start with the dal, a lentil stew or curry that is very filling.
- Use the raita, a yogurt-based sauce, for dipping your roti, chicken, and fish.
- Try the palak paneer, a spinach curry with mild cheese.
- Choose the mulligatawny if it's broth-based (the creamy version is made with coconut milk, which is very high in saturated fat). It's a stew of vegetables and lentils, sometimes with chicken or lamb added.
- Stick with the tandoori-cooked meats. Chicken or fish tikka, cooked tandoori-style, are very lean, and the cuts have been marinated in yogurt and healthy spices.

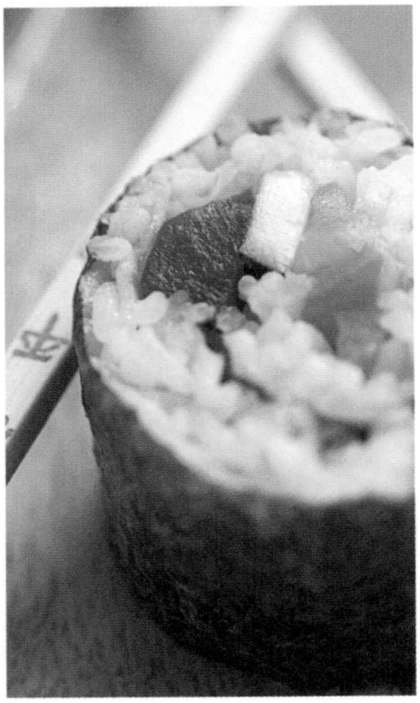

Japanese

Sushi-lovers rejoice: As a nation, Japan has the longest life expectancy on Earth. And when you look at the traditional Japanese diet, their longevity comes as no surprise—it includes plenty of fresh fish, vegetables, beans (mostly soy), and sensible portions. Green tea is typically served alongside the meal, and it's a great source of antioxidants that prevent bad cholesterol from building up in the arteries. But the Japanese have adopted some less-than-healthy cuisines in the last few decades, and these selections have become popular at Japanese restaurants around the world. Frying and deep-frying are the issue yet again. Key words to watch for—and avoid—on Japanese menus include "tempura" (deep-fried) and "*katsu*" (fried). Choose the low-sodium soy sauce, since regular soy contains shocking amounts of salt.

MIRACLE **ADVICE:**

- Start with miso soup, a soybean-based broth with chunks of tofu. The protein from the beans will help take the edge off your hunger.
- Edamame makes a good appetizer. These soybeans are boiled in a salty broth and served in the pods. Split a bowl amongst the table because you'll fill up fast.
- Sushi rolls are a great way to get fish. They contain a lot of rice, but the fish and nori (seaweed used to wrap the roll) balances out the carb hit. (Go easy on rolls made with tuna, swordfish, and other larger predatory fish since they can be high in mercury. But if you're only eating sushi occasionally—not more than two times a week—you don't have anything to worry about.) California rolls, which have avocado and crab, are a good choice if you're not a huge fan of raw fish.
- Try the sashimi—slabs of raw fish. You can order it with rice on the side, and then just take a chopstickful's worth of rice for every three to four mouthfuls of fish to ensure that your protein-to-carb ratio stays in the Healthy Heart Miracle Diet range.
- When you want noodles, soba are usually the best choice since they are made with whole-wheat grains. But freshly cooked udon are basically just thick spaghetti, and they can also fit into the Healthy Heart Miracle Diet approach, if the portion size is moderate.

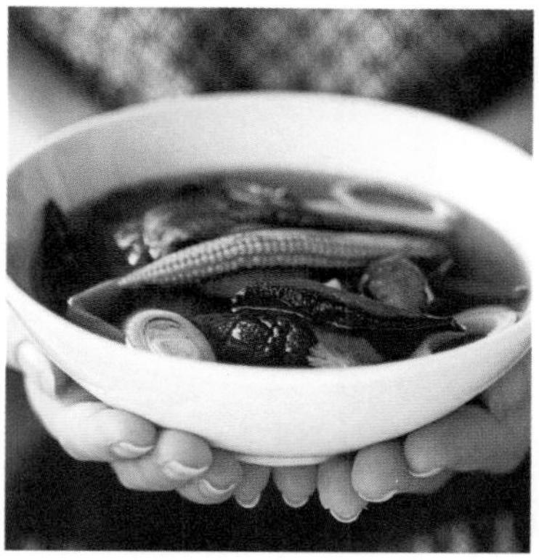

Thai

Thai food is a godsend for people interested in good health. The cuisine puts a strong emphasis on healthy food bursting with exotic flavor. Although some restaurants are offering more deep-fried versions of traditional staples, for the most part, Thai restaurants serve sensible portions of quality proteins, and fresh vegetables are in ready supply, often with surprising flavors. There is one pitfall: Some soups and curries have a coconut base, and coconut milk is absolutely loaded with saturated fat. A little won't hurt you, but don't go overboard.

MIRACLE **ADVICE:**

- Go for the summer rolls. You'll get veggies and pork or shrimp rolled in a thin sheet of rice paper—not fried—served with a sweet chili or peanut dipping sauce. They're a great way to take the edge off your hunger.
- Start with tom yum, a broth-based soup seasoned with lemongrass, cilantro, and Asian mushrooms. You can get it with pork, chicken, shrimp, or other types of seafood. This unique flavor blast will leave you wanting more—but since the soup doesn't contain a lot of calories, that's not necessarily a bad thing. And remember that starting a meal with a broth-based soup helps you eat less of the entrée.
- Give the sam tum salad a try. It's made with slivers of green papaya, green beans, chopped peanuts, lime juice, and fish sauce.

- For protein, consider the satay, grilled meat on a skewer served with peanut sauce.
- Look for other grilled meats on the menu. They're common in Thai food, and the Thai seasonings will ensure that these grilled items are distinct from other grilled dishes you've had.
- Ask for as much spice as you can stand. The spicy flavor in Thai (and Indian and Mexican, for that matter) means that you're getting capsaicin, an antioxidant that seems to tamp down inflammation. That will help protect you against heart disease and diabetes. And the spicier your food, the slower you'll eat it.
- Order lettuce wraps as an appetizer or a main course. You'll get a serving of ground or sliced beef or chicken (or whole shrimp) flavored with basil, chilies, and lime with lettuce leaves on the side. Spoon some of the fragrant meat into the leaves, then roll and eat.

Steakhouse

As you've learned by now, beef is okay on the Healthy Heart Miracle Diet as long as you choose lean cuts and watch your portion sizes—both difficult tasks at a steakhouse. Many such restaurants make their reputation by offering steaks that overlap the edges of your plate. A slab of prime rib that can feed a family as one portion? Yes. Steak sauces can make or break your meal as well: Béarnaise is mostly egg yolks and butter, while peppercorn sauces usually have a wine or brandy base and are much lighter. Avoid the creamed sides (cream spinach, creamed corn, creamy mashed potatoes) and deep-fried appetizers (blooming onions, wings, garlic fries).

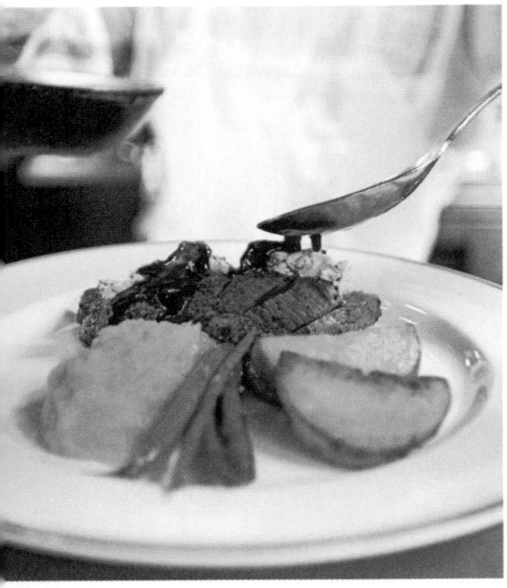

MIRACLE **ADVICE:**

- Check out the salads—more and more steakhouses are taking pride in their greens and offering a surprising range of options.
- Try the sirloin steak salad. Usually, you'll get admirably lean slices of sirloin arranged around greens with some chopped baked new potatoes in the skin. It can be a nearly perfect Healthy Heart Miracle Diet meal.
- Choose sirloin, filet mignon, and strip steaks to limit the amount of saturated fat. Order the smallest cut on the menu, or plan on splitting the steak and order an extra side dish for you and your dining partner.
- Order grass-fed beef, if you see it on the menu. Beef raised in the pasture tends to have less saturated fat and more heart-healthy omega-3 fats.
- For sides, look for steamed vegetables. These will provide a light counterpoint to your main course.

Fast Food

As long as you limit visits to no more than a couple of times a month, fast food can be okay. Just because you've pulled into the drive-thru doesn't mean that you can't make choices that fit with the Healthy

Heart Miracle Diet. Yes, fast food embodies most of what's wrong with modern cuisine. Loaded with sugar and salt and overstuffed with empty calories, it's the poster child for extreme eating. But if you stay away from the sodas and the deep-fried choices and watch how much food you order, you can limit the damage to your heart and waistline.

MIRACLE **ADVICE:**

- Avoid the so-called deals or value meals. That combination of sandwich, fries, and tub of soda is no deal when it comes to your blood sugar.
- Ask for water (or order bottled water) to drink with your meal. The sticky-sweet colas—regular and diet—spur your desire to eat more. Neutralize the extreme eating urge by taking sips of water between each bite.
- Recapture your youth by ordering the regular hamburger, not the quarter-pound or king size burger. Over the last 50 years, the size of what's considered an adult burger has inflated at roughly the same rate as our waistlines. The adult burger of the 1950s is now considered part of a child's meal. But don't let that deter you: Ask for a regular burger or cheeseburger, a small order of fries (if you must have fries), and a carton of milk (or water). It should be more than enough food to fill you up.
- Before you stray into healthier-sounding nonburger territory, such as the fish or grilled chicken sandwich, check the nutritional information that's posted somewhere in the restaurant (or look it up online ahead of time). Some chains offer a chicken sandwich that has more calories and fat than the burgers. And despite the important role of fish on the Healthy Heart Miracle Diet, you can pretty much forget about ordering fish at a fast-food place. Fried in the worst kinds of fat and loaded with an unbelievable number of calories, it simply doesn't count. Salads are always a better option.
- Slow down. Defy expectations (and undermine fast-food business plans) by actually stopping long enough between bites to chew and taste your food. Eaten quickly, the meal is soon forgotten except for the memory of the extreme salt/sweet taste; wolf it down, and it won't be long before you're craving more food. But if you slow down and taste your food, your gut and brain will have time to register that you've eaten.

REMEMBER THIS

Beef earns the "Prime" label after a federal inspector takes a look at the cuts and gauges the amount of marbling (fat) in the muscle. The theory is that the more fat, the more flavor—but in blind taste tests, people don't always pick the most marbled as the most flavorful. Aging and feed both play a big part in the way beef tastes. In the same blind taste tests, people often prefer grass-fed beef because it has a more pronounced flavor than beef that is fed corn to help fatten it up. Try both to see which you prefer, but skip the Prime-labeled cuts. You'll also save money while protecting your heart.

Having Healthy Holidays

Holidays are—or should be—times of joy and celebration, full of family, friends, and yes, food. In reality, they are also times of stress and anxiety. Joyous or stressful, holidays can also mark an eating marathon that begins a few days before the big event and lasts until the leftovers are consumed. It's no wonder that adults gain, on average, about 1 pound during the winter holidays—and most never lose it.

Overindulgence at holiday time seems to be hardwired into our behavior, probably because the earliest holidays celebrated harvest and plenty. And you'll almost certainly be faced with foods that don't fit nicely into the Healthy Heart Miracle Diet plan—candy, mashed potatoes (minus the skins), white dinner rolls, fatty appetizers, and sugary desserts. And holiday spirits—the alcoholic variety—can do a lot to break down your resolve.

Many of the tricks you've already learned for dealing with parties, such as taking just one small plate of appetizers and alternating alcoholic beverages with water and seltzer, will serve you well at these times. Also employ these strategies.

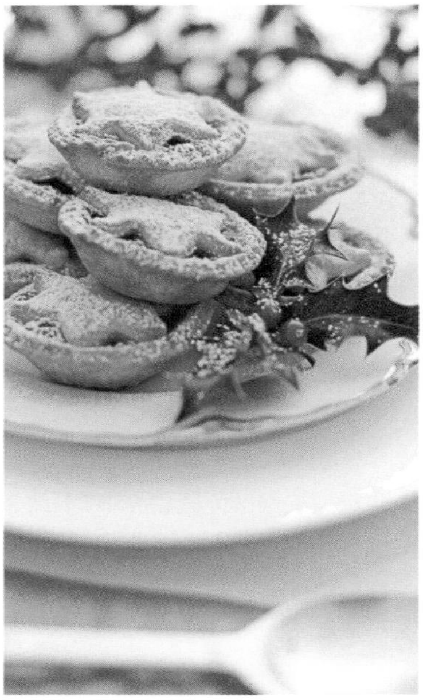

Have a little bit of everything. If you're facing a Thanksgiving or Christmas dinner where the side dishes outnumber the decorations, allow yourself a small sampling—really, a spoonful or two—of everything, including the mashed potatoes (even if they are skinless) and the stuffing (even though it was made with white bread). A few tastes will let you feel like you haven't missed anything. Really want more of those mashed potatoes? Go ahead—but then skip dessert.

Aim for a smaller portion of the main dish. At holidays, we tend to pile our plates as if we'll never eat again. In fact, an average Thanksgiving dinner contains an astounding 3,000 calories—more than a day's worth of food. No wonder we walk away feeling not just full but overstuffed and ready to fall asleep. Since you'll be sampling a variety of appetizers and side dishes, and also likely indulging in dessert, it's time to make your main dish smaller than usual, not larger. (And don't forget: If you're having turkey, choose the white meat over the dark.)

Stay out of the kitchen. Being in the kitchen during meal preparation often means you can sample enough food to equal an entire meal even before you sit down. If you're not hosting, see if you can help out somewhere besides the kitchen. Setting the table, running errands, playing bartender, cleaning up, keeping the young kids entertained, or spending time with the grandparents—all can be a huge help to your host and none will add calories.

Bring a healthy contribution. If you are hosting the holiday, you have the perfect opportunity to create a tasty, healthy holiday feast. You can keep the skins on the mashed potatoes, keep the extra sugar out of the yams, make the stuffing with whole-grain bread and add pistachios for extra protein, and put out plenty of salad and dishes of vegetables. But even if you aren't hosting, you can contribute a healthy dish. That way, you'll know there will be at least one item you can fill up on. Find a delicious healthy recipe that's low in carbs and calories and present it proudly.

Find tactful ways to say no thanks. The emotional atmosphere around the holidays can be especially charged. One common problem is that moms, dads, grandparents, or aunts and uncles may see your desire to manage your portion sizes as an insult. If your family is the type to say, "Eat, eat!" try these tricks. First, accept a plateful of food that may be a little larger than the one you had planned on eating just to assuage anyone's concerns that you don't like the food. A little extra on your plate is nothing compared to having seconds (and you don't have to finish the whole thing). Then, as you eat, engage all the people in earshot with conversation. Putting down your fork to chat will help you slow down and prevent you from matching the pace of those around you, who might be eager to go for another helping. And take sips of water after each bite.

If more food is pressed upon you, ask if you can take it with you instead of eating it now. That will reassure the host that you like the meal. Better still, explain that you're stuffed—but ask for the recipe. The same holds true with dessert: Ask for a small sliver of cake or pie now, and package a slice for home.

Walk it off. After the big meal, ask if anyone is up for a stroll. Not only will you burn calories but also the exercise can help blow off any steam created by the common holiday-dinner-table family tensions.

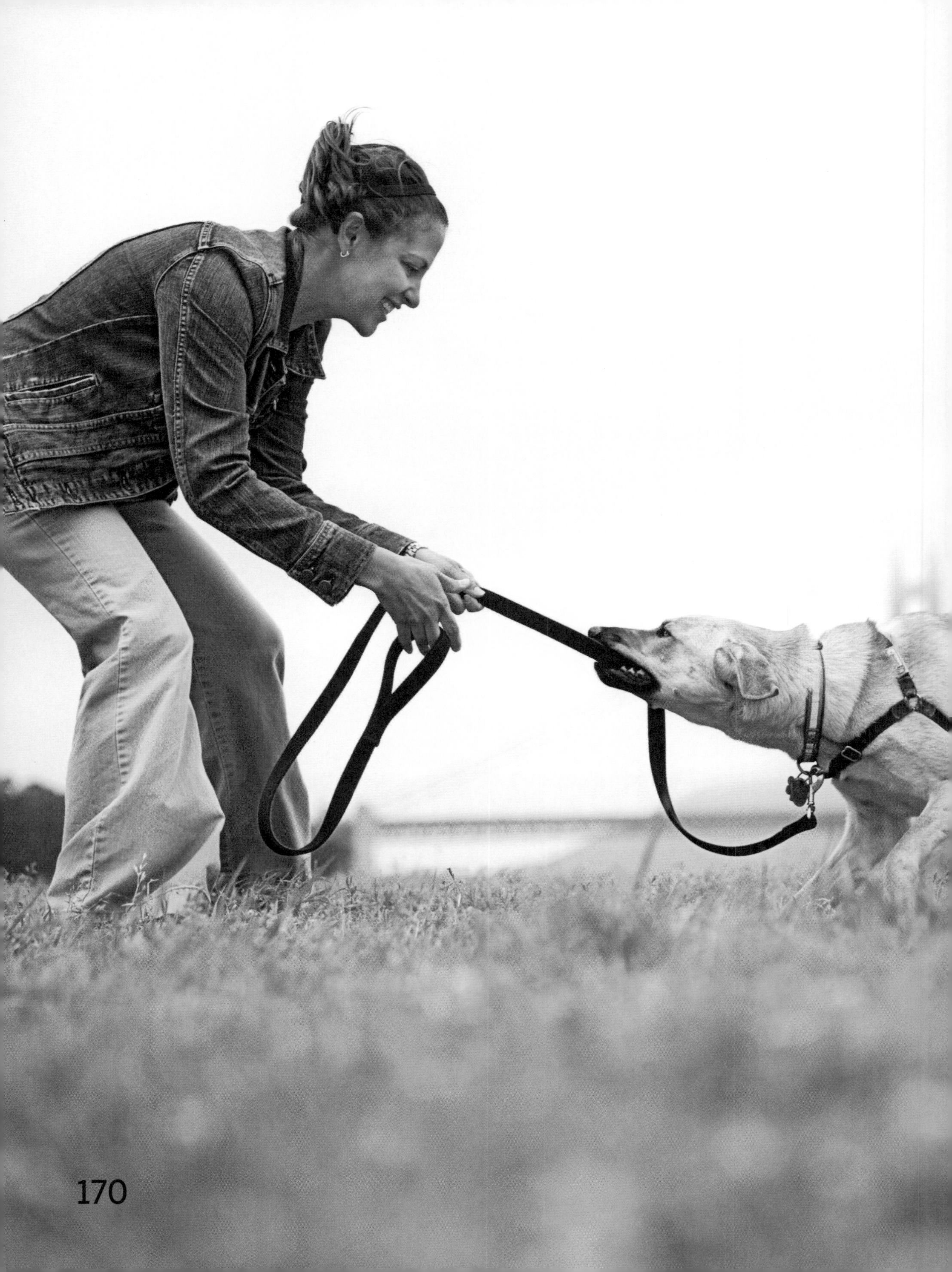

PART THREE

Living the Healthy Heart Miracle

When you eat healthy, you naturally start wanting to live healthy. Here's how to extend the healthy-heart philosophy to other parts of your life.

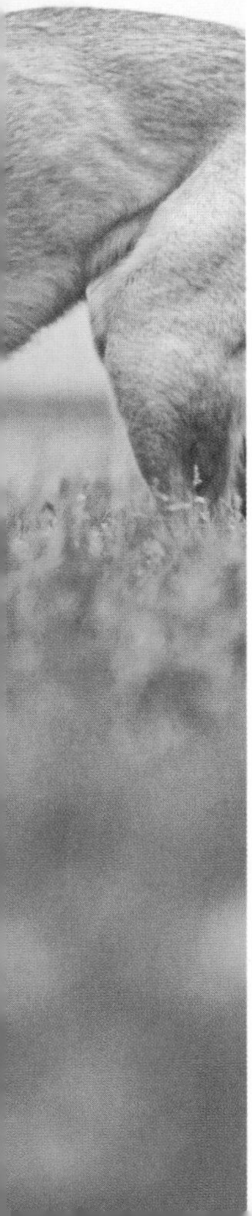

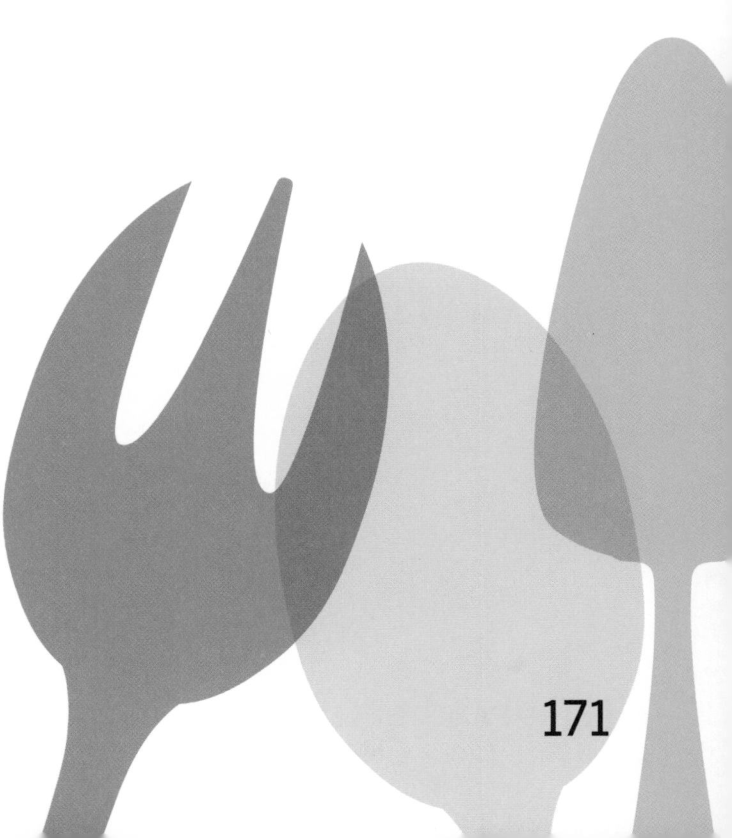

11

The Next Step: Exercise

Why didn't our ancestors get heart disease? For one reason, they spent their days on their feet. Simply building more movement into your day can lower high blood pressure. And more vigorous exercise is the original cholesterol cure.

By now you've read about all sorts of health problems that increase the risk for heart disease, from high cholesterol to insulin resistance to metabolic syndrome. There's one more to add to the list, and frightening numbers of people suffer from it. Fortunately, the cure rate is 100 percent with the right treatment—which, by the way, is free...and available everywhere. The condition? Sitting disease.

If people simply moved more during the day, millions could toss most of their medications away, while living longer with stronger hearts.

Consider the evidence: Exercise is one of the most effective ways to boost "good" HDL cholesterol. In one review of 37 studies on exercise and HDL, the researchers found that exercising three times a week for just 30 minutes could increase good cholesterol by as much as 18 percent. Staying active also reduces blood pressure and triglycerides, the blood fats that are linked to diabetes and increased risk of heart trouble. Lowering blood pressure is another reward: 500 men and women who were regularly active—even if they just golfed or gardened a couple of days a week—were far more likely to have arteries free of plaque and, as a result, lower blood pressure than people who were sedentary. On average, exercise can drop both your systolic and diastolic blood pressure numbers by 5 to 10 points, enough to allow people with borderline hypertension to go off medication.

Exercise also happens to be singularly effective in managing one of the biggest causes of heart trouble: excess weight. In 1994, diet and exercise researcher Rena R. Wing, PhD, established the National Weight Control Registry, one of the most remarkable ongoing health surveys in the United States. Dr. Wing has been recruiting people who have managed to lose more than 30 pounds (13 kg) and keep it off for at least a year. Some 5,000 people have registered with Dr. Wing's program, and she and her staff have interviewed and continued to follow the people in an attempt to figure out what a successful long-term weight-loss effort looks like.

In some respects, her findings are a mixed bag: Dr. Wing's volunteers have tried every type of diet imaginable. They've restricted their eating to one big meal a day or begun eating multiple small ones; they've gone vegetarian or become almost exclusively carnivorous. But nearly all of them (94 percent) have one thing in common: They exercise. Regularly. They exercised to lose the weight, and they continue to exercise to keep it off. They report that when they stop exercising, the weight starts to come back.

Do You Have Sitting Disease?

quiz

On most days, I:

1. Pass through the first 2 hours of the day without stretching, exercising, or walking strenuously **-1**

2. Do at least 30 minutes of active chores around the house **+1**

3. Watch at least 2 hours of TV **-2**

4. Spend at least 30 minutes outdoors **+2**

5. Cook dinner from scratch **+1**

6. Spend most of the workday sitting **-3**

7. Climb at least two flights of stairs **+1**

8. Spend at least 90 minutes in the car **-2**

9. Walk for at least 20 minutes total **+1**

10. Walk for at least 45 minutes total **+3**

11. Play a sport, ride a bike, or swim in the pool **+3**

12. Go to the gym or do a full workout at home **+3**

13. Have some playtime with the kids or other loved ones **+2**

14. Spend most my time after dinner in my den or living room **-2**

15. Spend time on a hobby that keeps me on my feet **+1**

Your Score

Add up your total to determine your score.

-10 TO -4: You have sitting disease. You urgently need to build more movement into your day for your heart's sake. Start slow—but do something.

-3 TO 5: You're fitting some movement into your day, but you're still leading a generally sedentary lifestyle that is hurting your health.

6 TO 12: You live an active, healthy lifestyle that keeps you on your feet a fair amount. Keep it up!

13 TO 18: Not only is your daily routine active, but you are fitting in lots of time for exercise and fun physical activity. Keep up the good work!

The benefits to your heart go on and on. It helps insulin become more efficient in processing sugar. It increases the flexibility of artery walls and it helps your body fight off the free radicals that contribute to plaque buildup. Moderate exercise even has a slight dampening effect on appetite. And it gives you the energy and confidence you need to make other healthy changes in your life.

Find Your Personal Cure for "Sitting Disease"

Although it has yet to be officially recognized by the World Health Organization, sitting disease is very real, and you may have it without even realizing it. Do you have a desk job? How much TV do you watch in the evening? What's your commute like? Without even thinking about it, you could be spending upward of 14 to 16 hours a day sitting. Add to that 6 to 8 hours of sleep, and you're talking about a nearly full day of inactivity.

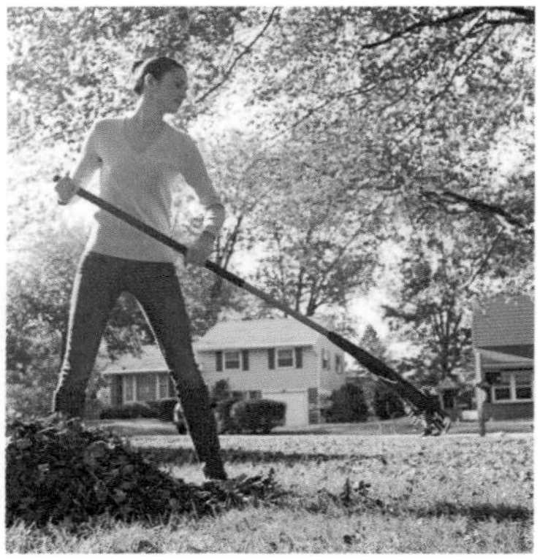

Things weren't always like this. Once upon a time, we had to hunt and gather our own food. We had to wash our clothes by hand. More recently, we had to walk across the office to check the mail (remember snail mail?). We had to go to an actual bricks-and-mortar store to do our shopping. We don't even walk to the counter to order our fast-food; instead, we use the drive-thru. In short, modern society has streamlined all the exercise out of our lives.

James Levine, MD, a researcher at the University of Minnesota, has calculated the cost of sitting disease by studying a concept called nonexercise activity thermogenesis, or NEAT. Thermogenesis means calorie burning, so NEAT is a term for the energy you expend when you're going about your daily life—for instance, when you walk up stairs, fidget, do chores around the house or in the garden. You might think that these calories don't count for much, but in fact, NEAT is critically important. That's because it has the potential to add up to many more calories than the burn you get during a half-hour at the gym.

For example, 30 minutes of walking on a treadmill would burn about 150 calories. Not bad—but not great. By comparison, the NEAT part of your daily burn can be five times higher than your gym efforts or more, depending on how active your day is. In studies of obese and normal-weight people, Dr. Levine has found that lean people burn as many as 2,000 NEAT calories more a day than those who are overweight.

Dr. Levine is a big proponent of reclaiming old habits to help increase your calorie burn. Thanks to modern conveniences like snow blowers, dishwashers, and the other advances we enjoy, we burn about 350 calories a day less than we did 40 years ago. That may not sound like much, but over a year, the difference could add up to a weight gain of 36 pounds. Our NEAT deficit alone could account for the obesity epidemic worldwide, according to Dr. Levine.

Declare War on Chairs, Couches, and Elevators

Rise up against sitting disease by finding new ways to be active. No one is asking you to give up your dishwasher or washing machine or to take up hunting and fishing. But if you're lucky enough to live near stores where you can shop, try walking or riding your bike there instead of driving. Are there stairs where you work or run errands? Can you take them instead of taking the escalator or elevator? If you must take the escalator, remember that even though they're moving, they're still stairs, you can still climb them (and get to the top that much faster). Even cooking homemade dinners—one of your goals on the Healthy Heart Miracle Diet—will get you on your feet.

> Are there stairs where you work or run errands? Can you take them instead of taking the escalator or elevator?

If you have the option of taking the subway, bus, or train to work, jump at it. Walking to and from the stop, both from home and stores or the office, adds up. Researchers at the Centers for Disease Control and Prevention found that the average public transportation ride requires 20 minutes of walking, and 30 percent of people who take public transportation to and from work get more than 30 minutes of walking daily. If you don't have the option, try parking a couple of blocks from work or the store.

Maintaining a home and yard or garden offers literally endless possibilities for physical activity. If you use a cleaning service to keep your house up, try letting them go, and dust and vacuum it yourself. If your lawn isn't too large, mow it yourself. If you're in decent shape, consider trading in your power mower for an old-school push mower, the kind with no engine. They're surprisingly efficient at cutting grass, and the extra resistance will add a lot to your calorie burn. Gardening can also provide substantial calorie-burning rewards.

Overcome sitting disease, and you'll be shocked at how quickly the extra pounds will melt away—and how easy it will be to keep them off.

That's NEAT!

Here's a list of common NEAT activities and how many calories a 150-pound person would burn in 30 minutes.

Raking leaves **147**

Gardening or weeding **153**

Vacuuming **119**

Cleaning the house **102**

Mowing the lawn **205**

Playing with the kids (moderate activity level) **136**

Strolling **103**

Biking to work (on a flat surface) **220**

quiz *Are You Ready to Be Active?*

Many people resist becoming more active without fully understanding why. If you're not active now, take this quiz adapted from the Centers of Disease Control and Prevention to discover what barriers hold you back. Read each statement and indicate how likely you are to make (or agree with) it.

HOW LIKELY ARE YOU TO SAY...	VERY LIKELY	SOMEWHAT LIKELY	SOMEWHAT UNLIKELY	VERY UNLIKELY
1. **My days are so busy I just don't think I can make the time to include physical activity.**	3	2	1	0
2. **None of my family members or friends likes to do anything active, so I don't have a chance to exercise.**	3	2	1	0
3. **I'm just too tired after work to get any exercise.**	3	2	1	0
4. **I've been thinking about getting more exercise, but I just can't seem to get started.**	3	2	1	0
5. **I'm getting older so exercise might be risky.**	3	2	1	0
6. **I don't get enough exercise because I have never learned the skills for any sport.**	3	2	1	0
7. **I don't have access to jogging trails, swimming pools, bike paths, and such.**	3	2	1	0
8. **Physical activity takes too much time away from other commitments like work and family.**	3	2	1	0
9. **I'm embarrassed about how I will look when I exercise with others.**	3	2	1	0
10. **I don't get enough sleep as it is. I just couldn't get up earlier or stay up later to get some exercise.**	3	2	1	0
11. **It's easier for me to find excuses not to exercise than to go out to do something.**	3	2	1	0
12. **I know of too many people who have hurt themselves by overdoing it.**	3	2	1	0
13. **I really can't see learning a new sport at my age.**	3	2	1	0
14. **It's just too expensive. You have to take a class or join a club or buy the right equipment.**	3	2	1	0
15. **My free times during the day are too short to include exercise.**	3	2	1	0

	VERY LIKELY	SOMEWHAT LIKELY	SOMEWHAT UNLIKELY	VERY UNLIKELY
16. My usual social time with family or friends does not include physical activity.	3	2	1	0
17. I'm too tired during the week and I need the weekend to catch up on my rest.	3	2	1	0
18. I want to get more exercise, but I can't seem to make myself stick to a plan.	3	2	1	0
19. I'm afraid I might injure myself or have a heart attack.	3	2	1	0
20. I'm not good enough at any physical activity to make it fun.	3	2	1	0
21. If we had exercise facilities and showers at work, I would be more likely to exercise.	3	2	1	0

Your Score

For each numbered question, enter the score you circled in the spaces provided. On the first line, for example, write down the scores you circled for questions 1, 8, and 15. Add the three scores on each line. Your barriers to physical activity fall into one or more of seven categories: lack of time, lack of social support, lack of energy, lack of motivation, fear of injury, lack of skill, and lack of resources. A score of 5 or above in any category shows that this is an important barrier for you to overcome.

______ + ______ + ______ = ______ **Lack of time**
Question 1 + Question 8 + Question 15

______ + ______ + ______ = ______ **Lack of social support**
Question 2 + Question 9 + Question 16

______ + ______ + ______ = ______ **Lack of energy**
Question 3 + Question 10 + Question 17

______ + ______ + ______ = ______ **Lack of motivation**
Question 4 + Question 11 + Question 18

______ + ______ + ______ = ______ **Fear of injury**
Question 5 + Question 12 + Question 19

______ + ______ + ______ = ______ **Lack of skill**
Question 6 + Question 13 + Question 20

______ + ______ + ______ = ______ **Lack of resources**
Question 7 + Question 14 + Question 21

Overcoming Exercise Hurdles

Take the quiz "Are Your Ready to Be Active?" above, then read up on any and all of the personal hurdles you face to make it easier for you to build more exercise into your life.

Lack of time. This is one of the most common excuses, and it's understandable given how crazy life can be. For many people, taking time to exercise feels almost self-indulgent. If that seems to be your barrier, consider this: If you don't make time for yourself, you won't be able to give your best to those who depend on you, from family and friends to the boss at work. Maybe you'll be more likely to make time for exercise if you realize that it's something you're doing for the people that count on you. And then, within a very short period of time, you'll realize how much you enjoy regular exercise. With the NEAT approach, you don't have to worry about scheduling trips to the gym or signing up for exercise classes. All you have to do is take every activity opportunity that presents itself, such as taking the stairs, strolling across the office to discuss work matters with a colleague (instead of calling or e-mailing), parking down the block from your destination, and so on.

Lack of energy? There's an easy solution: exercise.

Lack of social support. If your friends and family don't exercise, it can be hard to motivate yourself to do so. The solution: Find an exercise buddy. See if you can get your spouse or another family member or a friend to sign up for an activity with you or to join you for a regular evening walk. Setting aside even 20 minutes in the morning or evening to bicycle, swim, or stroll with family members will add considerably to everyone's well being and bring you closer together as a family. No takers? No problem. Enlist a neighbor or friend to start a new active habit with you.

Lack of energy. There's an easy solution to this problem because nothing boosts energy better than exercise. Surprised? Several studies have documented this phenomenon. By putting out some effort, your stamina and strength improve. Those benefits carry over into your daily life, whether you're carrying groceries, running an extra errand, or needing to put in some extra time at the office or cleaning around the house. But if low energy is keeping you from even beginning, schedule your exercise for the time of day when you feel the most energetic. If getting out of bed in the morning is a daily struggle, don't plan to exercise then—you'll never do it. Instead, set aside a half-hour in the middle of the day or early evening. Just choose a time when you're at a high point in your daily energy swing.

Lack of motivation. If you've never been one for physical activity, this is likely to be a problem. Why get all sweaty and out of breath? It's tough to convince yourself of the benefits when you've yet to experience them firsthand—which you will if you can only get yourself to start. Here's a trick: For one week, put on sneakers or walking shoes and head outside. Tell yourself you're going to walk for just 10 minutes. If that's all you do, okay. But chances are that once you get moving, you'll continue. After a week of walking, you'll probably be feeling better and sleeping better, and you won't want to go back to not walking. Need more motivation? Talk to you doctor about what kind of exercise it would take to get off of or lower your dose of whatever medication you take for high blood pressure or high cholesterol.

Fear of injury. This is a real concern. You don't want to run out the door, overdo it, and get laid up for a week or more. But most of the horror stories stem from weekend warrior syndrome: After years of inactivity, someone jumps into a football game and pulls a muscle or otherwise hurts himself. If you start slowly and gently, however, there's little cause for concern, especially if slow or moderate walking is your exercise of choice. Anytime you're planning a more vigorous workout, spend a few minutes warming up first by doing an easy version of the activity you have planned. Walking? Stroll slowly before you increase the pace. Bicycling? Pedal in a low gear on the flats before you try any hills. And be sure to cool down after you finish with a few minutes of slower activity.

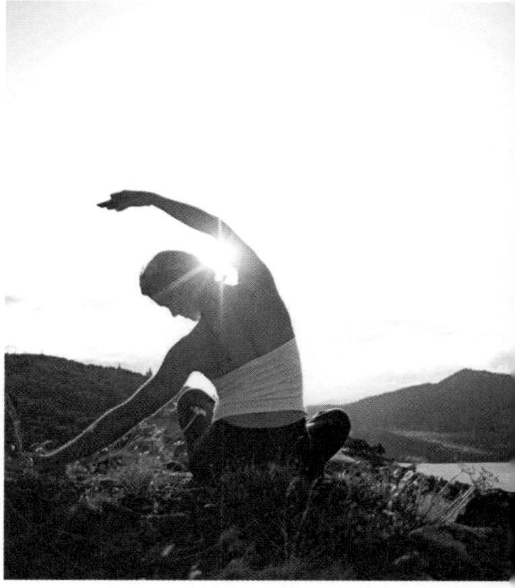

Lack of skill. If you stick to simple activities like walking, swimming, or bike riding, you really don't have to worry about skill. These are probably things you've done since you were a child. But if you're looking to add variety to your exercise by trying a new sport (say, tennis) or a regime like yoga, take a class or sign up with a trainer who can teach you the proper techniques. The investment will be well worth it should you find a sport that keeps you excited about exercising.

Lack of resources. Adopting regular exercise doesn't mean you have to join a gym or invest in expensive home equipment. With a jump rope and some elastic exercise bands you can get a full body workout and your total investment will be less than $30. Visit the American Council on Exercise site (www.acefitness.org) to find simple but effective workouts you can do at home.

How Much Activity Do You Really Need?

Most people should aim to accomplish at least 2.5 hours a week of moderate-effort activity. Some examples of moderate effort include brisk walking, water aerobics, riding a bike over gentle terrain, playing doubles in tennis, and pushing a lawn mower. A couple days a week, add strengthening moves like push-ups, sit-ups, and lunges, and you're done.

If you like more intense effort, you don't have to exercise as long. People who jog, swim laps, ride a bike over hilly terrain (or at a pace greater than 15 miles per hour), or play singles tennis or basketball can get many of exercise's benefits with only an hour and 15 minutes of activity each week.

But how do you know if you've hit your 2.5 hours a week if you're primarily pursuing NEAT activity? ("Hmm, how long did I fidget today? How many minutes did I spend climbing the stairs?") One handy way is to use a pedometer to track the number of steps you take.

The NEAT approach works well for managing heart-disease risk factors like high blood pressure and high blood sugar. But if you're looking to boost your good cholesterol or lose weight—especially in your midsection—research indicates that you'll have to raise your heart rate a bit higher. If you're in that group, you'll want to also pursue the interval training program on page 184.

To Control Blood Pressure, Inflammation, and Lower Your Risk of Diabetes

If your main concerns are high blood pressure and helping your body process sugar—which will help reduce inflammation and lower your risk of diabetes—you'll find that accumulating 2.5 hours of activity weekly works amazingly well. With a robust schedule of NEAT activities such as climbing the stairs, gardening, and cleaning the house, you should be able to give your heart the exercise it needs. But how can you be sure if you're doing enough?

The simplest way to is to wear a pedometer, or step counter, with the ultimate goal of taking 10,000 steps a day. In studies, people who achieve this number gain numerous benefits: not just lower blood pressure and heart disease risk, but improved mood and energy, stronger bones, a lower risk of cancer, relief from arthritis, and help in maintaining a healthy weight.

> With a robust schedule of NEAT activities such as climbing the stairs, gardening, and cleaning the house, you should be able to give your heart the exercise it needs.

Tracking your steps is easy. You can find a pedometer at any sporting goods store, most pharmacies, and even big box stores. Wear one as you go throughout your day and see where you are at the end of the day. Don't be dismayed if your total is less than 5,000 steps—that's typical when you're just starting out. Plan to add about 10 minutes of walking a day for the first week. That will give you an extra 1,200 steps. The following week, add another 10 minutes of walking per day; continue building in more walking each week until you reach 10,000 steps. You can also raise your count by incorporating more NEAT activities.

If you prefer to increase your count by means other than walking, refer to this conversion chart. It will help you translate your other activities into steps to help you reach your 10,000-step goal.

Physical Activity	Equivalent Steps (per minute)	Physical Activity	Equivalent Steps (per minute)
Aerobics, low-impact	125	Rowing, moderate effort	153
Aerobics, moderate	153	Sawing wood	113
Aerobics, high-impact	181	Shoveling heavy snow	278
Basketball	100	Skiing, downhill	109
Canoeing	72	Skiing, cross-country	114
Chopping wood	60	Snowshoeing	156
Dancing	133	Soccer	144
Football	133	Stationary bicycling, leisurely	100
Gardening	73	Stationary bicycling, moderate	181
Golf (walking)	100	Stationary bicycling, vigorous	250
Horseshoes	52	Swimming laps, light/moderate	200
Ice-skating, leisurely	84	Tennis	200
Judo and karate	236	Volleyball	90
Mopping	51	Walking	125
Painting	78	Water Aerobics	100
Racquetball	138	Waterskiing	136
Rollerblading	200	Weight lifting	100
Rowing, light effort	74	Yoga	50

To Lower Bad Blood Fats, Raise Good Cholesterol, and Lose Weight

Take 10,000 steps a day through moderate walks and NEAT activities and you'll go a long way toward lowering your risk of cardiovascular trouble. But if you'd like to lower your triglycerides or raise your "good" HDL cholesterol, you'll need to work your heart a little harder. In research, people who worked up a good sweat were able to drop their triglycerides by as much as 40 percent. And studies show that exercise that includes short bouts of higher-intensity efforts can raise HDL by as much as 8 points—enough to dramatically improve the ratio of good-to-bad cholesterol, an important marker of heart risk. You'll also want to pick up the pace if losing weight is part of your heart-health goals.

The nice thing about the Healthy Heart Miracle Diet program is that it targets visceral fat. That's the fat that accumulates deep in your midsection, enveloping internal organs. Visceral fat happens to be especially toxic to your arteries because it reenters the bloodstream on a regular basis, converting to "bad" LDL cholesterol and lodging in the narrow spaces in your arteries in the form of plaque.

Some reassuring news about this workout is that you won't have to exercise for longer than you would normally; you're just going to mix up your pace using a well-established method known as interval training. For short periods, you'll walk faster, swim harder, or spin quicker, then slow down again. During these bursts, you'll raise your heart rate to around 75 to 80 percent of your maximum heart rate, known as target heart rate (see "Determining Your Target Heart Rate" below). Or, if you'd rather, you can keep it very simple and go by how the effort feels.

it's a miracle! PUSH-UPS PROTECT YOUR HEART

Strength training is too often overlooked in exercise programs, but it's perhaps one of the easiest ways to speed your weight loss, improve the way your body looks, and lower your heart risk. A recent Danish study found that strength training reduced markers of heart risk as much as aerobic exercise did; stroke risk fell by 25 percent in both aerobic exercisers and people doing strength training. In a British study, regular strength training alone lowered "bad" LDL cholesterol by 14 percent. Even if you do just 10 minutes of push-ups, sit-ups, and lunges four times a week, you'll see a big improvement in your heart health and your overall fitness.

On page 184, you'll find a 6-week program that you can use whether you're walking, swimming, jogging, bicycling, rowing—nearly any endurance activity you can think of. If you're new to exercise and interval training, start by doing just 20 minutes with a 5-minute warm-up and cooldown (Week 1). Each week, add another interval and "rest" period (really, working at your normal pace) until you've reached the length of time you want to exercise (40 minutes five days a week is plenty to achieve the heart and weight-loss benefits you're after). If you find a particular week difficult, repeat it before moving on to the next. And if you find the workouts to be too easy, feel free to skip to the following week's workout.

Before You Begin

Exercise heals many ills, but you should still use a little caution before you dive in or, depending on your health, you could put yourself at risk for further heart complications. If you've had a heart

Heart Rate Monitors for Everyone

Heart rate monitors might seem as if they're designed only for triathletes and ultramarathoners, but you can put one to good use as well. They're incredibly handy for interval workouts. You can find a good one for around $50, and you can set it to alert you when you've reached your target heart rate. You can also set an alarm to go off when your heart rate drops out of your target zone—a helpful reminder to keep up the effort until the interval period is over. The monitor will also help keep you honest: It's easy to stop working as hard when you don't have any means of tracking your efforts. And a workout that was challenging in the beginning will become easier as you gain fitness. A monitor will ensure that you continue to push yourself and gain the most benefits from your exercise.

attack or have chest pain, seek your doctor's advice on appropriate activities and intensity levels. The same goes if anyone in your immediate family has a history of heart disease before the age of 55. If you're on medication for your heart, ask your doctor if it might interfere with your exercise. For instance, diuretics for high blood pressure can leave you light-headed or dizzy during activities that require balance.

People with high blood pressure should avoid holding their breath during any strength-training move—a common mistake that can trigger a sharp spike in blood pressure. Aerobic exercise in very hot or cold conditions can also adversely affect circulation. People who are overweight or obese should also take care during extreme weather. Try walking at a local mall when the conditions outside are too nasty.

Generally, though, if your primary exercise will come from NEAT activities, you can rest easy. As long as you don't add too much too soon, you won't overtax your heart. Just pay close attention to your body: When you're too short of breath, slow down. If you develop a rapid or irregular heartbeat, stop. Forget "no pain, no gain": If you don't feel good, take the rest of the day off. If you feel lousy again the next day, get a checkup and ask your doctor for advice on activities that make sense for you.

Determining Your Target Heart Rate

To determine your target heart rate during interval periods (70 to 85 percent of your maximum heart rate), use this formula.

1. **Subtract your age from 220. This is a rough estimate of your maximum heart rate.**
2. **Determine the lower end of your target heart rate by multiplying your maximum heart rate by 0.7.**
3. **Determine the upper end of your target heart rate by multiplying your maximum heart rate by 0.85.**

Remember these two numbers. While you're exercising, check your pulse. To check your pulse over your carotid artery, place your index and middle fingers on your neck to the side of your windpipe. To check your pulse at your wrist, place two fingers between the bone and the tendon over your radial artery, located on the thumb side of your wrist. When you feel your pulse, look at your watch and count the number of beats in 10 seconds. Multiply this number by 6 to get your heart rate, or heartbeats per minute.

The Healthy Heart Miracle Diet

6-Week Interval Workout

You can use this workout plan for any aerobic activity, including walking, swimming, rowing, and bike riding. It starts you out nice and slow, and builds up your endurance over time.

By Week 6, you'll have reached a workout that is challenging and that you can continue to follow indefinitely. As you become more fit, you'll have to work harder to keep your heart in the target zone, which will help keep this workout challenging. Or you can continue to push yourself by increasing your interval time to 2 minutes in Week 7, and then lower your rest time to 2 minutes in subsequent weeks.

KEY

Light: Easy effort; you should be able to carry on a conversation without any problems

Moderate: 45 to 60 percent of maximum heart rate (you should be able to say, but not sing, the words to a song)

Vigorous: 75 to 80 percent of maximum heart rate (you should not be able to say more than a few words without taking a breath)

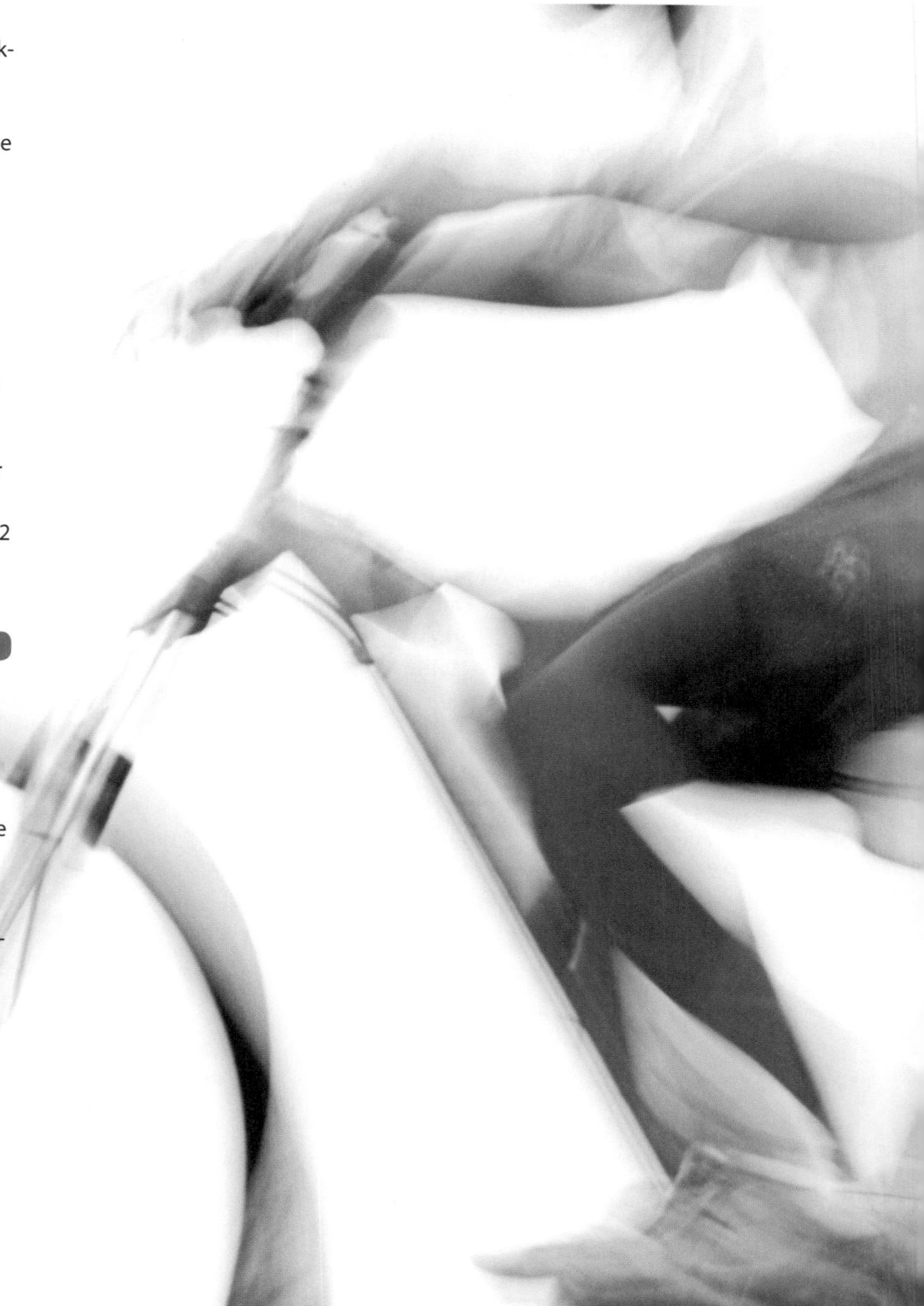

Week 1

20 MINUTES

Warm-up: 5 minutes

Baseline: 2 minutes

Interval: 30 seconds

Rest: 2.5 minutes

Interval: 30 seconds

Rest: 2.5 minutes

Interval: 30 seconds

Rest: 1.5 minutes

Cooldown: 5 minutes

Week 2

22 MINUTES

Warm-up: 5 minutes

Baseline: 2 minutes

Interval: 30 seconds

Rest: 2 minutes

Interval: 30 seconds

Rest: 2 minutes

Interval: 30 seconds

Rest: 2 minutes

Interval: 30 seconds

Rest: 2 minutes

Cooldown: 5 minutes

Week 3

30 MINUTES

Warm-up: 5 minutes

Baseline: 4 minutes

Interval: 1 minute

Rest: 4 minutes

Interval: 1 minute

Rest: 4 minutes

Interval: 1 minute

Rest: 5 minutes

Cooldown: 5 minutes

Week 4

35 MINUTES

Warm-up: 5 minutes

Baseline: 3 minutes

Interval: 1 minute

Rest: 3.5 minutes

Interval: 1 minute

Rest: 3.5 minutes

Interval: 1 minute

Rest: 3.5 minutes

Interval: 1 minute

Rest: 3.5 minutes

Interval: 1 minute

Rest: 3 minutes

Cooldown: 5 minutes

Week 5

40 MINUTES

Warm-up: 5 minutes

Baseline: 2 minutes

Interval: 1 minute

Rest: 3 minutes

Interval: 1 minute

Rest: 3 minutes

Interval: 1 minute

Rest: 3 minutes

Interval: 1 minute

Rest: 3 minutes

Interval: 1 minute

Rest: 3 minutes

Interval: 1 minute

Rest: 3 minutes

Interval: 1 minute

Rest: 3 minutes

Cooldown: 5 minutes

Week 6

40 MINUTES

Warm-up: 5 minutes

Baseline: 3 minutes

Interval: 1.5 minutes

Rest: 3 minutes

Interval: 1.5 minutes

Rest: 3 minutes

Interval: 1.5 minutes

Rest: 3 minutes

Interval: 1.5 minutes

Rest: 3 minutes

Interval: 1.5 minutes

Rest: 3 minutes

Interval: 1.5 minutes

Rest: 3 minutes

Cooldown: 5 minutes

12

Emotional Rescue

Your emotions don't literally come from your heart, but being happy and relatively stress-free sure can help it. In fact, joy, laughter, and relaxation are part of the Healthy Heart Miracle Diet prescription.

Hearts aflame with love. Lonely hearts. Broken hearts. Lion hearts. Light hearts. For thousands of years, poets have linked the human heart to all sorts of emotions. Turns out they were on to something. When it comes to keeping your heart healthy, 21st-century science shows that how you feel has a greater affect on your cardiovascular health than we ever imagined.

Until just a few years ago, the connection between heart health and feelings focused solely on stress. It all started in the 1970s, when scientists first announced that people with hard-charging "Type A" personalities were at higher risk for heart attacks. Today, that narrow view is as dated as disco music and bell bottoms.

The new thinking? Taming chronic, 24/7 stress—the kind brought on by overloaded work schedules, long commutes, financial worries, and difficult relationships or life situations—is still crucial. But equally important is lifting depression, an all-too-common condition that significantly raises the risk for heart disease and fatal heart attacks. Some of the solutions involve getting back to basics: spending time with friends, planning time to relax, and making sure you allow yourself enough opportunities for fun, all of which are emerging as powerful heart protectors in their own right.

Stress's Hidden Dirty Work

A little bit of stress is nature's way of kicking you into high gear—rushing you out the door to get to an appointment on time or pushing you to act fast in an emergency. In a flash, your body releases stress hormones including cortisol, norepinephrine, and adrenalin. As they race through your bloodstream, your heart beats faster, your blood pressure rises, and your body pumps sugar and fat into your bloodstream in case you need extra energy.

That's all well and good when your stress is short-lived—but these days, too many of our stressors stick around indefinitely. The nasty boss. The credit card balances. The family worries. Not only can they raise your blood pressure, they can even raise "bad" LDL cholesterol. Chronic stress is also linked with artery damage that opens the door to atherosclerosis—narrowed, hardened arteries.

Of course, stress affects more than your arteries. If you're living your life feeling anxious or overwhelmed, chances are you're relying on junk food or simple carbs as quick emotional fixes. (In one study in rats, University of California, San Francisco, researchers found that after a stressful event, the urge to eat sweet, fat-packed treats intensified—and that the cascade of stress hormones only shut itself off when the cravings were obeyed. The researchers think that something very similar happens in humans.) Or you're drinking too much alcohol. Almost certainly you're not taking time to prepare and enjoy healthy home-cooked meals. And you probably aren't exercising, either, which is too bad, since exercise is wonderfully effective at taming stress. All of this adds to the unfortunate fact that stress hormones encourage your body to deposit excess calories deep in your abdomen, where it's most dangerous to your heart.

Broken Heart Syndrome

A broken heart isn't just emotionally devastating. A big emotional or physical stress can "stun" cardiac muscle, triggering symptoms that look and feel just like a heart attack, such as excruciating chest pain, shortness of breath, and even temporary heart failure.

Cardiologists from Johns Hopkins University School of Medicine, whose research first identified "broken heart syndrome," say it's different from a full-fledged heart attack in one important way: People recover swiftly and fully, with no signs of blocked arteries or permanent damage to heart muscle. In one study of 19 people whose symptoms kicked in after stressful experiences such as a car accident or being a victim of an armed robbery, several ended up taking heart medications long-term that they didn't really need.

If you or a loved one has heart symptoms after a traumatic event, and if recovery is fast and complete, talk with your doctor about blood tests and scans to evaluate your heart health and risk for future events.

Which looks better to you when you're stressed?

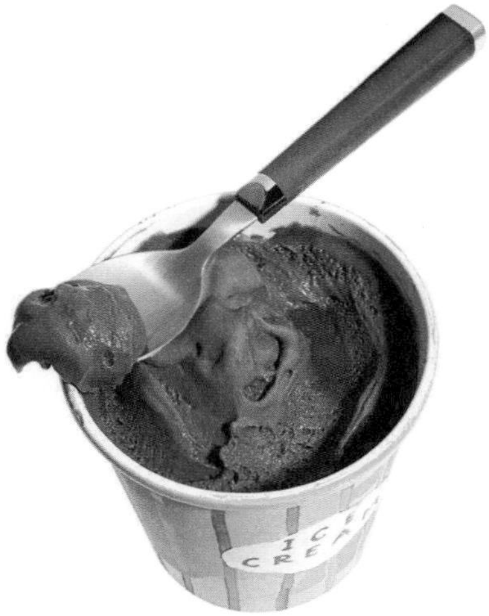

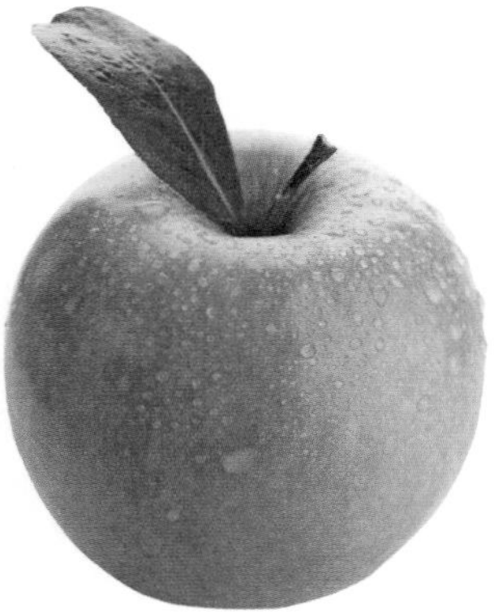

▲ The ice cream might appeal to your emotions, but the apple will do far more to relieve your tensions.

The trick to dealing with all this stress isn't so much to eliminate it, which may not be possible (although if one issue in particular is bothering you, write down three actions you can take to improve the situation—then take them, one at a time). It's more important that you learn how to cope better with what life throws at you—for instance, by building in time for relaxation, friends, and fun, not to mention getting more exercise, which is proven to help the body recover from surges of stress hormones faster.

Lifting stress is proven to help your heart. In one recent study, people with heart disease who cut their stress levels got a huge health bonus: They were 74 percent less likely to have a heart attack or need bypass surgery.

One of the reasons we're so stressed is that, even if we have dozens or hundreds of online friends, in person we live relatively isolated lives. Imagine life in prehistoric times, when it took a village, or at least a clan, to hunt for food, watch the kids, and fend off attackers. Back then, being alone was literally life-threatening. And it may be still: When Harvard School of Public Health researchers followed 3,000 women and men for 19 years, they found that women who said they felt extremely lonely were 76 percent more likely to develop heart disease than those who had plenty of friends. Loneliness raises cortisol levels, which can raise blood pressure. It also seems to nudge the heart into dangerous offbeat rhythms and make blood more likely to clot. Our brains even perceive social isolation as something very similar to physical pain.

The benefits of social contact are quite amazing. Studies show that women with more close friends have less heart-threatening plaque in their artery walls. Men who feel the least lonely have the lowest blood levels of an inflammatory chemical called interleukin-6 that's associated with heart attacks.

How Stressed Are You *Really*?

If you're thinking right now, "Gee, I don't feel very stressed. I'm handling the demands of life just fine. And I saw my best friend just a few weeks ago. Guess this isn't a problem for me," it's time to take a closer look. Chronic stress is insidious for yet another reason: Once it settles in, your mind and body tend to accept it as the new normal. In other words, you may simply have forgotten what it feels like to be free of stress. The first step in easing your body's heart-threatening reaction to stress is getting a handle on how much of it is hiding out in your life. To find it, ask yourself these seven questions.

#1 How cold are your fingertips?

Touch the back of your neck with the fingertips of both hands. Stress reduces blood circulation to your body's extremities. If your fingers feel chilly against the warm skin of your neck, it may signal extra tension. While your neck may register around 90°F (32°C), stress can cut finger temperature to as low as 60°F (15°C). (Mood rings—and relaxation techniques involving biofeedback—make use of this cold-hands-high stress/warm-hands-low-stress principle.)

#2 How often did you eat doughnuts, candy, chips, muffins, ice cream, or extra helpings of comfort foods yesterday?

More than once or twice could be a sign of chronic stress, not just a lack of willpower. A craving for treats packed with fat and refined carbohydrates like sugar and white flour is a hard-wired biochemical response to chronic stress, say University of California, San Francisco, researchers.

#3 How many colds did you have last winter? Did you get the flu?

We all get a couple of colds each year, and it can be tough fighting off the flu virus if it rampages through your workplace or community. But research shows that having high levels of stress doubles your odds for catching a cold. And a sunny outlook can reduce your risk by 40 percent.

What's going on? A growing stack of studies shows that chronic stress weakens immunity. At Ohio State University, researchers found that the caregivers of relatives with Alzheimer's disease had levels of a protein that signal immune-system problems four times higher than noncaregivers. The same researchers have also found that stress can limit the effectiveness of flu vaccines, too.

#4 Does your body hurt?

Yes, stress can lead to tension headaches, thanks to tension in your neck. But chronic stress also ignites aches in other parts of your body, thanks to the release of hormones that boost pain sensitivity, tighten muscles, and even slow digestion. Stress-related aches and pains often center on your neck and shoulders, face and jaw, lower back, and even your abdomen (where symptoms may include cramps, diarrhea, or constipation).

#5 How often do you laugh?

There's no correct answer to this one, but obviously, more is better. If you can't gauge this on your own, ask a friend or close colleague for an objective opinion. Laughter lowers stress and makes artery walls more supple, which reduces risk for high blood pressure and helps protect against damage that leads to plaque buildup. In a University of Maryland study of 300 people, researchers found that people with heart disease were 40 percent less likely to chuckle during potentially humorous situations.

The trick to dealing with all this stress isn't so much to eliminate it, but to learn how to cope better with what life throws at you.

#6 How wide—and deep—is your social life?

The more diverse your social circle, the lower your heart disease risk. Getting together not just with your spouse and kids but also with other family members, childhood friends, new acquaintances, and with coworkers (outside work—not in the company cafeteria) all count. And it's okay if some relationships are conducted by phone or email, Duke University researchers report. Deep friendships matter the most. In one study, women who were the most satisfied with their friendships had the lowest heart disease risk. Feeling you have friends who know you deep down may be especially important for women's hearts.

#7 How's your marriage?

From hot times between the sheets to friendship and respect, a healthy love relationship is great for your ticker—and a not-so-great one can create trouble. In one University of Utah study, couples who were the most hostile or demeaning while discussing difficult subjects (kids, money, the in-laws) had more calcifications—early signs of atherosclerosis—in their arteries.

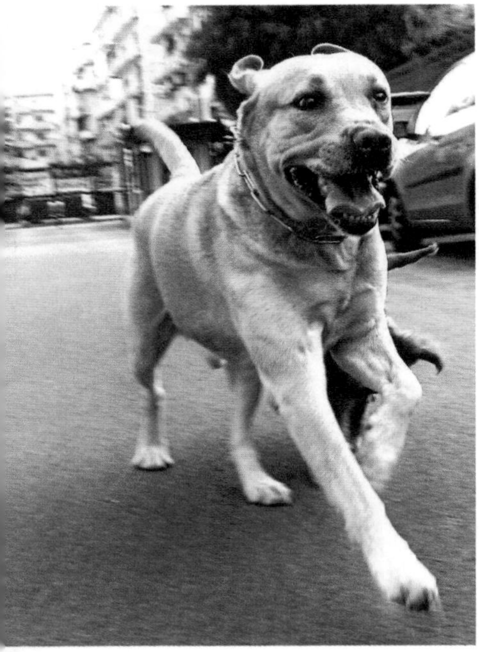

Your Antistress Prescription

Imagine what would happen if, when your doctor handed you a prescription for cholesterol or blood pressure medicine, he also gave you a prescription of 15 minutes of daily relaxation and 3 hours a week of fun time—and he told you to take it seriously. Most doctors don't actually do this (although some do), but you should take the advice to heart as if yours did.

Play Like a Dog

Have you ever watched dogs in a dog run? There's no mistaking the over-the-top excitement, evidenced by wagging tails and vigorous, joyous play. Dogs are inherently social creatures (they were originally pack animals)—and so are humans. Not only do we need contact with other humans but we also need play time, and many of us simply don't get enough. The message: Have more fun, especially with others.

When life gets hectic, it's easy to relegate your social life and hobbies to the back burner. You cancel lunch dates with friends in order to finish up a work project, fume over the checkbook instead of taking a walk with your spouse, finish the housework instead of catching the latest screwball comedy at the movie theater, gobble a high-fat snack to soothe your stress instead of enjoying time in the garden. But cutting-edge research shows that the kind of happiness your heart needs every day is way too important to skip—*especially* when life goes haywire. In fact, sometimes the stress we feel is a big red warning flag that we're missing out on basic, joyful experiences that boost cardiovascular health.

Think twice before skipping your book group meeting, bowling league, or family dinnertime. If you're not the social type, that's okay; even maintaining two or three close relationships will go a long way, especially if you can also find joy in the time that you do spend alone, whether it's from tending your tomato plants, knitting a sweater with the beautiful new yarn you found, or walking in the woods.

Physical contact is also important. Holding hands with a spouse led to lower levels of heart-threatening stress hormones in one study. In another study, men who make love once or twice a week had a 2.8 times lower risk for fatal heart attacks than those who got amorous just once a month.

it's a miracle! LAUGHTER OPENS THE ARTERIES

Popping in your favorite funny video could be almost as good for your heart as eating a serving of salmon or talking a walk. In a University of Maryland study of 20 healthy adults, watching part of a funny movie (in this case, the 1996 comedy *Kingpin*) relaxed the endothelium—the fragile lining of blood vessels—enough to increase blood flow 22 percent. In contrast, viewing part of a stressful film (the opening battleground scene of *Saving Private Ryan*) made blood vessels stiffer and decreased blood flow by 33 percent. Laughter boosts levels of feel-good brain chemicals called endorphins. These chemicals lock into receptors in the endothelium that release nitric oxide, which relaxes blood vessels. Of course, all you feel is the a-a-ah of a good laugh!

Do a Little Advance Planning

Our days get filled with tasks before we know it, and suddenly there's no time left for leisure. Or maybe you simply didn't plan for a fun activity, so your day got filled with chores and TV and dead time instead. Prioritize so you can focus on what's most important to you. When there's too much to do, say "no" to the less important stuff, delegate where possible (yes, your kids can load the dishwasher and set the table), or find shortcuts so that low-priority tasks don't use up precious time. Instead of cooking on a night when you want to be sure to fit in a walk with your favorite neighbor, why not pick up a rotisserie chicken (remove the skin before eating) and a bag of salad greens at the supermarket? When there's not enough to do, schedule something. Sign up for a class that sounds like fun, whether it's pottery making or ballroom dancing. Or join a local film club. Or simply get up the courage to ask that friendly neighbor to join you for a walk or a cup of coffee.

Think Positive

Life hands us lemons all the time. Your job is to make lemonade. Simply looking at the positive side of a situation can make obstacles, challenges, and setbacks seem smaller—and maybe even look like opportunities. Often, the difference between one person's stress level and another's isn't what happens to them in life but how they choose to react. You can dwell on your problems and indulge in some serious self-pity or make a conscious decision to make the best of it. Letting optimism triumph over pessimism is proven to reduce stress and to help people recover from the physical and emotional aftermath of high-tension experiences.

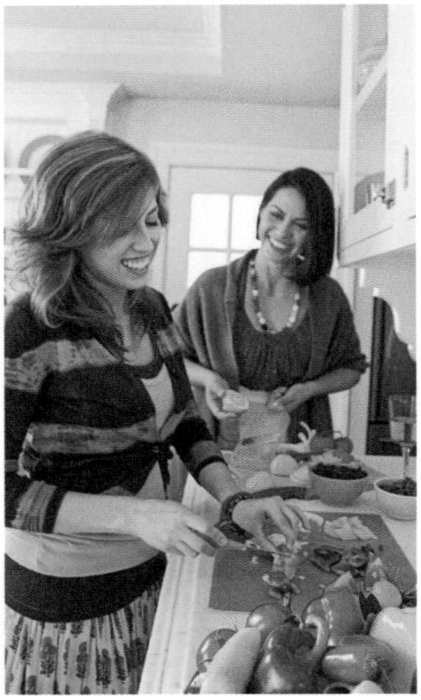

Not born to see the glass half full? It doesn't matter. Anyone can learn to see things in a more balanced, realistic way. Start by simply tuning into what your inner critic is saying. Psychologists say we color our world grimly in three common ways:

- **Sifting out the good stuff.** This critic forgets the positive and focuses on the negative—ignoring the fact that you sent a gift on time or got a phone call from an old friend, and honing in on the fact that you forgot a doctor's appointment or got stuck in a traffic jam.
- **Interpreting events as a bad reflection on you.** Your inner doomsayer may assume that you're responsible for anything negative or inconvenient that happened today ("They canceled lunch because they don't like me!").
- **Catastrophizing.** Your grown-up daughter is 15 minutes late meeting you for dinner, and you begin calling local hospital emergency rooms, convinced that she's had an accident. You find termites and assume that the house is about to fall down.

Once you've met your own inner skeptic, be ready to stop and silence it next time it pipes up. Take a breath and give it a gentle yet firm response. "Yes, my daughter's late, but I know traffic's bad at rush

it's a miracle! FRIENDSHIP FIGHTS HEART DISEASE

It's great spending time with your spouse and immediate family, but it may be time to branch out. In one Duke University study, people who had the largest variety of social contacts—including relatives who aren't immediate family, neighbors, new friends, childhood friends, and friends from work you see outside the office—were 40 percent less likely to have heart disease than those with just one or no contacts.

hour. That's all it probably is." Or "I'm very disappointed about not getting the promotion. I'll go find out why, and what I can do to get one next time." Or "Too bad Paula canceled our movie plans, but I won't take it personally. In fact, I'll call someone else and still go!" Positive thinking can help you develop flexibility and resilience—the ability to stay calm and optimistic even when none of your plans are quite working out.

Another way to build a more positive world view is to stop and be thankful for something every day—the beautiful weather, a good night's sleep, a phone call from your daughter, the fact that you avoided an accident on the highway. You can use a gratitude journal to record these thoughts, or simply note them to yourself.

Working Mom Syndrome

More than a decade ago, Duke University researchers found that stress hormone levels in working mothers stayed high from morning till night, putting them at higher risk than other working women for heart attacks. Yet despite this and dozens of other well-publicized studies over the last 20 years, doctors often overlook tension. In one University of Michigan study of 457 women with heart disease, only 1 in 5 got stress-reduction advice from their doctors. Without a medical test to identify stress, it's up to you to find it—and tame it.

Practice Relaxing

Your body's fight-or-flight reaction to stressful events is automatic. Eventually the reaction fades once the stress recedes, but you can speed up that process by training yourself to elicit the "relaxation response." It's the a-a-ah you feel after a week's vacation, when a loved one gives you a long hug, when holding a sleeping baby, or even while petting your dog or cat. It doesn't just make you feel good, it also reduces levels of stress hormones in your bloodstream, lowers blood pressure, and even helps restore artery flexibility.

There are plenty of ways to get to this level of relaxation without the vacation or the purring pet. One simple method is to sit in a comfortable chair or lie on your bed or floor and shut your eyes. Pay attention to your breath as you inhale and exhale. When your mind wanders, return your attention to your breath. You'll soon find yourself breathing slower and deeper, signs of the relaxation response in action.

A more structured version of this exercise is called mindfulness meditation. It's one of the core techniques used in a relaxation

it's a miracle! A PET CAN LOWER YOUR BLOOD PRESSURE

There's evidence that your pet can buffer you from dangerous, stress-driven spikes in blood pressure. Pet it, play with it, walk it, and talk to it. Furry four-legged friends are proven stress-reducers that buffered against blood pressure spikes in studies involving hard-charging Wall Street stockbrokers and caregivers for spouses with brain injuries.

method called mindfulness-based stress reduction. You can find training in this method at many local hospitals, or find a class near you by logging onto www.umassmed.edu/cfm/mbsr/. This lists classes in Canada, too.

Another trick is called progressive muscle relaxation. It's especially helpful for people who tend to hold tension in their bodies without realizing it. Lie down on the floor or your bed, close your eyes, and breathe slowly. Now, starting with your feet, tense and relax one group of muscles at a time. Count to 5 when you tense the muscles, then relax and let tension ebb away as you count to 10. Move on to your lower legs, upper legs, hips and buttocks, back, abdomen, chest, hands and arms, shoulders and neck, and finally your face.

Any time you feel stress, whether you're at work, at home, or in the car, you can also take even just 1 minute to practice deep breathing. Count a steady rhythm to yourself—perhaps 1-2-3 on each inhale, 1-2-3 on each exhale. After a while, lengthen your breaths a little (count to 4) or try pausing for a second after each exhalation to deepen the relaxing effect.

Move More

Exercise is a key component of the Healthy Heart Miracle Diet, and you'll read a lot more about it in chapter 11. But for now, know that just about any kind of exercise you do will help combat stress. Working up a sweat is effective. So is slower, rhythmic exercise, such as walking, swimming, or t'ai chi. And yoga may be especially beneficial, both for your heart and your state of mind. Sign up for a class at your local YMCA. You'll get a double bonus of getting out of the house and meeting other people. In one study, people with heart disease who took a 6-week yoga class saw artery flexibility improve by 69 percent. In another study, a year of regular yoga sessions lowered levels of "bad" LDL cholesterol by 26 percent.

Strike a Better Work/Life Balance

Long work hours raise your odds for high blood pressure, report University of California, Irvine, researchers. Putting in 41 to 51 hours per week doubled the risk for high blood pressure compared to those who logged only 40 hours. A tense job, a toxic boss, plus a vending machine (or other easy source of high-fat, high-sugar snacks) added up to a 68 percent higher risk for heart disease in one study that tracked 10,000 British white-collar workers for 12 years.

If you can't work fewer hours, or you're stuck in a difficult work situation, recognize the health risk and take control where you can—by promising that you won't let a bad boss or unfriendly colleagues affect your heart. Pack some healthy snacks to have on hand (almonds are perfect, as is fruit), take a walk at lunchtime, and give yourself a real break from work once you leave the office: Do some creative gardening, cook a new dish, or visit a local attraction you've never seen before. In a 28-year study from Finland, people who used weekends to get away from work stress were three times less likely to have fatal heart attacks than those who didn't really unwind. Bonus points for booking a vacation: Regular vacations can cut heart attack risk by 30 percent.

Stress: How Well Are You Protected?

quiz

Do you have the tools to keep tension under control? Ask yourself these questions and write down "yes" or "no."

1. When life gets busy, I plan my time more carefully so I won't feel overwhelmed.

2. I have no trouble saying "no" when someone asks me to do something that's inconvenient or that I'm not interested in doing.

3. I turn to close friends and family frequently for emotional support.

4. I'm fairly flexible—when plans change, I adapt easily.

5. Seeing the funny side helps me cope when things aren't going my way.

6. I rarely use alcohol in order to unwind.

7. I have a hobby in which I regularly engage.

8. When someone makes me angry, I'm quick to recover and brush it off, especially when the affront was minor.

9. Even when life is hectic, I try to fit in some exercise almost every day.

10. If I start blaming myself or expecting the worst when things go wrong, I try to catch myself and try to think more positively.

Your Score

Give yourself 1 point for every "yes" answer, 0 points for every "no."

7 TO 10 POINTS: You're well-equipped to keep stress under control (though feel free to work on any questions to which you answered "no").

4 TO 6 POINTS: Sometimes you beat stress, sometimes it beats you. Learning and practicing a tension-melting stress-reduction exercise can help counteract elevated stress hormone levels even if you can't always keep tension away.

0 TO 3 POINTS: Your lifestyle and outlook are putting your heart in danger. It's time to make some changes. Start with something simple, like a daily walk or some deep breathing to remind you what it feels like to relax.

Depression: A Silent Epidemic

Depression doesn't just make life more difficult, it makes *health* more difficult.

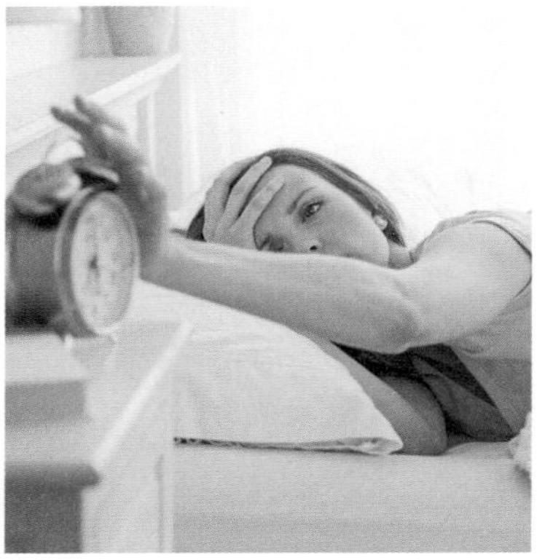

Depression has an uncanny ability to hide in plain sight. It's easy to convince yourself that you'll snap out of that stubbornly grim, low mood any day now, and it's easy to avoid talking about what's bothering you or even admitting to yourself that you're in the grip of a shadow that's stealing the pleasure and the energy from your life.

If you're feeling depressed, you're hardly alone. Today, at least 1 in 10 Americans takes an antidepressant—double the number of a decade ago—making these pills and capsules the most prescribed medications in the United States. So if you think you may be depressed, don't be afraid to bring it up with your doctor. Getting treated is more important than you realize.

Depression doesn't just make life more difficult, it makes *health* more difficult. Like stress, depression has physical effects on the body, including increased inflammation. But what's worse is the fact that feeling down in the dumps makes you less likely to exercise and eat well and more likely to smoke and drink too much. Depression quadrupled heart disease risk in one Johns Hopkins University study that tracked 1,500 people for 13 years. And it increases the odds of a fatal heart attack six- to eightfold.

If you're a heart attack survivor hoping to avoid a repeat attack, pay close attention: Up to one in three people who've had a heart attack are coping with depression (likely thanks in part to temporary changes in the brain brought on by the event). Taking it seriously could be a matter of life or death, since depression raises the risk of dying in the first 6 months after a heart attack 3 percent to 17 percent. It also increases the chances that you'll have a second heart attack or develop congestive heart failure.

While cardiologists are increasingly aware of the mind-body connections that influence heart health, they often overlook depression in the rush of treating someone who's had a heart attack or is at high risk for a heart attack. That means it's up to you and your loved ones to stay tuned for signs that your mood and outlook are heading south—and to speak up about it.

Experts now have solid proof that dealing with depression protects your heart. People with heart disease and depression who took antidepressants to ease depression lowered the odds for a fatal heart attack by 42 percent, for example. Other research shows that lifting depression will also make it easier to exercise and eat right, which are both obviously important to your heart health.

Getting Help

About 70 percent of depressed adults try to deal with painfully low moods on their own, without getting help from a doctor or counselor. You may be among them if you are downplaying your feelings, feel too ashamed to ask for help, or think that nothing can help you feel better. Even your doctor may miss the warning signs.

If you think you're depressed, ask your doctor for an evaluation—and for help getting relief. It may take a combination of antidepressants, therapy, and lifestyle changes to lift your spirits, so be patient. The keys to beating depression are patience and high expectations. In the largest-ever American study of depression treatments, 67 percent of the 3,671 volunteers eventually got relief, though some had to try different combinations of antidepressants and cognitive behavioral therapy to get there.

Meanwhile, a recent review of dozens of studies concludes that physical activity may be a missing link for many people looking for depression relief. It helps by lowering levels of stress hormones and boosting levels of feel-good brain chemicals. Plus, exercise provides a mental break from negative thinking—and a chance to start noticing the good things in your life. All it takes is 30 minutes of activity most days of the week. Some types of depression may respond to exercise alone, while others need a combination of treatments.

Are You Depressed?

On your own, it can be tricky knowing whether you're depressed enough to need help or you're just a little low. It's worth figuring it out, so that you can feel like your old self again and reduce your risk for heart disease, too.

Depression feels different for different people. If you have one or more of these warning signs, you may have depression and should talk with your doctor about the best way to start feeling better.

- Persistent sad, anxious or "empty" feelings
- Feelings of hopelessness and/or pessimism
- Feelings of guilt, worthlessness, and/or helplessness
- Irritability, restlessness
- Loss of interest in activities or hobbies once pleasurable, including sex
- Insomnia, early-morning wakefulness, or excessive sleeping
- Fatigue and decreased energy
- Difficulty concentrating, remembering details, and making decisions
- Overeating or appetite loss
- Thoughts of suicide, suicide attempts
- Persistent aches or pains, headaches, and/or cramps or digestive problems that do not ease with treatment

13

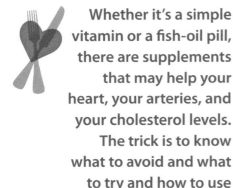

Supplements for Your Heart

Whether it's a simple vitamin or a fish-oil pill, there are supplements that may help your heart, your arteries, and your cholesterol levels. The trick is to know what to avoid and what to try and how to use supplements safely.

You're faithfully following the Healthy Heart Miracle Diet—heck, you're even exercising more frequently. But is it enough? Could you be doing more?

It is part of these modern times that we want our medical cures to come in pill form. And so a booming business has developed around not only prescription drugs for heart health but also supplements that claim to offer myriad heart and health benefits.

To be clear: There is no off-the-shelf supplement that can protect your heart from a bad diet or a sedentary lifestyle. Research is scant on many supplements, and oversight of the supplements industry is light, so you never know exactly what you're getting in the pill you just swallowed.

But there's more to this story. As people increasingly seek more natural ways to improve their health (and devote an increasing amount of their money toward natural and alternative healing and prevention), the medical world has gained interest. Increasingly, researchers and doctors are coming out in support of some (though certainly not all) of the supplements now available.

For example, fish-oil capsules are increasingly recommended by doctors for people with heart disease or high triglycerides. Doctors are also recommending vitamin D supplements to their patients more often, whether or not they have heart disease, since many of us are low in the vitamin, which is proving to be important to overall health. And if you have low "good" HDL cholesterol, you might get a prescription for niacin, a B vitamin available as a prescription medicine.

Based on your personal needs, it may be that a couple of these vitamins, herbs, and other supplements will give you some extra support to help keep your heart in peak condition. Here are those that are standing up to medical review and that are getting the increasing support of the scientific and medical communities.

FOR GENERAL HEART HEALTH

Fish Oil (Omega-3 Fatty Acids)

It's an indisputable fact: Fish-eaters have healthier hearts and tend to live longer than folks who eat lots of red meat. Chalk it up to two things: One, eating less red meat means eating less saturated fat. And two, eating more fish means getting more omega-3 fatty acids. Taking fish-oil supplements (or eating several weekly servings of fish) can lower your levels of bad cholesterol, help keep your arteries free of plaque, and protect you against heart attacks and strokes.

REMEMBER THIS

Always tell all your medical providers about every drug and supplement you're taking. They can keep an eye out for related side effects and advise you about dangerous interactions. Just because something is natural doesn't mean it's safe or safe in combination with something else.

What It Does

Fish oil's heart benefits come from two omega-3 fatty acids known as EPA and DHA (eicosapentaenoic acid and docosahexaenoic acid). Their actions are many. They aid in the production of prostaglandins, hormonelike substances that play a role in regulating blood pressure and blood-clotting. They help prevent arteries from thickening and help keep blood vessels supple. Omega-3s also improve blood flow and tamp down inflammation, a major contributor to heart attacks.

People who take fish-oil supplements or eat fish regularly have a 62 percent lower risk of having a fatal heart attack than those who don't, according to a new study published in the *Journal of Nutrition*. In the study, Dutch researchers followed more than 20,000 people ages 20 to 65 for 9 to 14 years and monitored their fish-oil consumption. In addition to slashing their fatal heart attack risk, folks who ate the most fish or who took fish-oil supplements also lowered their chances of dying from coronary artery disease by 49 percent.

Recent studies also show that fish-oil supplements can:

- Lower the risk of heart failure by 30 percent in middle-age and elderly women
- Keep heart attack survivors alive longer and lessen their risk of future hospitalizations
- Help prevent heart attacks in people who have high cholesterol
- Help prevent coronary artery disease and reduce the chances of dying from coronary heart disease by 29 percent
- Reduce atherosclerosis (also known as hardening of the arteries)
- Improve heart function and lessen the risk for having a fatal heart attack
- Lower high triglyceride levels by 30 to 40 percent (at doses of 3 to 4 grams a day)
- Lower LDL cholesterol, even in people already taking cholesterol-lowering medication
- Reduce blood pressure

Who Might Benefit

If you don't eat at least two to three servings of fatty fish each and every week, it could make sense to take a fish-oil supplement, even if you have no known risk factors for heart disease. Strongly consider taking fish oil you if you do have heart disease, high blood pressure, high cholesterol, high triglycerides, or diabetes.

it's a myth. FLAXSEED-OIL SUPPLEMENTS ARE AS GOOD AS FISH-OIL SUPPLEMENTS

Fish oil is good for you because of its omega-3 fatty acids, specifically, types called DHA and EPA. Flaxseed contains omega-3s, too, but a different kind, called ALA. The body converts ALA to DHA and EPA, but not very efficiently. (ALA may also offer health benefits, but they aren't as well-researched as those of EPA and DHA.) Get your omega-3s from seafood or fish-oil supplements.

How To Use It

Dose: The dose used most often in the studies is 1 gram of omega-3, containing both EPA and DHA. Doses up to 4 grams daily are used to lower high triglyceride levels.

Cautions: Fish oil can cause mild gastrointestinal problems such as loose stools. Because of fish oil's blood-thinning properties, high doses may increase the risk of bleeding, so talk with your doctor before taking it if you're taking a blood-thinning medication such as warfarin (Coumadin) or aspirin. Some people experience fishy-tasting burps after taking fish oil. If you're among them, try buying enteric-coated capsules, freezing the capsules, taking them at the beginning of a meal, or switching brands. Finally, if you have allergies to seafood, avoid fish-oil capsules.

Buying tips: The dosage listed on the front label is the total amount of fish oil per serving, *not* the amount of DHA and EPA. Fish oil contains other fatty acids, so buy products that list the amount of DHA and EPA on the ingredient list. Some fish-oil supplements contain as little as 30 percent DHA and EPA; more-expensive brands contain up to 90 percent.

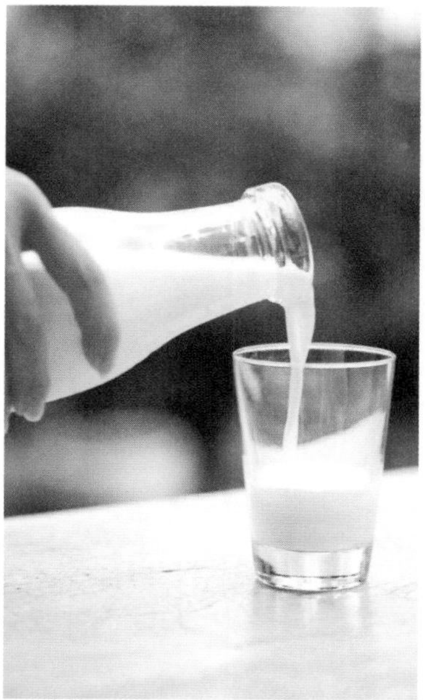

FOR HEALTHIER BLOOD VESSELS AND LONGEVITY

Vitamin D

In many Northern countries, vitamin D deficiency has reached nearly epidemic proportions, and that's very bad news for your heart. In the United States, for example, more than 40 percent of men and 50 percent of women have low vitamin D levels, which puts you at risk for coronary artery disease and heart failure, report doctors at the Cleveland Clinic. Studies have shown that people in Northern Europe tend to have similarly low D levels.

What It Does

Vitamin D helps prevent high blood pressure, suppresses inflammation (by protecting the cells that line your blood vessels), and maintains blood vessel flexibility, among its many other benefits.

In a very recent study published in the *American Journal of Cardiology*, researchers who pored over data from a landmark health and nutrition study reported that low levels of vitamin D make your heart work harder. This may be why adequate vitamin D levels protect you against cardiovascular disease, they suggested. A flurry of other recent studies pointed to vitamin D's other heart-protective benefits: In one, researchers noted that vitamin D supplements could protect you from congestive heart failure. In another, after German and Austrian researchers reviewed several studies about vitamin D's heart benefits, they concluded that people with low vitamin D levels, or those who are at high risk for heart disease, should take 1,000 IU (international units) of vitamin D every day. And Italian researchers discovered that older people with chronic heart failure often have severe vitamin D deficiencies.

Who Might Benefit

If your doctor says that your vitamin D levels are low, you'll want to add a vitamin D supplement to your healthy-heart program.

According to the most recent research, most people who live in the Northern Hemisphere—especially people over age 50 and people who are overweight—could benefit from taking D supplements.

How To Use It

Dose: Though the current official recommendation calls for 400 IU for those ages 51 to 70 and 600 IU for people over 71, many vitamin D researchers recommend taking from 1,000 to 4,000 IU per day. Doctors will sometimes prescribe special vitamin D supplements containing 50,000 IU, usually for elderly patients.

Cautions: Steroids such as prednisone can impair the way your body uses vitamin D, so have your doctor check your vitamin D levels regularly if you're on long-term steroid therapy. Other drugs, including orlistat (taken for weight loss), and phenobarbital and phenytoin, which control epileptic seizures, interfere with vitamin D absorption.

Buying tips: Look for vitamin D supplements in the form of vitamin D_3, which is three times more effective at raising blood levels of vitamin D than supplements containing the D_2 form.

TO LOWER HOMOCYSTEINE

B-Complex Vitamins

Under the umbrella of vitamins marked with a "B" are eight different nutrients. Several have powerful heart benefits, including folate (B_9) and vitamin B_6 (pyridoxine), which researchers recently discovered can help protect people from dying from various forms of heart disease. Here's everything you need to know about how certain B vitamins keep your heart functioning at its peak capacity.

What It Does

Vitamin B_1 (thiamine) and vitamin B_2 (riboflavin) help your body produce energy and influence enzymes that affect your heart. If you're taking water pills (diuretics) for heart disease, you could be at risk for B_1 or B_2 deficiencies, because the pills make your body excrete these vitamins along with excess water. People who have heart failure may also be deficient in B_1 and B_2. In fact, two recent Canadian studies show that 25 to 33 percent of people hospitalized for heart failure had low thiamine and riboflavin levels.

Vitamin B_6 (pyridoxine) is a workhorse vitamin responsible for manufacturing hemoglobin and enabling your red blood cells to function properly.

In chapter 2, you read about homocysteine, the amino acid that's been pegged as a risk factor for heart disease, stroke, and peripheral vascular disease. Vitamin B_6 is one of the Bs that help break homocysteine down so it can't do its dirty work, which includes wrecking artery walls and making blood platelets "sticky" and more likely to clot.

it's a myth. B_{12} IS AN ALL-PURPOSE ENERGY-BOOSTER

Vitamin B_{12} has a legendary reputation as an energy-booster. True, B_{12} deficiencies do make you feel exhausted. But unless you're deficient (ask your doc to check your levels), there's absolutely no science to suggest that you'll rev up your engine by taking extra B_{12}.

Researchers have discovered that men who consume lots of vitamin B_6 and folate die less often from heart failure than men who get low levels. They also learned that men and women die less often from strokes and coronary heart disease, and that women are less likely to have heart disease, if their diets are rich in B_6 and folate.

Vitamin B_9 (folate) occurs naturally in foods; folic acid is the synthetic form found in supplements and added to food. When U.S. dietary surveys revealed that most Americans were deficient in this essential B vitamin, the government launched a folic acid fortification program in 1998 to make sure that most Americans get enough of this extremely essential vitamin.

Folate lowers your levels of homocysteine and improves the way your blood vessels function. It also helps build cells from the ground up (which is why it's considered an especially vital vitamin during pregnancy).

Researchers know that if you don't get enough folate in your diet, you're more likely to have heart problems. But the jury's still out as to whether taking folic acid supplements will actually prevent heart disease, and studies to confirm the connection are currently underway.

Vitamin B_{12} helps your body maintain healthy nerve cells and, along with folate, assists with red blood cell formation and helps lower high levels of homocysteine.

Who Might Benefit

If you take diuretics or have had heart failure, it makes sense to take a B-complex vitamin. Heavy drinkers and smokers should follow suit, since these unhealthy activities lead to B-vitamin deficiencies.

Ten to 30 percent of older people may be unable to absorb naturally occurring B_{12}, and vegetarians might not get enough B_{12} unless they eat fortified breakfast cereals or take a supplement. Health problems like celiac and Crohn's disease, weight loss, or stomach surgery can also lead to deficiencies, as can pernicious anemia. The Institute of Medicine recommends a B_{12} supplement to people older than age 50.

How To Use It

Dose: A daily B-complex vitamin or good multivitamin containing all the B vitamins will guard against most deficiencies.

Buying tips: The folic acid in B-vitamin supplements or folic acid supplements can break down and lose effectiveness when they are poorly manufactured or become old. Be sure to buy supplements from large, reputable companies, shop at stores with a high product turnover rate, and check the expiration date on the product's label.

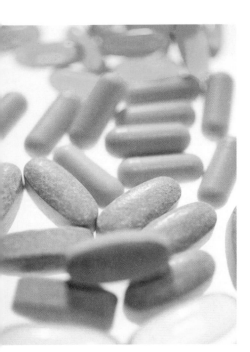

TO LOWER BAD CHOLESTEROL AND RAISE THE GOOD

Vitamin B_3 (Niacin)

Considered a giant among heart-helpers, niacin can help lower your triglycerides and "bad" LDL cholesterol. What's more, it also raises levels of healthy HDL cholesterol and helps improve your circulation. However, to achieve these results with niacin, you'll need to take a very high dose, which requires a doctor's supervision. Niacin comes in many different forms and doses; your doctor will choose a version that's right for you.

What It Does

Cardiologists at the Walter Reed Army Medical Center in Washington, D.C., recently pitted high-dose niacin against the cholesterol-lowering drug, ezetimibe. They discovered that niacin reduced the thickness of the carotid artery wall, which is a very good thing: Wider arteries mean better blood flow and less chance that stray globs of plaque will clog things up (clogged blood flow equals a heart attack). Ezetimibe had no such effect. Other niacin studies show that niacin helps prevent coronary artery disease by shielding blood vessels from inflammation.

Who Might Benefit

Niacin is sometimes prescribed for people with high LDL cholesterol or triglycerides, low HDL, or circulation problems. It may be used in conjunction with statin medicines.

How To Use It

Dose: The official daily niacin recommendation is 14 milligrams for women and 16 milligrams for men. However, studies show that doses as high as 3 grams reduce cholesterol, triglycerides, and nonfatal heart attacks. At this dosage, niacin is considered a drug and should only be taken under a doctor's supervision.

Cautions: Some 60 percent of people who take niacin experience mild to moderate flushing, which can include feeling warm, itching and tingling, and turning a lobstery red color. You can lessen your chances of this side effect by taking niacin with meals or a bedtime snack, avoiding alcohol and hot beverages near dosing time, and taking a 325-milligram aspirin 30 minutes before you take the niacin (with your doctor's okay).

Buying tips: A B-complex vitamin will contain all the niacin you normally need, unless your doctor advises you to take it at prescription strength.

TO REDUCE INFLAMMATION IN ARTERIES

Coenzyme Q10

Coenzyme Q10, called CoQ-10 for short, is a vitamin-like compound found naturally in every cell of your body. It's responsible for producing an essential energy-generating substance called ATP (adenosine triphosphate). What's more, CoQ-10 is a powerful antioxidant that helps fight damage from inflammation.

What It Does

Since heart cells demand especially high levels of energy, and since CoQ-10 fuels cellular energy, some researchers suspect that low CoQ-10 blood levels could damage your heart. If you think about how bad it is for your car's engine to run when the gas tank is nearly empty, you begin to get the picture. Researchers also suspect that CoQ-10 hinders the formation of blood clots.

Those actions aren't verified. Here's what we know for sure: People who have high cholesterol, high blood pressure, or heart failure have low CoQ-10 levels. We also know that cholesterol-lowering statin drugs deplete your natural CoQ-10 levels. That's why some cardiologists advise their patients to take CoQ-10, especially if they're also taking a statin. The supplements will boost your CoQ-10 levels and may also help ease the side effects, such as muscle and joint aches, that some people experience when they take statins.

When Italian researchers studied men in their fifties with coronary artery disease who took either 300 milligrams of CoQ-10 or a sugar pill, they discovered that the men in the CoQ-10 group had much better heart function after 1 month of treatment. Those men also lowered their blood pressure levels by 19 percent, compared with the men in the placebo group.

Who Might Benefit

If you take a statin drug to lower your cholesterol, or if you're being treated for any form of heart disease, consider taking a CoQ-10 supplement.

How To Use It

Dose: Doctors usually recommend 100 to 400 milligrams a day. Since it's fat-soluble, take CoQ-10 with a meal or snack containing fat. Finally, taking CoQ-10 at night may help your body utilize it better.

Buying tips: Soft gels may be better absorbed than other forms of CoQ-10.

TO HELP TREAT ANGINA AND HEART FAILURE

Hawthorn

In Germany, Austria, and Switzerland, hawthorn (*Crataegus monogyna*) ranks as a top herbal treatment for hearts that aren't functioning up to par. But it's not just a modern European heart medicine. In America, 19th- and early 20th-century physicians used hawthorn to ease angina, high blood pressure, hardening of the arteries, and other heart problems.

What It Does

Hawthorn leaves and flowers contain antioxidants that may help improve circulation by dilating blood vessels and protecting them from the ravages of inflammation. European researchers say that the herb can improve symptoms of heart failure—in one study, 900 milligrams of hawthorn extract taken twice a day was as effective as low doses of captopril, a drug treatment for high blood pressure and heart failure. In 2009, British researchers scrutinized every well-conducted, placebo-controlled hawthorn study. Their bottom line? Hawthorn has significant benefits for people with chronic heart failure, and has few side effects.

Who Might Benefit

Clinical herbalists recommend hawthorn as a preventive therapy to people who are at risk of developing heart disease. They also suggest that the herb can help treat symptoms of angina, mild high blood pressure, and heart failure.

How To Use It

Dose: Take 240 to 480 milligrams daily of a hawthorn supplement that is standardized to contain 18.75 percent oligomeric procyanidins (OPCs). Avoid products that don't list this percentage on the label.

Note: Hawthorn only works if you take it regularly for at least 6 weeks.

Cautions: Hawthorn may interact with certain heart medications, including digoxin, beta-blockers, and calcium channel blockers. Discuss hawthorn with your doctor if you're taking these or other heart drugs.

Buying tips: The German extract used in many hawthorn studies is sold in the United States as HeartCare by Nature's Way.

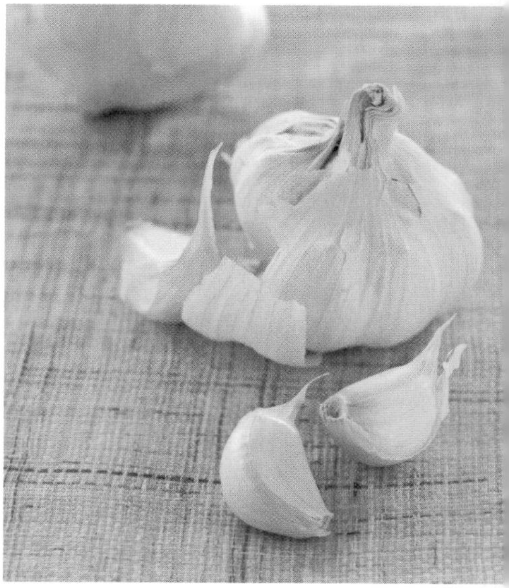

TO PREVENT ARTERY BLOCKAGES

Garlic

Here's something you probably didn't know: Garlic was the world's first performance-enhancing drug. Ancient Greek physicians dosed Olympian athletes with garlic to boost their strength and endurance. Egyptians fed it to pyramid-building slaves to increase their work capacity, and the Romans gave it to their hard-fighting soldiers and sailors. Fascinating historical note: Dioscorides, the first century's great Greek physician, wrote that garlic "cleans the arteries" hundreds of years before scientists unraveled the mysteries of blood circulation.

What It Does

Today, we know that garlic's ability to fight heart disease is largely powered by allicin, a sulfur compound that reduces "bad" LDL cholesterol and raises healthy HDL cholesterol. Garlic contains compounds that thin the blood, which helps stave off heart-busting clots. In studies, garlic has lowered homocysteine and C-reactive protein, two markers of heart disease, and has also lowered high blood pressure.

In one recent year-long study, aged garlic extract reduced arterial plaque by 7.5 percent in a small group of people at high risk for heart disease; plaque deposits increased by 22 percent in the placebo group.

And in another year-long placebo-controlled study of 65 people in their sixties, a garlic supplement slowed the advance of plaque deposits and lowered the volunteers' total cholesterol, LDL cholesterol, and homocysteine levels, while raising their levels of "good" HDL cholesterol and other heart-healthy markers.

Who Might Benefit

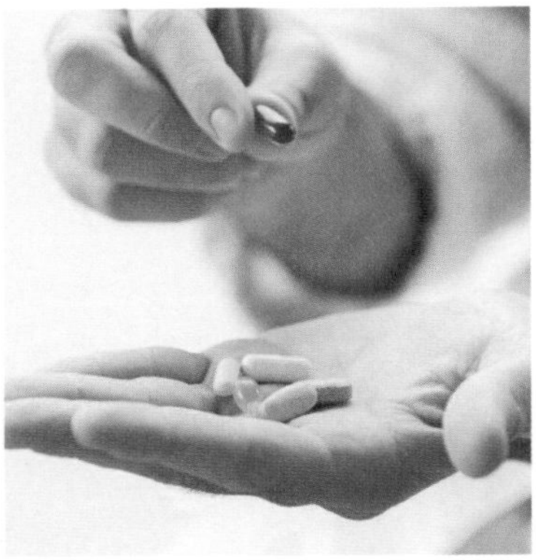

People who have high cholesterol, high blood pressure, or other heart disease markers could benefit by taking a daily garlic supplement.

How To Use It

Dose: Doses used in studies range from 250 milligrams to 1,200 milligrams. Clinical herbalists recommend taking up to three 500 to 600 milligrams capsules a day.

Cautions: Since garlic is a blood thinner, it can increase the risk of bleeding. Stop taking garlic before having surgery or dental procedures, and avoid it if you have bleeding disorders or take other blood-thinning drugs.

Buying tips: Choose garlic supplements containing at least 5,000 micrograms of allicin, or choose aged garlic supplements. Aged garlic is high in sulfur compounds that are easily absorbed.

TO LOWER CHOLESTEROL

Red Yeast Rice

The Chinese have used red yeast rice for centuries as a food (it's used to make rice wine and Peking duck) and as a medicine. It's created when a yeast called *Monascus purpureus* is fermented on a special red rice. Chinese physicians use red yeast rice to lower cholesterol and promote circulation.

What It Does

Red yeast rice contains substances that are chemically similar to prescription statin drugs. In a recent study conducted at the University of Pennsylvania School of Medicine, cardiologists tested red yeast rice against the cholesterol-lowering drug pravastatin. They gave 43 people with high cholesterol either 4,800 milligrams of red yeast rice or 40 milligrams of pravastatin. Cholesterol levels of people in the red yeast rice group dropped by 30 percent, and by 27 percent in the pravastatin group. What's more, neither group of volunteers experienced muscle pain, a known statin side effect; all volunteers had previously had muscle pain when they'd taken other statin drugs.

Two other studies further confirm red yeast rice's ability to lower "bad" LDL cholesterol and raise "good" HDL levels. Finally, another study showed that red yeast rice significantly lowered total cholesterol, LDL cholesterol, and triglycerides, although it didn't change levels of good HDL cholesterol.

Who Might Benefit

A 2010 study concluded that red yeast rice is an acceptable statin alternative for the 10 to 15 percent of people who experience muscle pain when they take these drugs.

How To Use It

Dose: In studies, red yeast rice doses ranged from 1,800 to 4,800 milligrams.

Cautions: Be sure to tell your doctor that you're taking red yeast rice. Many doctors are critical of this supplement because of their concern over its manufacturing quality. This supplement is often imported from the Far East, where manufacturing oversight is minimal.

Buying tips: The cardiologist who conducted some of the red yeast rice studies recommends the supplement Cholestene. He suggests taking one capsule twice a day.

TO FIGHT INFLAMMATION

Turmeric

The spice that colors curries, ballpark mustard, and even bread-and-butter pickles vividly yellow has been generating intense research interest in labs all over the world. That's because recent turmeric studies have shown considerable promise for its ability to keep hearts healthy and potentially fight cancer and its anti-inflammation power, which may keep diseases like arthritis, diabetes, asthma, and skin problems at bay.

What It Does

Turmeric's active compound, curcumin, is a superhero antioxidant that plays a role in turning off the switch that triggers inflammation, says one of the world's leading turmeric researcher, Bharat B.

Aggarwal, professor of cancer research at the University of Texas M.D. Anderson Cancer Center. That's good news for your heart, because preventing inflammation keeps heart cells healthy and shields your heart and blood vessels from damage. What's more, says Aggarwal, curcumin may also slow the progress of atherosclerosis.

In a recent study, researchers from India pitted the cholesterol-lowering drug atorvastatin, better known as Lipitor, against a curcumin supplement. Their goal was to figure out how well the treatments reduced inflammation and improved blood vessel function in people with type 2 diabetes. So they gave 72 people with type 2 diabetes curcumin, atorvastatin, or a placebo for 8 weeks. At the end of the study, researchers concluded that curcumin and atorvastatin were equally effective treatments.

Who Might Benefit

Curcumin is proven to reduce heart disease markers in people with type 2 diabetes and reduce inflammation that contributes to heart disease.

How To Use It

You can simply add ground turmeric directly to foods (yes, it's the same yellow powder you find in the spice aisle of your supermarket). To get its benefits, though, you need to consume about a teaspoon a day, and take it regularly over time. It blends nicely with egg, rice, and bean dishes and is a good addition to curries and stir-fries. It

Pills with Promise

Although the jury's not in as to whether taking the following supplements will improve your heart's health, some doctors who practice integrative medicine often recommend them.

Carnitine Your body naturally produces this chemical, which helps turn fat into energy. Several clinical trials suggest that supplements help reduce angina symptoms and help people with angina exercise without chest pain. Your doctor may recommend it if you're being treated for angina. What's more, some studies point to carnitine's ability to reduce heart failure symptoms and to reduce symptoms of peripheral vascular disease.

Alpha-lipoic acid (ALA) An antioxidant found in every cell, ALA helps turn glucose into energy. It has an interesting action: It actually reactivates other antioxidants as they're depleted by killer free radicals. It may provide your heart with an extra layer of protection against inflammation and cell damage.

Arginine Because your body normally makes enough of it, arginine is considered a semi-essential amino acid. But some people need to take an arginine supplement because burns, infections, dialysis, and other problems can cause deficiencies. Arginine changes into nitric oxide, which makes blood vessels relax. It may be helpful for treating problems that improve with vasodilation (widening that occurs when blood vessel walls relax), including chest pain, coronary artery disease, and heart failure.

has a warm, exotic (but not spicy hot), slightly citrusy flavor. Or, you can simply take a supplement.

Dose: Clinical herbalists recommend taking 350 milligrams of a turmeric extract that is standardized to contain 95 percent curcumin twice a day.

Cautions: Don't take curcumin supplements if you have gallstones; high doses of turmeric or curcumin may inhibit fertility in women.

Buying tips: Of the 14 curcumin products tested and listed on consumerlab.com, an independent laboratory that tests dietary supplements and health products, 5 products were rated as "unapproved." Two products contained high levels of lead, two didn't contain as much active ingredient as claimed, and one failed to identify the ingredients properly. Buy from major, reputable supplement-makers, and check online to see which brands are considered the most reliable.

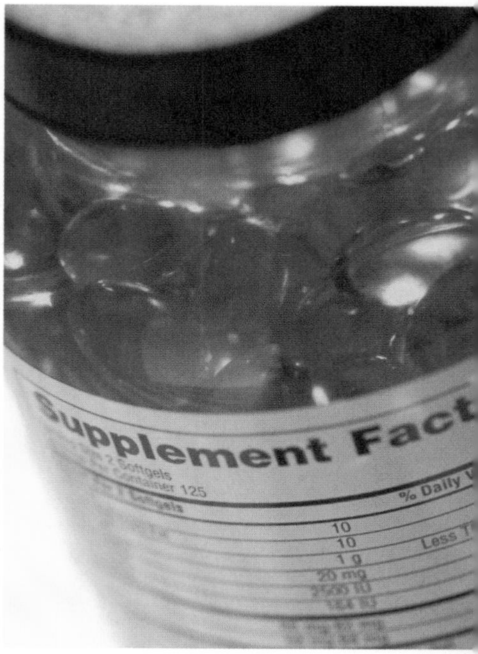

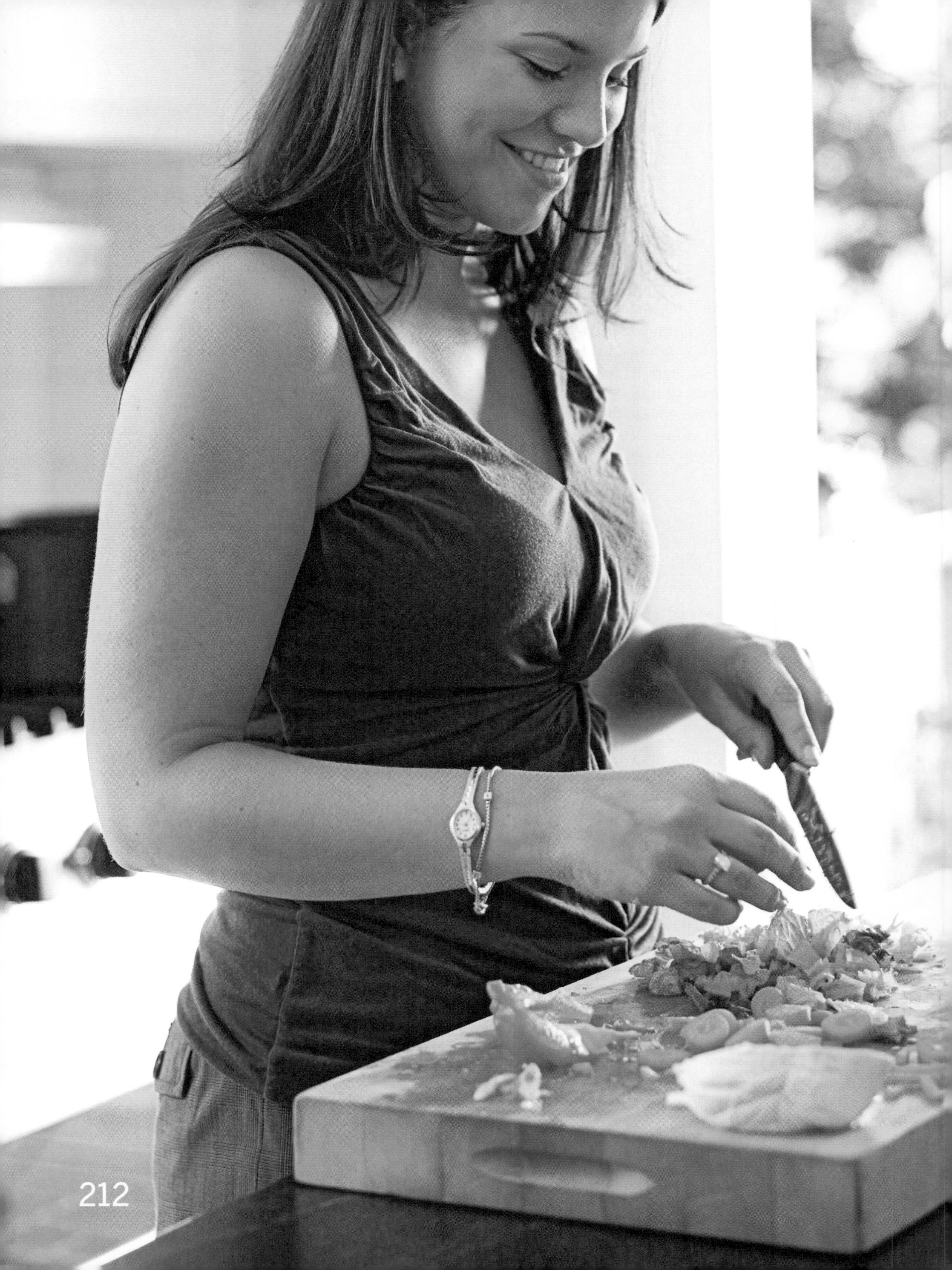

PART FOUR

Healthy Heart Recipes

These 102 recipes are simple to cook and a pleasure to eat. You'll love the freshness, the flavors, the creativity. Try one today!

Breakfast **214**

Appetizers and Snacks **224**

Salads
Main Dish **236**, Side Dish **242**

Soups **252**

Entrées
Poultry **262**, Lamb **269**,
Pork **272**, Beef **274**,
Seafood **278**,
Pasta **289**, Vegetarian **295**

Vegetables and Grains **300**

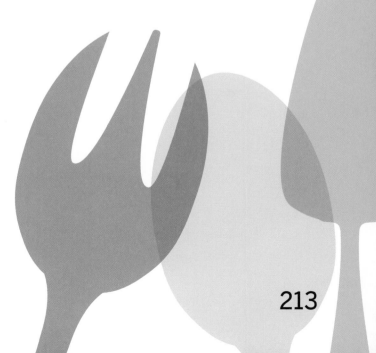

Desserts **328**

Walnut-Topped Blueberry-Bran Muffins

Makes 18–20

PREP TIME: **18 minutes**
COOK TIME: **20 minutes**

250 mL	1 cup shredded bran cereal (All-Bran)
250 mL	1 cup plain low-fat yogurt
250 mL	1 cup whole-wheat pastry flour
10 mL	2 teaspoons baking powder
5 mL	1 teaspoon baking soda
5 mL	1 teaspoon ground cinnamon
250 mL	1 cup fresh blueberries
1	1 large egg
125 mL	1/2 cup dark molasses
50 mL	1/4 cup light olive oil or vegetable oil
5 mL	1 teaspoon vanilla extract
125 mL	1/2 cup finely chopped walnuts

Moist and flavorful, plus sweet and nutty—muffins don't get much better than this! This muffin is so wonderful-tasting that you'll want to make extra to store in the freezer so you can pop one in the toaster oven to enjoy even on a busy morning. Plus they're high in fiber and antioxidants as well.

1. Preheat the oven to 400°F (200°C). Coat a muffin pan with nonstick cooking spray or use paper cupcake liners.
2. Stir the cereal and yogurt together in a small bowl and set aside.
3. Stir the flour, baking powder, baking soda, and cinnamon in a large bowl until blended. Add the blueberries and gently toss to coat.
4. Whisk the egg, molasses, oil, and vanilla in small bowl until blended. Fold into the dry ingredients along with the yogurt mixture until evenly moistened. Spoon into the prepared pan, filling each cup about three-quarters full. Sprinkle the tops with the walnuts.
5. Bake until a toothpick inserted in the center of a muffin comes out clean, about 20 minutes. Cool slightly before turning out onto a wire cooling rack.

Per muffin: 116 calories, 6 g total fat, 1 g saturated fat, 16 g carbohydrate, 3 g protein, 2 g fiber, 11 mg cholesterol, 127 mg sodium, 96 mg calcium

Blueberry-Orange Yogurt Smoothies

Serves 2

PREP TIME: **5 minutes**

This naturally sweet and creamy smoothie will get you off to a good start in the morning. Blueberries and fresh orange juice are high in vitamin C, antioxidants, and fiber.

3 or 4	3 or 4 ice cubes, optional
250 mL	1 cup plain low-fat yogurt
250 mL	1 cup fresh orange juice
250 mL	1 cup fresh or frozen blueberries (if frozen, omit ice cubes)
2 mL	1/2 teaspoon vanilla extract

1. In a blender, puree the ice (if using), yogurt, orange juice, blueberries, and vanilla until smooth. Pour into two tall glasses.

Per serving (12 ounces/375 mL): 180 calories, 2 g total fat, 1 g saturated fat, 33 g carbohydrate, 6 g protein, 2 g fiber, 10 mg cholesterol, 86 mg sodium, 205 mg calcium

Strawberry, Pineapple, and Almond Smoothies

Serves 2

PREP TIME: **10 minutes**

Sure, the strawberries and pineapple juice make this smoothie fruity and sweet, but the real surprise is in the almonds. They add fiber and healthy fats, making a good smoothie great.
Note: If the strawberries are naturally sweet, you may not need the maple syrup.

3 or 4	3 or 4 ice cubes, optional
250 mL	1 cup hulled and sliced fresh or frozen strawberries (if frozen, omit ice cubes)
250 mL	1 cup low-fat (1%) milk
175 mL	3/4 cup unsweetened pineapple juice
20	20 whole almonds (skin on)
15 mL	1 tablespoon maple or agave syrup, optional
2 mL	1/2 teaspoon ground cinnamon

1. In a blender, puree the ice (if using), strawberries, milk, pineapple juice, almonds, syrup (if using), and cinnamon until smooth. Pour into two tall glasses.

Per serving (12 ounces/375 mL): 216 calories, 7 g total fat, 1 g saturated fat, 32 g carbohydrate, 7 g protein, 3 g fiber, 6 mg cholesterol, 57 mg sodium, 214 mg calcium

Whole-Grain French Toast with Sautéed Apples

Serves 4

PREP TIME: **30 minutes**
COOK TIME: **8 minutes**

Nutty French toast served with apples simmered in maple syrup is decadent, but this version is superhealthy, thanks to its good fats and high thiamin, zinc, and fiber counts.

250 mL	1 cup low-fat (1%) milk
50 mL	1/4 cup maple syrup, divided
2	2 large eggs
5 mL	1 teaspoon vanilla extract
6 mL	1 teaspoon plus 1/4 teaspoon ground cinnamon
4	4 slices (1/2-inch/1-cm thick) crusty multigrain bread
500 mL	2 cups cored, peeled, and thinly sliced Golden Delicious or Granny Smith apples
45 mL	3 tablespoons water
50 mL	1/4 cup chopped pecans

1. Whisk the milk, 2 tablespoons (25 mL) of the syrup, the eggs, vanilla, and 1 teaspoon (5 mL) of the cinnamon in medium bowl. Arrange the bread in a baking dish and pour the egg mixture over top. Let it stand, turning at least twice, until the egg mixture is absorbed, about 15 minutes.
2. Combine the apples, water, the remaining 2 tablespoons (25 mL) of syrup, and the remaining 1/4 teaspoon (1 mL) of cinnamon in a large saucepan. Cover and cook over low heat, stirring occasionally, until the apples are softened, about 15 minutes.
3. Heat a nonstick griddle over medium heat. Reduce the heat to medium-low, add the bread, and cook until browned, 3 to 4 minutes. Turn with a wide spatula and cook until browned on the other side, 3 to 4 minutes longer. Spoon the apples onto the French toast and sprinkle with the nuts.

Per serving: 262 calories, 9 g total fat, 2 g saturated fat, 37 g carbohydrate, 9 g protein, 4 g fiber, 93 mg cholesterol, 173 mg sodium, 143 mg calcium

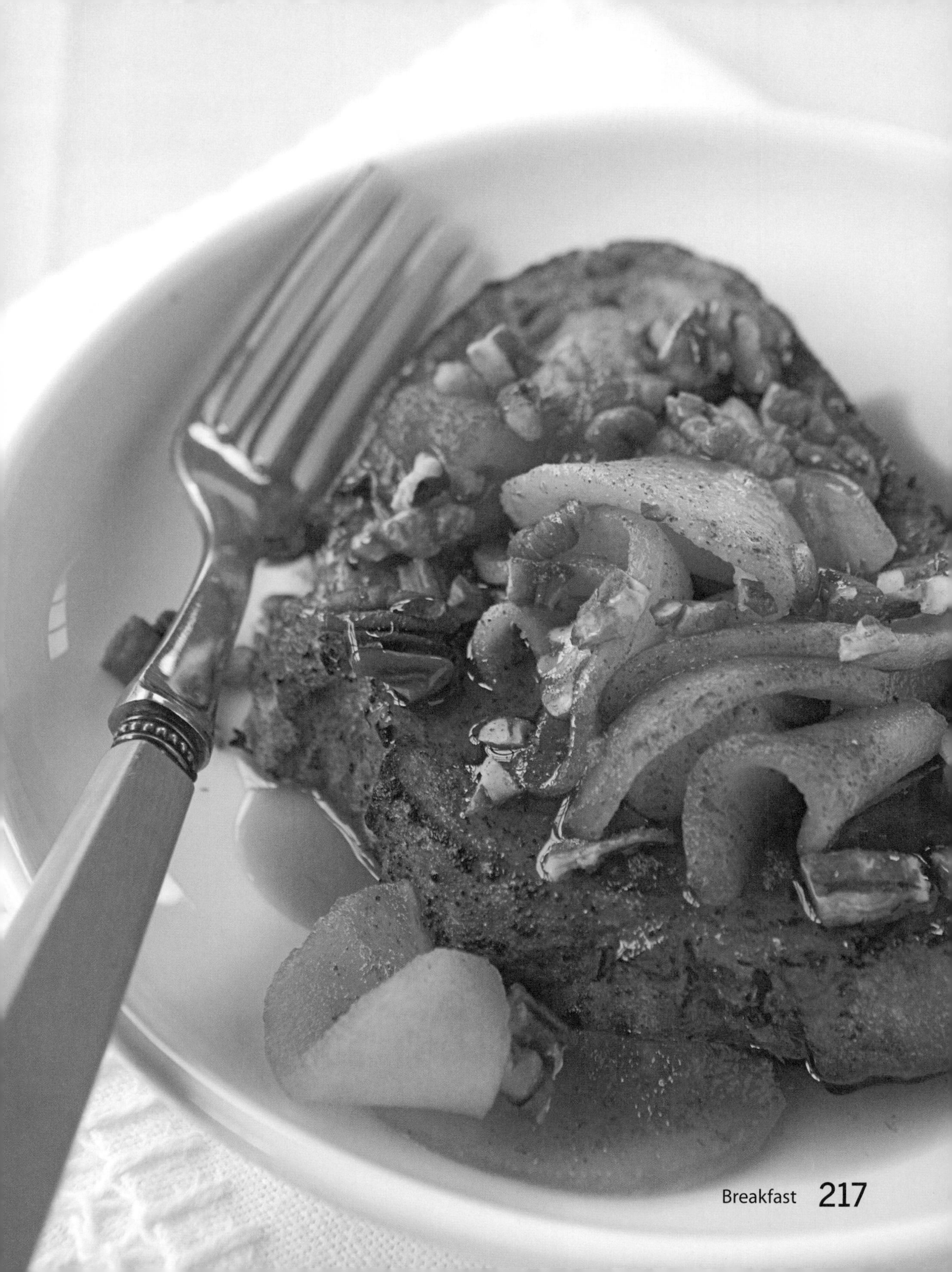

Cooked Oatmeal-and-Bulgur Cereal with Apples and Dates

Serves 4

PREP TIME: **10 minutes**
COOK TIME: **10 minutes**

Cooked cereal is a special treat no matter what the season. This healthy combination of bulgur and oatmeal is dressed up with the naturally sweet flavors of apples and dates, which are rich in potassium and fiber.

375 mL	1 1/2 cups low-fat (1%) milk
375 mL	1 1/2 cups water
250 mL	1 cup unpeeled apple pieces (1/4 inch/0.5 cm)
125 mL	1/2 cup old-fashioned oatmeal
125 mL	1/2 cup coarse bulgur
3	3 dates, pitted and snipped
2 mL	1/2 teaspoon ground cinnamon

1. Stir together the milk, water, apples, oatmeal, bulgur, dates, and cinnamon in a medium saucepan and heat, stirring frequently, until boiling. Cover, reduce the heat to low, and cook, stirring occasionally, until the grains are tender, about 10 minutes.

Per serving: 185 calories, 2 g total fat, 1 g saturated fat, 37 g carbohydrate, 7 g protein, 6 g fiber, 5 mg cholesterol, 44 mg sodium, 135 mg calcium

Strawberry, Oatmeal, and Whole-Wheat Pancakes with Strawberry Maple Syrup

Serves 6

(each pancake about 6 inches/15 cm)

PREP TIME: **15 minutes**

COOK TIME: **30 minutes**

Hearty, filling, and naturally sweet, these pancakes are winners on all fronts. They are sweetened with maple syrup and fresh berries and filled with nutrients and fiber from oatmeal and whole-wheat flour.

300 mL	1 1/4 cups maple syrup, divided
375 mL	1 1/2 cups strawberries, rinsed, hulled, and thinly sliced, divided
250 mL	1 cup whole-wheat pastry flour
125 mL	1/2 cup old-fashioned or quick-cooking (not instant) oatmeal
10 mL	2 teaspoons baking powder
5 mL	1 teaspoon ground cinnamon
175 mL	3/4 cup low-fat (1%) milk
1	1 large egg
5 mL	1 teaspoon vanilla extract

1. Heat 1 cup (250 mL) of the syrup and 1/2 cup (125 mL) of the strawberries in a small saucepan over medium-low heat, stirring, until the mixture boils. Let cool, then puree in a blender or food processor. Return to the saucepan and keep warm.
2. Stir the flour, oatmeal, baking powder, and cinnamon together in a large bowl. In a small bowl, whisk together the milk, the remaining 1/4 cup (50 mL) of maple syrup, the egg, and vanilla. Pour into the dry ingredients and fold to blend. Let stand for 10 minutes.
3. Heat a large nonstick griddle or skillet over medium heat until hot enough that a drop of water sizzles. Reduce the heat to medium-low, then pour the batter onto the griddle, using 1/2 cup (125 mL) for each pancake. Cook until the tops are covered with small bubbles, about 3 minutes. Place 4 or 5 of the remaining berry slices on top of each pancake and cook 1 minute longer. Flip the pancakes and cook until lightly browned on the other side, 3 to 4 minutes more. Repeat with the remaining batter. Top with the syrup.

Per serving: 274 calories, 1 g total fat, 0 g saturated fat, 62 g carbohydrate, 4 g protein, 3 g fiber, 32 mg cholesterol, 215 mg sodium, 141 mg calcium

Individual Breakfast Tortilla

Makes 1

PREP TIME: **12 minutes**
COOK TIME: **4 minutes**

1	1 large egg
0.5 mL	1/8 teaspoon chili powder
1	1 corn or whole-grain tortilla (6-inch/15-cm)
15 mL	1 tablespoon shredded Monterey Jack, provolone, or cheddar cheese
30 mL	2 tablespoons cooked or canned black beans, drained and mashed with a fork
1	1 thin slice tomato, halved
5 mL	1 teaspoon chopped fresh cilantro
1	1 thin slice avocado
7 mL	1 1/2 teaspoons fat-free sour cream

Satisfy your morning hunger by biting into an explosion of flavors and textures wrapped up in a soft, warm tortilla. This is one cheesy and hearty breakfast that's bursting with nutrition.
Note: It's better to prepare all ingredients before scrambling the egg and heating the tortilla.

1. Whisk together the egg and chili powder in a small bowl until well-blended.
2. Heat a small, heavy skillet over medium heat until hot enough that a drop of water sizzles. Coat with nonstick cooking spray and pour in the egg. Cook, stirring with a rubber spatula, until set, 5 to 15 seconds. Transfer to a plate and keep warm. Wipe out the skillet and respray.
3. Increase the heat to medium-high. Heat the tortilla in the skillet, turning, until heated, about 1 minute. Turn, sprinkle with the cheese and heat until it melts, about 10 seconds. Transfer to a serving plate.
4. Spread the beans on half of the tortilla. Add the egg, tomato, cilantro, avocado, and sour cream. Fold the tortilla to make a "sandwich."

Per tortilla: 238 calories, 10 g total fat, 3 g saturated fat, 25 g carbohydrate, 12 g protein, 5 g fiber, 188 mg cholesterol, 229 mg sodium, 110 mg calcium

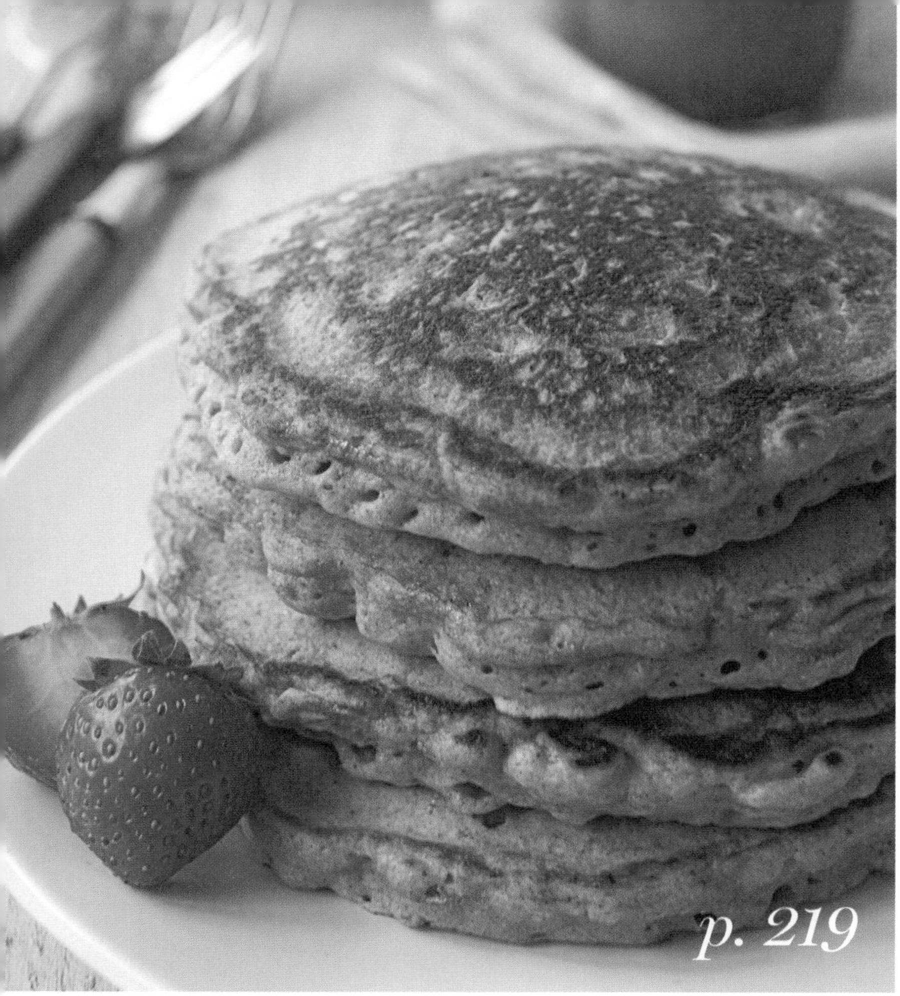
p. 219

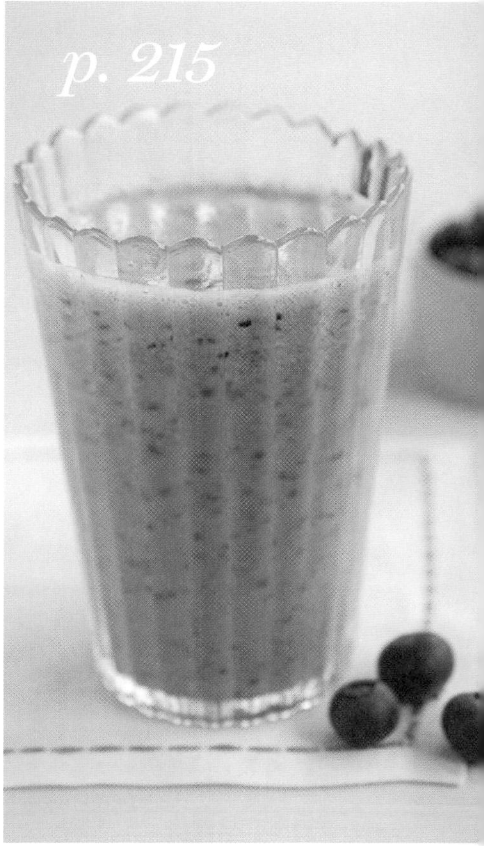
p. 215

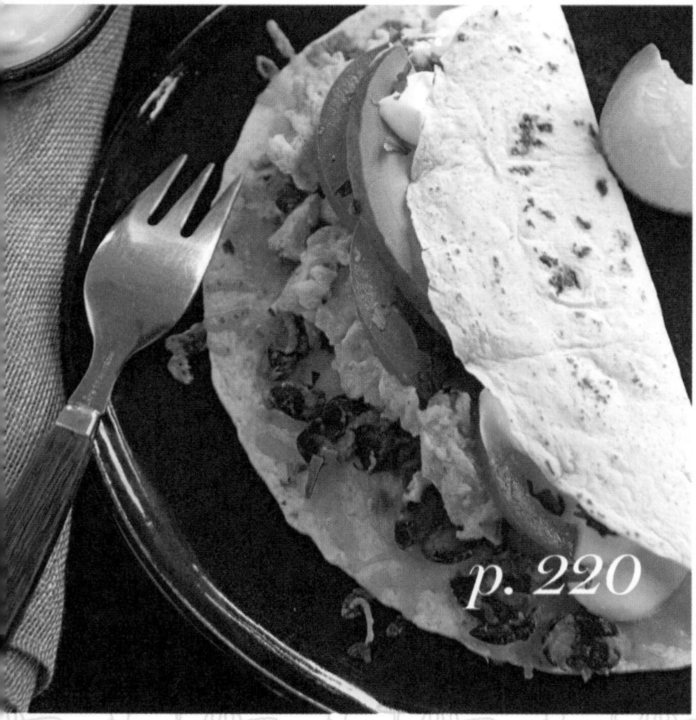
p. 220

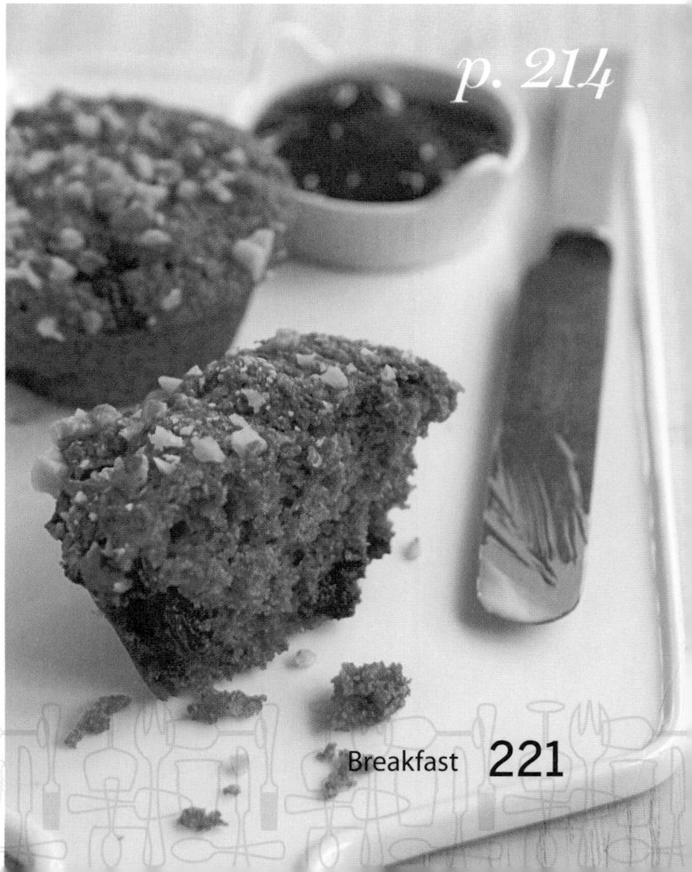
p. 214

One-Egg Omelets with Chopped Broccoli, Tomatoes, and Cheddar

Makes 4

PREP TIME: **10 minutes**
COOK TIME: **12 minutes**

These are quick-and-easy omelets filled with a delicious mélange of broccoli, tomato, and garlic and made using a "pancake" technique. The egg provides excellent protein and a wide range of vitamins and minerals for its caloric content. So enjoy—guilt-free!

375 mL	1 1/2 cups chopped broccoli florets
30 mL	2 tablespoons water
50 mL	1/4 cup chopped tomato
15 mL	1 tablespoon chopped fresh basil or cilantro
5 mL	1 teaspoon virgin olive oil
1	1 clove garlic, crushed or grated
1 mL	1/4 teaspoon coarse salt
0.5 mL	1/8 teaspoon freshly ground black pepper
4	4 large eggs
4	4 shavings cheddar cheese (about 1 ounce/30 g)

1. Cook the broccoli together with the water in a small covered saucepan over medium-low heat until the broccoli is fork-tender, about 4 minutes. Drain off the excess moisture, then add the tomatoes, basil or cilantro, oil, garlic, salt, and pepper. Stir to blend. Keep warm over low heat.
2. Heat a small, heavy nonstick skillet over medium heat until hot enough that a drop of water sizzles. Coat with nonstick cooking spray. Beat 1 of the eggs until frothy and add to the pan, tilting the pan to let the egg run to the edges. Cook, undisturbed, until the egg is set along the edges and the center is moist but not runny, about 2 minutes.
3. Slide the egg "pancake" onto a plate. Place 1/4 cup (50 mL) of the broccoli mixture on half of the egg and top with a sliver of the cheese. Fold the egg over to make an omelet. Repeat with the remaining eggs.

Per serving: 129 calories, 7 g total fat, 3 g saturated fat, 4 g carbohydrate, 9 g protein, 1 g fiber, 188 mg cholesterol, 269 mg sodium, 91 mg calcium

Smoked Salmon and Asparagus Frittata

Serves 4

PREP TIME: **15 minutes**
COOK TIME: **10 minutes**

Perfect to share for brunch or a special breakfast treat, the frittata is easy on the cook and lends itself to endless variations. Low in fat and high in fiber, asparagus is a good source of folate, other B vitamins, iron, and vitamin C, while a bit of goat cheese adds just the right zing.

15 mL	1 tablespoon extra-virgin olive oil
375 mL	1 1/2 cups trimmed asparagus pieces (1/2-inch/1-cm diagonals)
50 mL	1/4 cup water, divided
50 mL	1/4 cup thinly sliced scallions
0.5 mL	1/8 teaspoon freshly ground black pepper
4	4 large eggs
15 mL	1 tablespoon chopped fresh dill
4	4 slices (about 2 1/4 ounces/67 g) smoked salmon, cut into 1/4-inch/0.5-cm strips
60 g	2 ounces crumbled fresh goat cheese (about 1/4 cup/50 mL)

1. Heat an ovenproof 9-inch (22-cm) skillet over medium heat. Add the oil and asparagus and toss to coat. Add 1 tablespoon (15 mL) of the water and cook, covered, until the asparagus is crisp-tender, about 3 minutes. Stir in the scallions and pepper.
2. Move the oven rack so that the top of the skillet will be about 2 inches from the broiler. Preheat the broiler.
3. Whisk the eggs, the remaining 3 tablespoons (15 mL) of water, and the dill until frothy. Pour the eggs over the asparagus mixture and cook over medium heat until the edges begin to set, about 2 minutes. Top the eggs with strips of salmon, and dot with the cheese. Lift the edges of the frittata to allow any remaining liquid egg to run underneath. Cook until the bottom is lightly browned, about 5 minutes.
4. Slide the skillet under the broiler and broil until the frittata is set, about 2 minutes. Slice into four wedges.

Per wedge: 184 calories, 11 g total fat, 4 g saturated fat, 5 g carbohydrate, 15 g protein, 2 g fiber, 190 mg cholesterol, 254 mg sodium, 70 mg calcium

Deviled Eggs with Black Olives

Serves 4

PREP TIME: **20 minutes**
COOK TIME: **15 minutes**

4	4 large eggs
50 mL	1/4 cup extra-virgin olive oil, divided
25 mL	2 tablespoons minced pitted Kalamata olives, divided
15 mL	1 tablespoon minced flat-leaf parsley
2 mL	1/2 teaspoon Dijon-style mustard
	Ground paprika (optional)

Made creamy with poly- and monounsaturated heart-healthy olive oil instead of mayonnaise, these unique deviled eggs are deliciously addictive. Not to worry, though...research has affirmed that eggs are an incredibly nutritious food and should be, albeit in moderation, a part of a heart-healthy diet.

1. Place the eggs in small saucepan in a single layer and cover with water. Heat over medium-high heat, just until the water begins to boil. Immediately remove from the heat, cover, and let stand for 13 minutes. Drain the water and fill the pan with cold water. Crack the eggs against the side of the pan and gently remove the shells underwater.
2. Halve the eggs and place the whites, cut side up, on a plate.
3. In a small bowl, mash the yolks together with 2 tablespoons (25 mL) of the oil until blended. Gradually beat in the remaining 2 tablespoons (25 mL) of oil until smooth and fluffy. Stir in 1 tablespoon (15 mL) of the olives, the parsley, and mustard until blended.
4. Stuff the egg whites using a teaspoon, dividing the filling evenly. Top each with a pinch of the remaining 1 tablespoon (15 mL) of olives. Sprinkle lightly with paprika (if using).

Per serving: 85 calories, 5 g total fat, 1 g saturated fat, 2 g carbohydrate, 6 g protein, 0 g fiber, 180 mg cholesterol, 140 mg sodium, 29 mg calcium

Avocado, Tomato, and Cucumber Dip with Steamed Shrimp

Serves 8

PREP TIME: **8 minutes**

1	1 large ripe Hass avocado (about 8 ounces/250 g), peeled, halved, and pitted
15 mL	1 tablespoon fresh lime juice
15 mL	1 tablespoon chopped fresh cilantro
5 mL	1 teaspoon seeded, deveined, and minced jalapeño (wear gloves when handling), or to taste
2 mL	1/2 teaspoon coarse salt
125 mL	1/2 cup chopped, seeded plum tomato
125 mL	1/2 cup seeded, chopped Kirby cucumber or seedless cucumber
50 mL	1/4 cup chopped red onion
16	16 large frozen pre-cooked shrimp, thawed, rinsed, and patted dry

Think guilt-free guacamole when you try this recipe. Made with good-fat-rich avocado bulked up with chopped tomatoes and crisp Kirby cucumbers (more crunch and less water than regular cukes)—adding vitamins, minerals, and fiber—you can give yourself permission to take another dip. This is also great with celery, red pepper strips, or pita chips.

1. In a small bowl, roughly mash the avocado with a fork or pastry blender. Stir in the lime juice, cilantro, jalapeños, and salt until blended. Fold in the tomatoes, cucumbers, and onions. Serve with the shrimp, Pita Chips (page 234), or raw vegetables.

Per serving (2 teaspoons/10 mL dip per shrimp): 87 calories, 5 g total fat, 1 g saturated fat, 5 g carbohydrate, 7 g protein, 3 g fiber, 43 mg cholesterol, 191 mg sodium, 22 mg calcium

Crisped Potato Skins with Veggie Salsa

Serves 6–8

PREP TIME: **12 minutes**
COOK TIME: **1 hour 10 minutes**

Crunchy and crisp are two textures for which we yearn, especially when it comes to snacks. Potato skins are high in vitamin C and are an excellent source of fiber. Paired with flavor-rich and nutrient-packed vegetable salsa with just a small amount of shredded cheese melted on top, this snack is a win-win on all fronts.

2	2 large (about 15 ounces/450 g each) russet potatoes, washed and skins pierced with a knife
250 mL	1 cup cored, chopped tomato
125 mL	1/2 cup corn kernels
50 mL	1/4 cup chopped green bell pepper
50 mL	1/4 cup chopped red onion
25 mL	2 tablespoons minced fresh cilantro or basil
15 mL	1 tablespoon seeded, deveined, and chopped jalapeño (wear gloves when handling), or to taste
10 mL	2 teaspoons fresh lime juice
50 mL	1/4 cup shredded part-skim mozzarella

1. Preheat the oven to 400°F (200°C). Place the potatoes directly on the oven rack and bake until tender, about 55 minutes. Let cool.
2. Stir together the tomatoes, corn, bell peppers, onions, cilantro or basil, jalapeños, and lime juice in a small bowl until blended.
3. Halve the potatoes lengthwise and scoop out the cooked potato flesh, leaving about 1/4 inch (0.5 cm) potato and skin intact. Reserve the potato flesh for another use. Cut the potato shells into 3 lengthwise strips. Lightly coat both sides of the strips with nonstick cooking spray. Place the potatoes skins, cut side down, on a baking sheet.
4. Position an oven rack so that the potatoes are 3 to 4 inches (7 to 10 cm) from the broiler. Preheat the broiler. Broil the potatoes until crisp, 2 to 3 minutes. Turn them cut side up and broil until browned and crisp, about 2 minutes longer. Remove the baking sheet from the oven and spoon the salsa evenly into the potato skins. Sprinkle with the cheese, dividing evenly. Broil until the cheese is melted, about 1 minute.

Per serving: 140 calories, 1 g total fat, 1 g saturated fat, 29 g carbohydrate, 5 g protein, 3 g fiber, 3 mg cholesterol, 35 mg sodium, 58 mg calcium

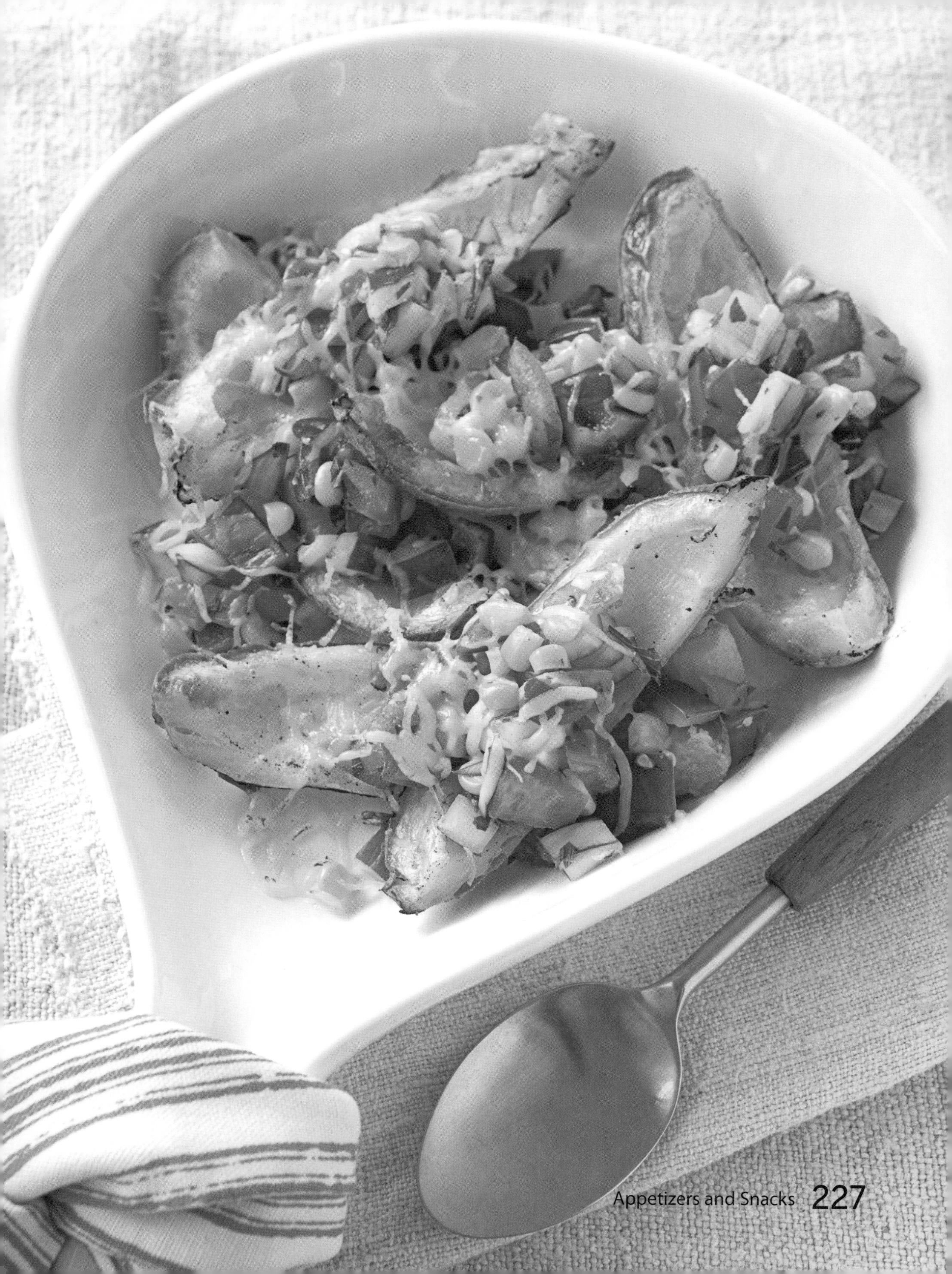

Cranberry-Peanut Cereal Bars

Makes 25 squares

PREP TIME: **10 minutes**
COOK TIME: **15 minutes**

Irresistible little morsels of crunch and sweetness, these snacks have lots going for them. Peanuts are an excellent source of protein, iron, and fiber, while flaxseed has a wide range of health benefits including being rich in alpha-linolenic acid, an essential fatty acid that contributes to heart health. Beyond that, they are a fun and convenient snack on-the-run or anytime.

750 mL	3 cups puffed whole-grain cereal, like Kashi
125 mL	1/2 cup chopped dry-roasted unsalted peanuts
50 mL	1/4 cup chopped unsweetened dried cranberries
25 mL	2 tablespoons ground flaxseed
75 mL	1/3 cup creamy peanut butter
125 mL	1/2 cup agave syrup

1. Preheat the oven to 350°F (180°C). Coat an 8-inch (20-cm) square metal baking pan with nonstick cooking spray.
2. Stir together the cereal, peanuts, cranberries, and flaxseed in large bowl.
3. In a small saucepan over low heat, stir together the peanut butter and syrup until the mixture boils, about 1 minute. Stir into the cereal mixture until well-blended. Scrape into the prepared pan and press down firmly with the back of spatula to compact.
4. Bake until the edges are golden, about 15 minutes. Cool thoroughly before cutting into squares.

Per square: 112 calories, 4 g total fat, 1 g saturated fat, 19 g carbohydrate, 3 g protein, 2 g fiber, 0 mg cholesterol, 78 mg sodium, 9 mg calcium

Endive with Curry-Walnut Cream Cheese

Serves 16

PREP TIME: **10 minutes**

10 mL	2 teaspoons Madras curry powder
250 mL	1 cup 1/3 less fat cream cheese
75 mL	1/3 cup walnut pieces
1 mL	1/4 teaspoon hot red-pepper sauce
4 to 5	4 to 5 heads Belgium endive
25 mL	2 tablespoons thinly sliced scallions

Madras curry powder adds a pleasant spiciness and a hint of sweetness to this creamy spread made with calcium-rich, reduced-fat cream cheese and walnuts, which are a heart-healthy source of polyunsaturated fats.

1. In a small skillet set over low heat, heat the curry until warm and fragrant, about 2 minutes.
2. Pulse the curry, cream cheese, walnuts, and red-pepper sauce in a food processor until blended.
3. Cut the stems from the endive and separate the leaves (32 total) without breaking. Rinse in cold water and pat dry. Place a 1/2-tablespoon (10-mL) dollop of the cream cheese mixture in the center of each leaf and garnish with a few slices of scallion.

Per tablespoon (15 mL): 48 calories, 4 g total fat, 1 g saturated fat, 2 g carbohydrate, 2 g protein, 1 g fiber, 8 mg cholesterol, 69 mg sodium, 28 mg calcium

Olive and Dried Fig Tapenade

Serves 16

PREP TIME: **15 minutes**

Dried Black Mission figs and black olives pureed together make an exotic sweet-and-savory spread that is luscious on celery sticks or crackers. Dried figs have more heart-healthy fiber than any other fruit, plus vitamin E, calcium, iron, and antioxidants.

250 mL	1 cup moist pack Black Mission figs, stems trimmed
50 mL	1/4 cup chopped and pitted Kalamata olives
15 mL	1 tablespoon extra-virgin olive oil
5 mL	1 teaspoon chopped fresh rosemary
1	1 small clove garlic, crushed or grated
2 mL	1/2 teaspoon grated orange zest
1 mL	1/4 teaspoon freshly ground black pepper
16	16 celery pieces (3-inch/7.5-mL) or 16 small rye crisps

1. Snip the figs into small pieces with kitchen shears. Puree them, along with the olives, oil, rosemary, garlic, orange zest, and pepper, in a food processor until well-blended.
2. Transfer to a small bowl and serve spread on the celery or crackers.

Per tablespoon (15 mL): 26 calories, 1 g total fat, 0 g saturated fat, 4 g carbohydrate, 0 g protein, 1 g fiber, 0 mg cholesterol, 66 mg sodium, 21 mg calcium

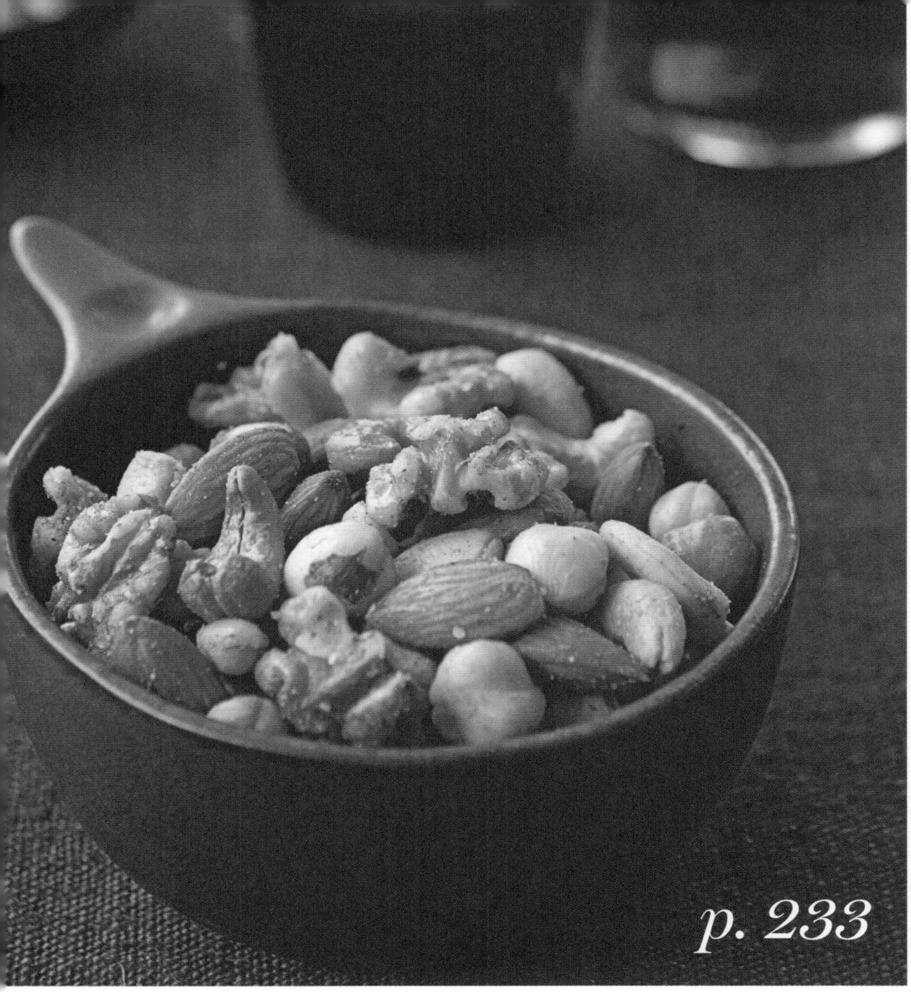
p. 233

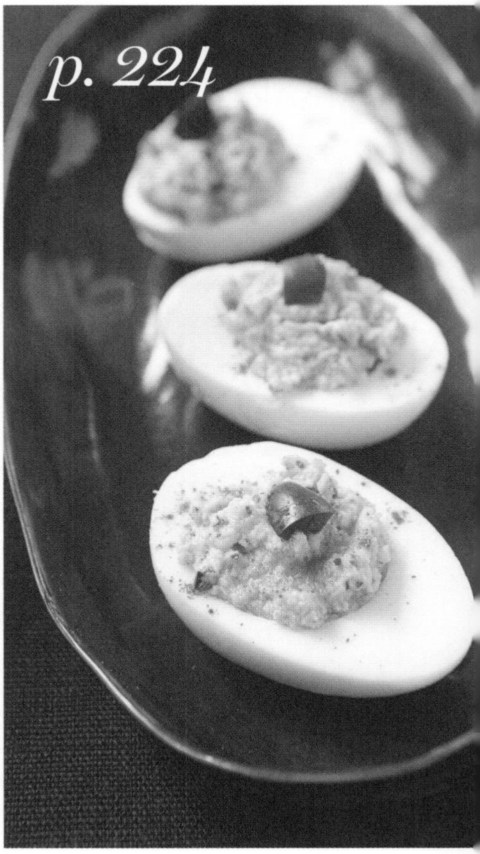
p. 224

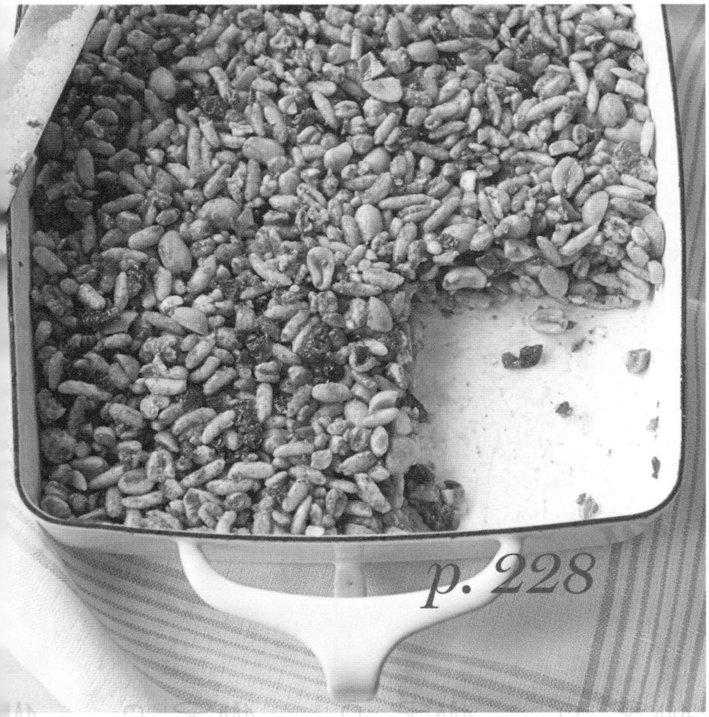
p. 228

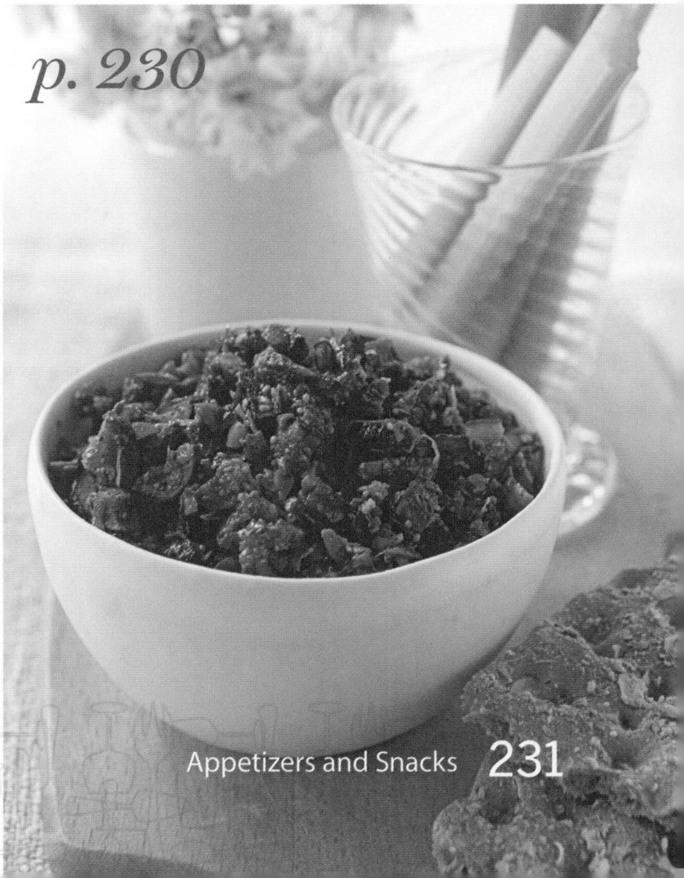
p. 230

Smoked Trout Pâté with Dill

Serves 12

PREP TIME: **10 minutes**
CHILL TIME: **30 minutes**

Trout, a freshwater fish high in the fatty acids essential to heart health, is excellent when smoked. Though smoked trout is higher in sodium, you can enjoy it worry-free in this delicious spread that stretches a small amount into 12 luscious servings.

125 g	4 ounces smoked trout, skinned and coarsely chopped (about 3/4 cup/175 mL)
250 mL	1 cup fat-free sour cream
25 mL	2 tablespoons fresh lemon juice
25 mL	2 tablespoons chopped fresh dill, divided
7 mL	1 1/2 teaspoons horseradish
1 mL	1/4 teaspoon freshly ground black pepper
24	24 no-salt-added whole-grain crackers or unpeeled seedless cucumber slices (1/4-inch/0.5-cm)

1. Pulse the trout, sour cream, lemon juice, 1 tablespoon (15 mL) of the dill, the horseradish, and pepper in a food processor just until blended.
2. Scrape into a serving bowl and sprinkle with the remaining 1 tablespoon (15 mL) of dill. Refrigerate, covered, until thoroughly chilled, about 30 minutes. Serve with the crackers or cucumbers.

Per serving (2 tablespoons/25 mL): 59 calories, 1 g total fat, 0 g saturated fat, 7 g carbohydrate, 4 g protein, 0 g fiber, 9 mg cholesterol, 31 mg sodium, 38 mg calcium

Curry-Spiced Nuts

Serves 8

PREP TIME: **5 minutes**
COOK TIME: **15 minutes**

250 g	8 ounces walnuts, whole almonds (skin on), raw unsalted cashews, and shelled and skinned hazelnuts
15 mL	1 tablespoon extra-virgin olive oil
10 mL	2 teaspoons Madras curry powder
2 mL	1/2 teaspoon coarse salt

Walnuts, almonds, cashews, and hazelnuts dusted with curry powder and oven roasted are a special treat. Nuts, which are high in good fats, supply good-quality plant protein and an array of vitamins and minerals. Put out a small bowl with drinks or sprinkle them on a salad—any way you serve them, they are always delicious.

1. Preheat the oven to 350°F (180°C).
2. Spread the nuts on a jelly-roll pan and drizzle with the oil. Toss to coat. Sprinkle with the curry powder and salt. Roast, stirring once or twice, until golden and fragrant, about 15 minutes.

Per ounce (30 g): 195 calories, 18 g total fat, 2 g saturated fat, 5 g carbohydrate, 5 g protein, 3 g fiber, 0 mg cholesterol, 146 mg sodium, 16 mg calcium

Stuffed Dried Apricots with Chopped Pistachios

Serves 6

PREP TIME: **10 minutes**
CHILL TIME: **30 minutes**

90 mL	6 tablespoons fresh goat cheese
12	12 moist-pack dried apricot halves
50 mL	1/4 cup shelled, peeled, and chopped natural pistachios

This tangy combination of sweet-and-sour dried apricots topped with creamy goat cheese and studded with bright green pistachios is as much a joy to look at as it is to devour. Dried apricots, although high in calories, are nutrient-rich, supplying iron, potassium, beta-carotene, and fiber.

1. Form a 1/2-tablespoon (7.5-mL) mound of goat cheese in the center of each apricot half. Press about 1 teaspoon (5 mL) of the pistachios into the cheese. Refrigerate, covered, at least 30 minutes before serving.

Per serving (2 apricot halves): 103 calories, 5 g total fat, 2 g saturated fat, 10 g carbohydrate, 4 g protein, 1 g fiber, 7 mg cholesterol, 54 mg sodium, 32 mg calcium

Roasted Red Pepper and Chickpea Dip with Pita Chips

Serves 12

PREP TIME: **10 minutes**
CHILL TIME: **1 hour**
COOK TIME: **15 minutes**

The versatile chickpea goes from soups to salads to stews and now to a flavorful dip by just opening a can. The chickpea is a near-perfect food: delicately flavored and rich in protein, fiber, folate, iron, and zinc.

7 mL	1 1/2 teaspoons ground cumin
1	1 can (14.5 ounces/540 mL) no-salt-added chick-peas, rinsed and drained
125 mL	1/2 cup rinsed, drained, and coarsely chopped jarred roasted red bell peppers
25 mL	2 tablespoons extra-virgin olive oil
25 mL	2 tablespoons fresh lemon juice
2 mL	1/2 teaspoon minced garlic
1 mL	1/4 teaspoon ground red pepper
2	2 whole-wheat pita breads

1. In a small skillet set over low heat, heat the cumin until it becomes fragrant, about 2 minutes.
2. Puree the cumin, chickpeas, bell peppers, oil, lemon juice, garlic, and ground red pepper in a food processor until smooth. Scrape into a container and refrigerate until the flavors are blended, about 1 hour.
3. Preheat the oven to 350°F (180°C). Coat a jelly-roll pan with nonstick cooking spray. Separate the pitas along the edges to make four flat circles. Stack and cut them into six pie-shaped wedges. Spread in a single layer on the prepared pan and bake until golden, 12 to 15 minutes. Serve with the dip.

Per serving (2 tablespoons/25 mL): 33 calories, 1 g total fat, 0 g saturated fat, 4 g carbohydrate, 1 g protein, 1 g fiber, 0 mg cholesterol, 33 mg sodium, 8 mg calcium

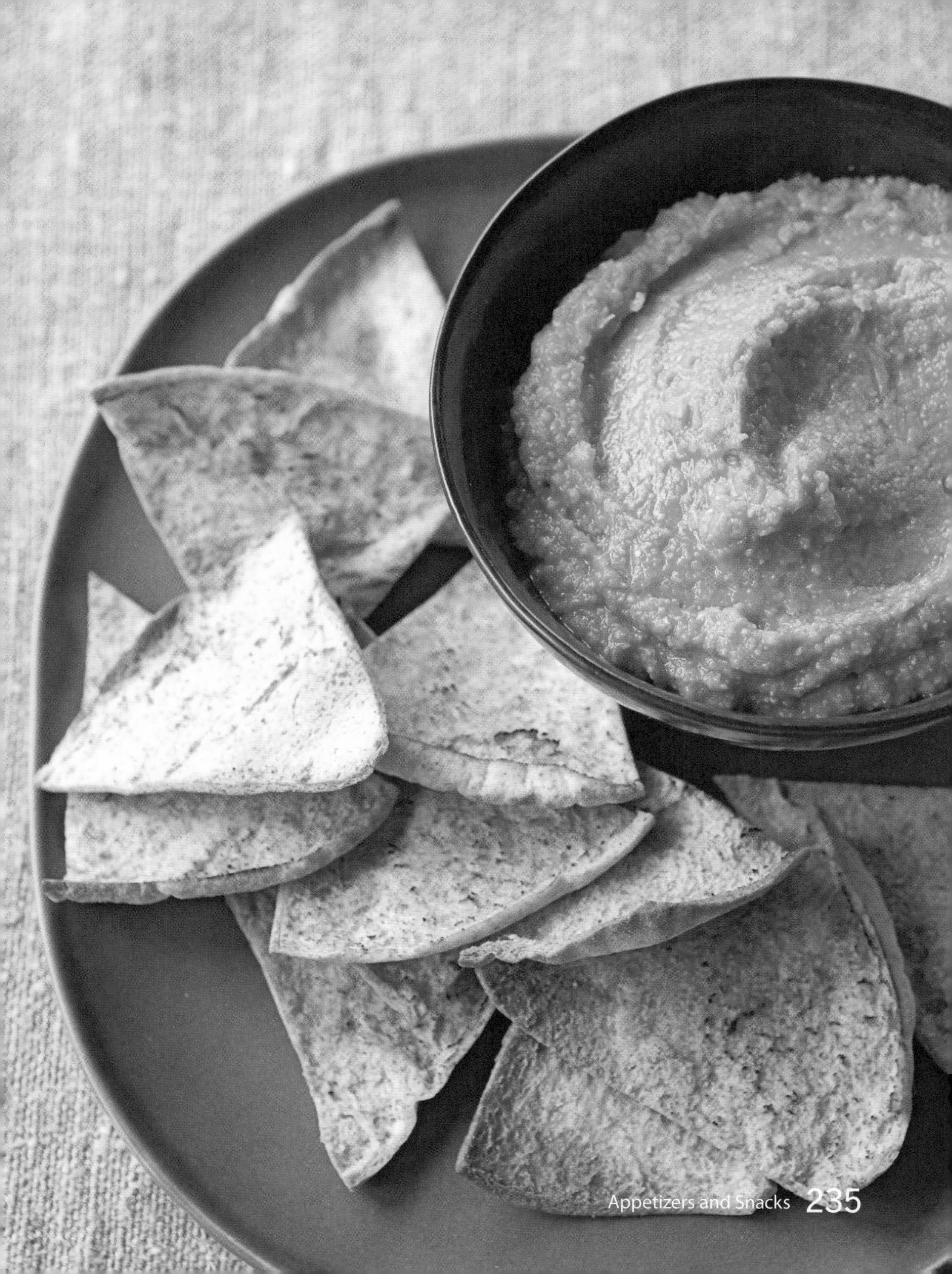

Salads | MAIN DISH

Tuna, Red Cabbage, Green Bean, and Caper Salad

Serves 4

PREP TIME: **30 minutes**

250 mL	1 cup trimmed and diagonally sliced green beans
1 L	4 cups chopped red cabbage (about 8 ounces/250 g)
125 mL	1/2 cup chopped red onion
125 mL	1/2 cup chopped flat-leaf parsley
1	1 can (6 1/2 ounces/170 g) olive-oil-packed tuna, rinsed with cold water, well-drained, and flaked with a fork
25 mL	2 tablespoons red-wine vinegar
15 mL	1 tablespoon extra-virgin olive oil
15 mL	1 tablespoon capers, rinsed and drained
0.5 mL	1/8 teaspoon freshly ground black pepper

Crunch plus a rich and satisfying balance of flavors makes this pretty red cabbage and tuna salad a favorite. Take advantage of the availability of preshredded red and green cabbage. Cabbage is high in vitamin C, fiber, and B vitamins, plus cancer-fighting phytochemical compounds, but red cabbage is much higher in vitamin C than its relatives.

1. Heat a small saucepan half-filled with water to boiling. Add the beans and cook until crisp-tender, about 3 minutes. Drain and rinse with cold water. Pat dry with paper towels.
2. Toss the beans in a large serving bowl with the cabbage, onions, parsley, tuna, vinegar, oil, capers, and pepper.

Per serving: 162 calories, 8 g total fat, 1 g saturated fat, 11 g carbohydrate, 14 g protein, 3 g fiber, 14 mg cholesterol, 277 mg sodium, 67 mg calcium

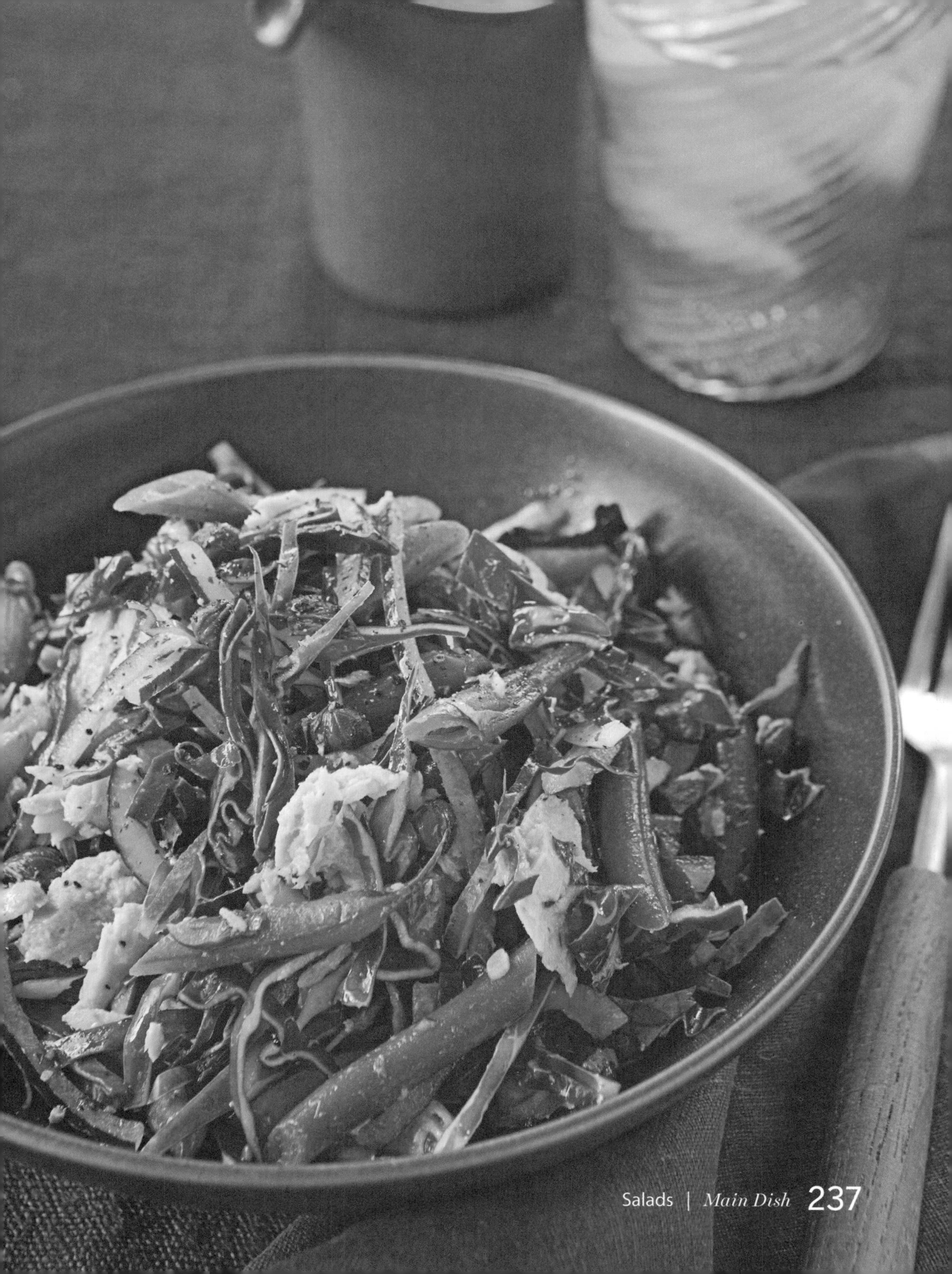

Chicken, Arugula, Avocado, and Tomato Salad with Lemon-Garlic Dressing and Black Olives

Serves 4

PREP TIME: **30 minutes**
COOK TIME: **6 minutes**

Pleasantly seasoned with fresh basil and lemon juice, quick-cooking and convenient strips of chicken make a welcome main-dish salad. Although avocados are high in fat, most of it is the good monounsaturated kind, plus they are high in folate, potassium, niacin, and vitamin B_6.

500 g	1 pound chicken tenders or skinless, boneless chicken breasts cut into 1/2-inch/1-cm strips
45 mL	3 tablespoons fresh lemon juice, divided
25 mL	2 tablespoons chopped fresh basil leaves, divided
25 mL	2 tablespoons extra-virgin olive oil
1	1 small clove garlic, crushed or grated
0.5 mL	1/8 teaspoon freshly ground black pepper
1.5 L	6 cups lightly packed arugula leaves
1	1 medium tomato, cored and cut into thin wedges
1/2	1/2 small avocado, peeled, pitted, and cut into thin wedges
125 mL	1/2 cup thin slivers of red onion
15 mL	1 tablespoon pitted and chopped Kalamata olives

1. Heat a large nonstick skillet over medium heat until hot enough that a drop of water sizzles. Coat with nonstick cooking spray. Add the chicken and cook, turning, until golden and cooked through, about 2 minutes per side. Add 1 tablespoon (15 mL) of the lemon juice and 1 tablespoon (15 mL) of the basil. Stir to coat and set aside to cool.
2. Whisk the remaining 2 tablespoons (25 mL) of lemon juice, the oil, garlic, and pepper in a large bowl until blended. Add the arugula, tomatoes, avocado, onions, and the remaining 1 tablespoon (15 mL) of basil and toss to coat evenly.
3. Divide among four plates and divide the chicken on top of the salads. Sprinkle with the olives.

Per serving: 264 calories, 14 g total fat, 2 g saturated fat, 8 g carbohydrate, 26 g protein, 3 g fiber, 73 mg cholesterol, 185 mg sodium, 75 mg calcium

Sardine and New Potato Salad with Spinach and Dill-Mustard Dressing

Serves 4

PREP TIME: **35 minutes**
COOK TIME: **10 minutes**

A tangy dressing of mustard and dill, tender chunks of potato, and canned sardines are combined to make a deliciously satisfying meal. Because the canning process softens the tiny sardine bones and makes them edible, you'll get significant amounts of calcium.

500 g	1 pound unpeeled small new potatoes, halved
45 mL	3 tablespoons fresh lemon juice
45 mL	3 tablespoons extra-virgin olive oil
5 mL	1 teaspoon Dijon-style mustard
500 mL	2 cups packed baby spinach leaves (about 3 ounces/90 g), rinsed and dried
125 mL	1/2 cup unpeeled chopped seedless cucumber
50 mL	1/4 cup chopped fresh dill
50 mL	1/4 cup thinly sliced scallions
2	2 cans (3.5 ounces/125 g each) sardines in olive oil, rinsed, drained, patted dry, and cut into 1-inch/2.5-cm pieces
1	1 tomato, cored and cut into wedges
4	4 lemon wedges
4	4 sprigs of dill

1. In a medium saucepan, cook the potatoes in boiling water until tender, about 10 minutes. Drain and cool.
2. Whisk together the lemon juice, oil, and mustard in a large bowl until blended. Add the potatoes, spinach, cucumbers, dill, scallions, and sardines and toss to blend.
3. Spoon onto a serving platter, then place the tomato and lemon wedges along the side. Top with the dill.

Per serving: 319 calories, 20 g total fat, 4 g saturated fat, 23 g carbohydrate, 14 g protein, 3 fiber, 59 mg cholesterol, 246 mg sodium, 179 mg calcium

Quinoa, Shrimp, and Fresh Corn Salad on Curly Leaf Lettuce with Toasted Cumin-Lime Dressing *Serves 4*

PREP TIME: **25 minutes**
COOK TIME: **20 minutes**

Crunchy bites of quinoa, sweet shrimp, and chopped vegetables tossed with a lively dressing makes a delicious salad meal. Quinoa has a very high level of lysine, an amino acid necessary for the synthesis of protein, which makes it one of the best sources of plant protein. Enhance the already nutty taste of quinoa by toasting it in a hot skillet before cooking it in water.

250 mL	1 cup quinoa
500 mL	2 cups water
7 mL	1 1/2 teaspoons ground cumin
45 mL	3 tablespoons fresh lime juice
25 mL	2 tablespoons extra-virgin olive oil
500 g	1 pound frozen cooked peeled small shrimp, thawed, rinsed, and drained (about 3 1/2 cups/750 mL)
250 mL	1 cup fresh corn kernels, cut from 1 to 2 ears corn
125 mL	1/2 cup chopped red bell pepper
125 mL	1/2 cup trimmed and thinly sliced scallions
50 mL	1/4 cup chopped fresh cilantro leaves and stems
15 mL	1 tablespoon seeded, deveined, and minced jalapeño (wear gloves when handling), or to taste
4	4 large curly leaf lettuce leaves
4	4 leafy sprigs of cilantro

1. Rinse the quinoa in a strainer under running water or swish in a bowl of water and strain. Shake dry. Heat in a deep skillet or wide saucepan over medium-low heat, stirring, until it begins to darken slightly, about 8 minutes. Add the water and heat to a boil. Reduce the heat to low. Cook, covered, until the liquid is absorbed and the quinoa is fluffy, 12 to 18 minutes. Set aside to cool.

2. Heat the cumin in a small skillet set over low heat, stirring, until warmed and fragrant, about 2 minutes. Remove from the heat and stir in the lime juice and oil. Pour into a large bowl.

3. Add the quinoa, shrimp, corn, peppers, scallions, cilantro, and jalapeños to the bowl and mix until well-blended.

4. Line each of four plates with a lettuce leaf. Spoon the quinoa on top. Add cilantro to each.

Per serving: 380 calories, 12 g total fat, 2 g saturated fat, 37 g carbohydrate, 31 g protein, 5 g fiber, 172 mg cholesterol, 201 mg sodium, 102 mg calcium

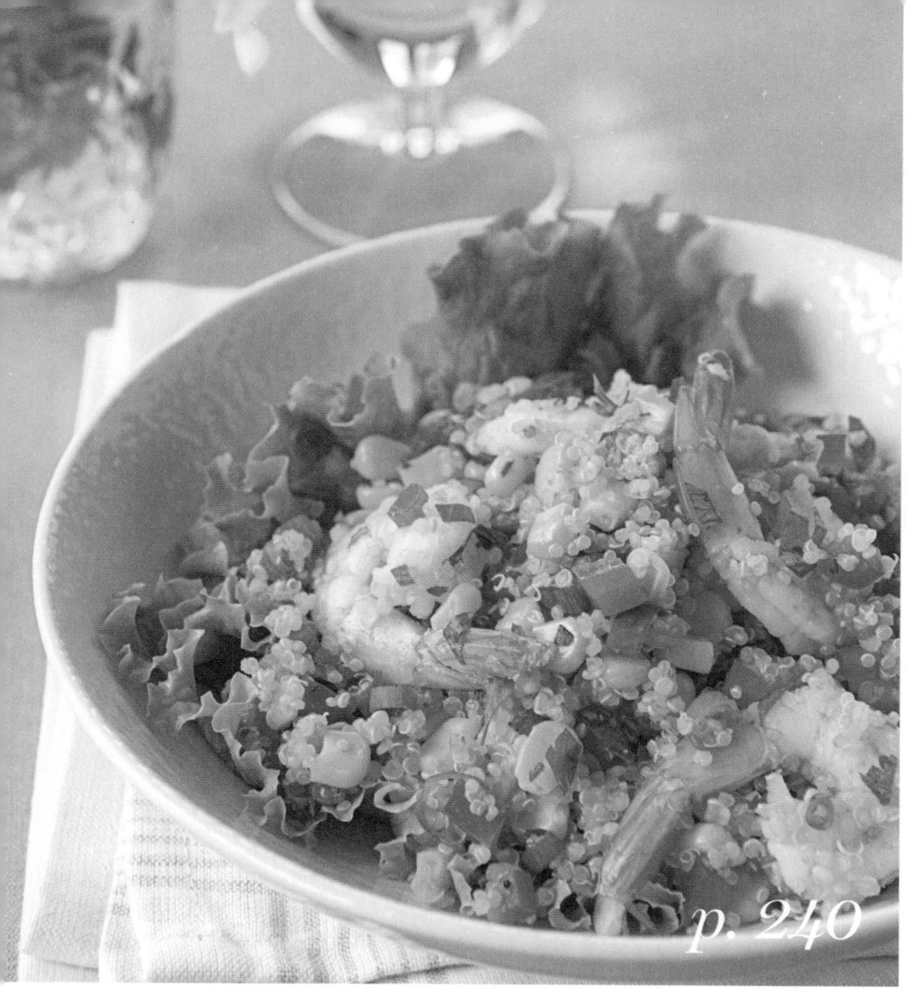

p. 240

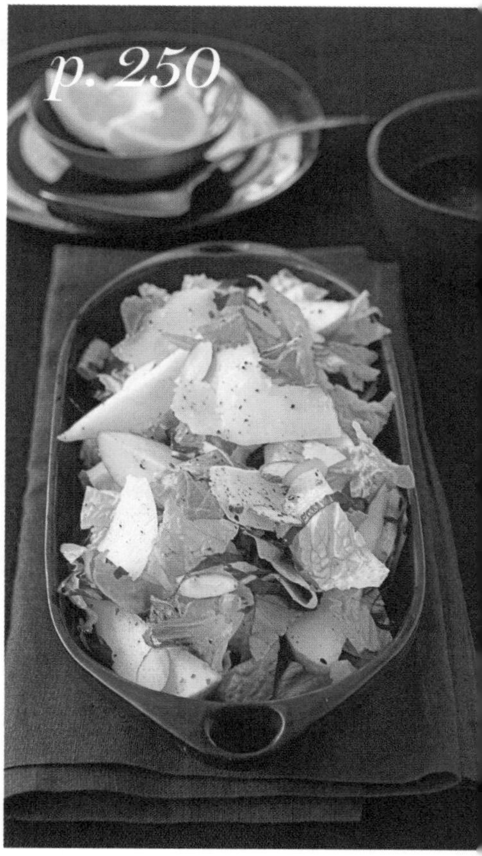

p. 250

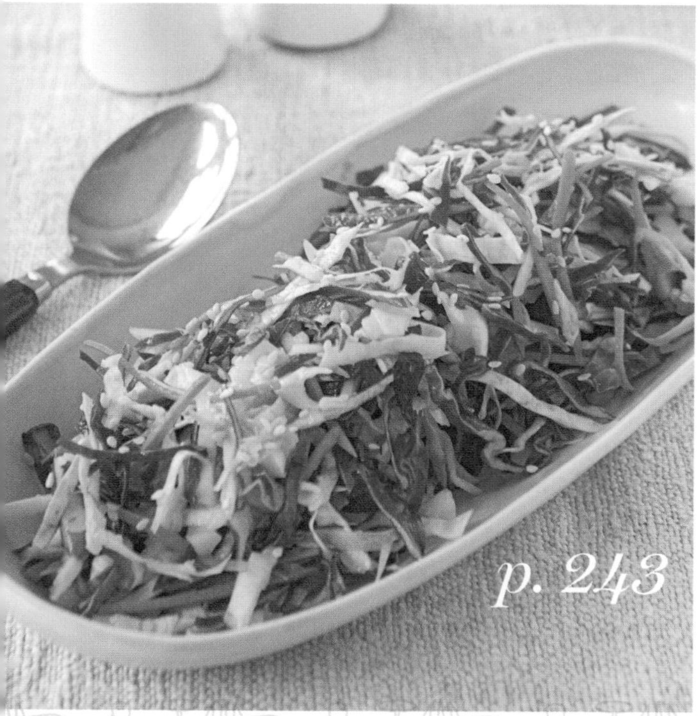

p. 243

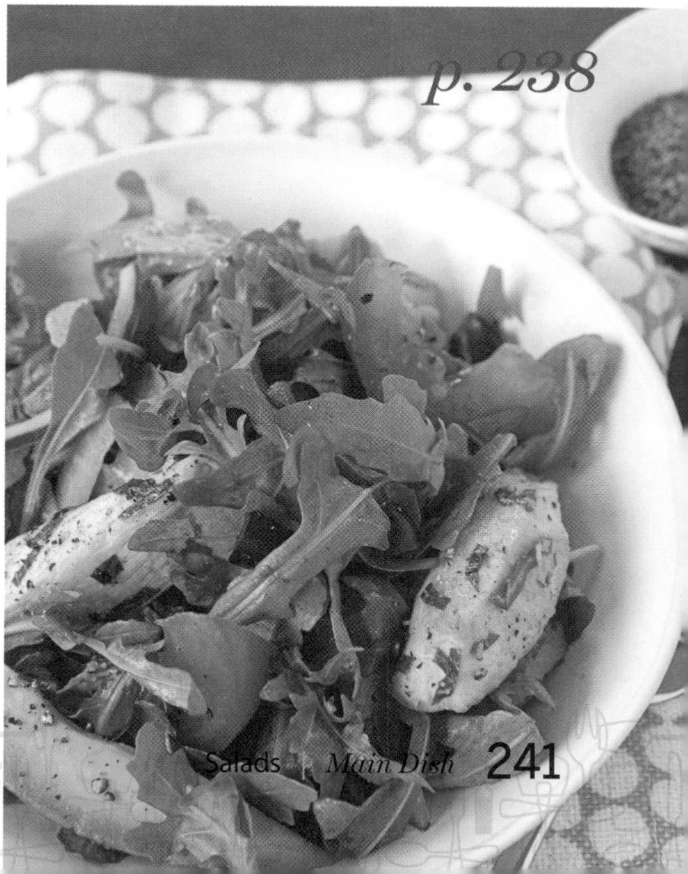

p. 238

Salads | SIDE DISH

Sweet Potato, Green Apple, and Peanut Salad with Apple-Cider-Vinegar Dressing

Serves 4

PREP TIME: **20 minutes**
COOK TIME: **35 minutes**

Roasted sweet potatoes and green apples offer a perfect balance of soft and crunchy and sweet and tangy in this delightful salad. The salad is lively with a bright apple-cider-vinegar dressing and topped with the favored heart-healthy peanut.

2	2 small unpeeled sweet potatoes (about 8 ounces/250 g each), scrubbed and pierced with a knife tip
25 mL	2 tablespoons apple-cider vinegar
25 mL	2 tablespoons extra-virgin olive oil
1	1 clove garlic, crushed or grated
0.5 mL	1/8 teaspoon freshly ground black pepper
2	2 Granny Smith apples, quartered, cored, and cut into 1/2-inch/1-cm pieces (about 2 cups/500 mL)
125 mL	1/2 cup diagonally sliced scallion
15 mL	1 tablespoon moist pack raisins
25 mL	2 tablespoons chopped unsalted dry-roasted peanuts, divided

1. Preheat the oven to 400°F (200°C).
2. Place the sweet potatoes in a baking pan and roast until tender, about 45 minutes. Cool completely. Cut into 1/2-inch/1-cm-thick slices and cut each slice in half.
3. Whisk the vinegar, oil, garlic, and pepper in a large bowl until blended. Add the potatoes, apples, scallions, raisins, and 1 tablespoon (15 mL) of the peanuts. Toss to blend. Sprinkle with the remaining 1 tablespoon (15 mL) of peanuts.

Per serving: 196 calories, 9 g total fat, 1 g saturated fat, 27 g carbohydrate, 2 g protein, 5 g fiber, 0 mg cholesterol, 39 mg sodium, 32 mg calcium

Asian Coleslaw with Ginger and Two Sesame Flavors

Serves 4

PREP TIME: **15 minutes**

45 mL	3 tablespoons unseasoned rice vinegar
25 mL	2 tablespoons unflavored vegetable oil
5 mL	1 teaspoon toasted sesame oil
5 mL	1 teaspoon grated fresh ginger
1	1 small clove garlic, crushed
500 mL	2 cups coarsely shredded green cabbage
500 mL	2 cups coarsely shredded red cabbage
250 mL	1 cup coarsely shredded carrots
15 mL	1 tablespoon seeded, deveined, and thinly sliced jalapeño (wear gloves when handling), or to taste
10 mL	2 teaspoons white sesame seeds, toasted, or brown sesame seeds, divided

Pretty, crunchy, and tangy with rice vinegar, fresh ginger, and spicy jalapeños, this will become your favorite slaw to pair with grilled seafood. Look for brown sesame seeds where Asian or Indian groceries are sold. Research suggests that cabbage, which is high in phytochemicals, may play a part in cancer prevention...so enjoy the flavor and the benefits!

1. Whisk together the vinegar, vegetable oil, sesame oil, ginger, and garlic in a large serving bowl until blended. Add the green and red cabbage, carrots, jalapeños, and 1 teaspoon of the sesame seeds (if using white sesame seeds, heat them in a small skillet set over low heat, stirring, until golden, about 2 minutes). Toss to blend. Sprinkle the remaining 1 teaspoon (5 mL) of sesame seeds on top.

Per serving: 116 calories, 9 g total fat, 1 g saturated fat, 9 g carbohydrate, 2 g protein, 3 g fiber, 0 mg cholesterol, 36 mg sodium, 63 mg calcium

Chopped Mango, Broccoli, Tomato, and Romaine Salad with Herbed Buttermilk Dressing

Serves 4

PREP TIME: **20 minutes**
COOK TIME: **5 minutes**

500 mL	2 cups chopped broccoli florets
75 mL	1/3 cup buttermilk
75 mL	1/3 cup packed chopped curly leaf parsley
25 mL	2 tablespoons chopped fresh dill
25 mL	2 tablespoons sliced scallion
1	1 small clove garlic, chopped
15 mL	1 tablespoon extra-virgin olive oil
0.5 mL	1/8 teaspoon freshly ground black pepper
1 L	4 cups coarsely chopped romaine lettuce leaves, including crisp center ribs
1	1 medium mango, peeled, pitted, and diced
250 mL	1 cup small grape or tiny cherry tomatoes

Every forkful of this brightly colored chopped salad presents a surprising medley of textures and tastes. Soft, sweet, and full of flavor, mangos are an excellent source of beta-carotene, vitamin C, soluble fiber, and pectin, which research indicates help to reduce cholesterol.

1. Cook the broccoli in a small saucepan half-filled with boiling water until crisp-tender, about 3 minutes. Drain and rinse with cold water. Pat dry with paper towels and place in a large bowl to cool.

2. Puree the buttermilk, parsley, dill, scallions, garlic, oil, and pepper in a blender, then pour over the broccoli. Add the lettuce, mangoes, and tomatoes and toss until blended.

Per serving: 102 calories, 4 g total fat, 1 g saturated fat, 14 g carbohydrate, 3 g protein, 3 g fiber, 1 mg cholesterol, 43 mg sodium, 68 mg calcium

White Bean, Fennel, and Onion Salad with Red-Wine Vinaigrette

Serves 4

PREP TIME: **20 minutes**
COOK TIME: **1 to 1 1/2 hours**

Crisp fennel and crunchy red onions paired with creamy white beans is a perfect trio, especially when tossed with a lively red-wine vinaigrette. Versatile beans are mostly nutritional superstars contributing impressive amounts of low-fat protein, B vitamins, and minerals. If you're short on time, you can use a can (15 ounces/540 mL) of no-salt-added beans that are rinsed and drained instead of using dried beans.

175 mL	3/4 cup dried white kidney or cannellini beans
1	1 leafy celery top
1	1 slice onion
1	1 bay leaf
1	1 clove garlic, finely chopped
2 mL	1/2 teaspoon coarse salt (optional)

SALAD

50 mL	1/4 cup red-wine vinegar
25 mL	2 tablespoons extra-virgin olive oil
1	1 clove garlic, finely chopped
0.5 mL	1/8 teaspoon freshly ground black pepper
250 mL	1 cup chopped fennel
250 mL	1 cup chopped red onion
50 mL	1/4 cup chopped flat-leaf parsley
50 mL	1/4 cup finely chopped fernlike fennel tops (optional)
4	4 Boston lettuce leaves

1. Place the beans in a medium bowl. Add enough water to cover the beans and soak in the refrigerator overnight. Drain them and place them in a deep ovenproof casserole with the celery, onion slice, bay leaf, and garlic. Add water to cover by at least 1 inch (2.5 cm). Bake, covered with a lid or foil, until tender, 1 to 1 1/2 hours, checking every 15 minutes after 1 hour to prevent overcooking. Drain liquid, if necessary, and reserve for soup. Discard the celery, onion, and bay leaf. Stir in the salt (if using). Cool.
2. Prepare the salad. Whisk the vinegar, oil, garlic, and pepper in a large bowl. Fold in the beans, chopped fennel, red onions, parsley, and fennel tops (if using) until coated.
3. Place a lettuce leaf on each of four plates and place a scoop of bean salad in the center.

Per serving: 181 calories, 8 g total fat, 1 g saturated fat, 22 g carbohydrate, 6 g protein, 6 g fiber, 0 mg cholesterol, 65 mg sodium, 76 mg calcium

Black Bean, Corn, Tomato, Avocado, and Cilantro with Lime and Jalapeño Dressing

Serves 4

PREP TIME: **20 minutes**

45 mL	3 tablespoons fresh lime juice
25 mL	2 tablespoons extra-virgin olive oil
5 mL	1 teaspoon seeded, deveined, and minced jalapeño (wear gloves when handling), or to taste
1	1 can (15 ounces/540 mL) no-salt-added black beans, rinsed and drained
250 mL	1 cup corn kernels removed from 1 ear of corn
125 mL	1/2 cup cored, seeded, and diced tomato
1	1 scallion, trimmed and thinly sliced
1/2	1/2 medium avocado, peeled, pitted, and diced (about 1/2 cup/125 mL)
45 mL	3 tablespoons chopped fresh cilantro
4	4 Boston lettuce leaves

The rich, earthy taste of black beans complements the sweet crunch of corn kernels and the bright flavors in the Southwest-inspired lime and jalapeño dressing. Black beans, like all beans, are rich in heart-healthy, cholesterol-reducing, soluble fiber.

1. Whisk the lime juice, oil, and jalapeños in a large bowl until blended. Add the beans, corn, tomatoes, scallions, avocados, and cilantro. Gently toss until blended.
2. Place a lettuce leaf on each of four plates and fill each with bean salad, dividing evenly.

Per serving: 218 calories, 11 g total fat, 2 g saturated fat, 24 g carbohydrate, 7 g protein, 8 g fiber, 0 mg cholesterol, 40 mg sodium, 57 mg calcium

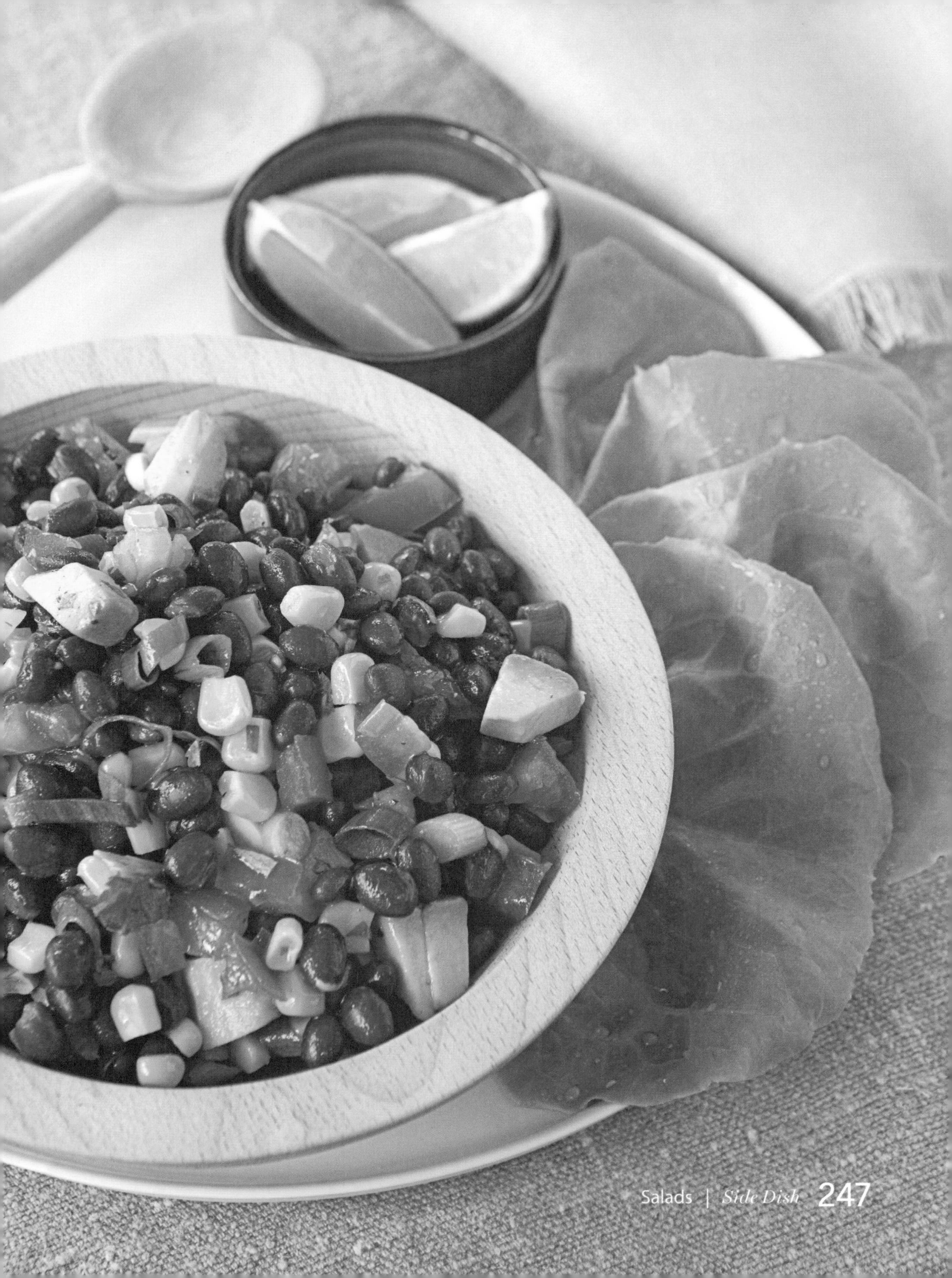

Hot Smoked Salmon, Celery, and Egg Salad with Creamy Mustard Dressing

Serves 4

PREP TIME: **10 minutes**
COOK TIME: **20 minutes**

Hot smoked salmon has a wonderful rich taste that goes well with hard-cooked eggs. Eggs in moderation are an excellent, heart-healthy vitamin source. Yogurt adds just the right balance of creamy flavor to this mustardy dressing.

50 mL	1/4 cup nonfat plain yogurt
50 mL	1/4 cup low-fat mayonnaise
15 mL	1 tablespoon fresh lemon juice
2 mL	1/2 teaspoon Dijon-style mustard
0.5 mL	1/8 teaspoon freshly ground black pepper
4	4 hard-cooked eggs, peeled and cut into 1/2-inch/1-cm pieces
125 g	4 ounces hot smoked salmon, broken into 1/2-inch/1-cm pieces
125 mL	1/2 cup chopped celery
125 mL	1/2 cup chopped red onion
25 mL	2 tablespoons chopped fresh dill
500 mL	2 cups packed torn chicory (curly endive) leaves
25 mL	2 tablespoons thinly sliced radishes

1. Whisk the yogurt, mayonnaise, lemon juice, mustard, and pepper in a large bowl until blended. Add the eggs, salmon, celery, onions, and dill and fold to blend.
2. Spread the chicory leaves evenly among four salad plates. Top each with egg salad and add the radishes.

Per serving: 184 calories, 12 g total fat, 2 g saturated fat, 7 g carbohydrate, 13 g protein, 1 g fiber, 224 mg cholesterol, 447 mg sodium, 71 mg calcium

Lentil, Roasted Red Pepper, and Spinach Salad with Walnuts, Olives, and Sherry Vinaigrette

Serves 4

PREP TIME: **10 minutes**
COOK TIME: **15–20 minutes**

Inexpensive, nutritious, and quick-cooking, tender, earthy lentils and roasted red peppers make a great side-dish salad with a light meal. High in protein, lentils are also a good source of fiber.

250 mL	1 cup dried lentils, rinsed and picked over
25 mL	2 tablespoons extra-virgin olive oil
25 mL	2 tablespoons sherry vinegar
1	1 clove garlic, crushed or grated
2 mL	1/2 teaspoon Dijon-style mustard
0.5 mL	1/8 teaspoon freshly ground black pepper
500 mL	2 cups packed baby spinach (about 3 ounces/90 g), rinsed and dried
125 mL	1/2 cup chopped jarred roasted red peppers, rinsed, drained, and patted dry
125 mL	1/2 cup chopped celery
50 mL	1/4 cup chopped red onion
50 mL	1/4 cup chopped flat-leaf parsley
25 mL	2 tablespoons pitted and chopped green olives
25 mL	2 tablespoons chopped walnuts

1. Cook the lentils in plenty of boiling water in a medium saucepan until tender, 15 to 20 minutes. Drain and rinse. Set aside to cool.
2. Whisk the oil, vinegar, garlic, mustard, and black pepper in a large bowl until blended. Add the lentils, spinach, red peppers, celery, onion, parsley, and olives and toss until coated. Sprinkle with the walnuts.

Per serving: 275 calories, 11 g total fat, 1 g saturated fat, 33 g carbohydrate, 12 g protein, 8 g fiber, 0 mg cholesterol, 248 mg sodium, 58 mg calcium

Mixed Greens with Sliced Pears, Toasted Almonds, and Shaved Parmesan

Serves 4

PREP TIME: **15 minutes**

25 mL	2 tablespoons sliced almonds
1	1 large ripe Bosc or Bartlett pear, quartered, cored, and cut into thin wedges
45 mL	3 tablespoons fresh lemon juice, divided
25 mL	2 tablespoons extra-virgin olive oil
1	1 clove garlic, crushed or grated
0.5 mL	1/8 teaspoon freshly ground black pepper
1	1 bag Italian mix (Romaine and radicchio) salad greens (10 ounces/300 g), rinsed and dried
8	8 shavings (about 1 ounce/30 g) Parmesan

Aromatic, juicy slices of pear add a pleasant crunch to this simple but elegant salad. Pears are high in fiber, including cholesterol-lowering pectin. Use a vegetable peeler to shave thin curls from a nice wedge of authentic Parmesan.

1. Heat the almonds in small heavy skillet over medium-low heat, stirring, until golden, 3 to 4 minutes. Set aside.
2. Toss the pears and 1 tablespoon (15 mL) of the lemon juice in a small bowl until the pears are coated. Set aside.
3. Whisk the remaining 2 tablespoons (25 mL) of lemon juice, the oil, garlic, and pepper in a large bowl until blended. Add the greens, pears, and almonds and toss until blended.
4. Divide among four salad plates. Top with the cheese shavings.

Per serving: 169 calories, 11 g total fat, 3 g saturated fat, 15 g carbohydrate, 5 g protein, 4 g fiber, 7 mg cholesterol, 120 mg sodium, 127 mg calcium

Cantaloupe and Watercress Salad with Feta Cheese

Serves 4

PREP TIME: **20 minutes**

1/2	1/2 cantaloupe, halved, seeded, and cut into 1/2-inch/1-cm chunks
500 mL	2 cups packed trimmed and chopped watercress
250 mL	1 cup chopped unpeeled seedless cucumber
125 mL	1/2 cup halved cherry tomatoes
125 mL	1/2 cup chopped sweet onion
25 mL	2 tablespoons fresh lime juice
25 mL	2 tablespoons extra-virgin olive oil
0.5 mL	1/8 teaspoon freshly ground black pepper
30 g	1 ounce feta cheese, rinsed and crumbled (about 1/4 cup/50 mL)

The ingredients in this salad offer a perfect balance of sweetness, crunch, and both peppery and salty with every bite. Cantaloupe, low in calories and filled with flavor, is an excellent source of vitamin C, potassium, and B_6 and is a good source of beta-carotene. Treat yourself to this refreshing flavor combination.

1. Toss the cantaloupe, watercress, cucumbers, tomatoes, onions, lime juice, oil, and pepper together in a large bowl until blended. Sprinkle with the cheese.

Per serving: 150 calories, 9 g total fat, 2 g saturated fat, 15 g carbohydrate, 4 g protein, 2 g fiber, 8 mg cholesterol, 134 mg sodium, 88 mg calcium

Mushroom, Spinach, and Wild Rice Soup

Serves 4

PREP TIME: **15 minutes**
COOK TIME: **1 hour 10 minutes**

20 mL	1 tablespoon plus 1 teaspoon extra-virgin olive oil, divided
300 g	10 ounces white button mushrooms, trimmed and chopped
125 mL	1/2 cup chopped onion
2	2 cloves garlic, minced
1 L	1 quart reduced-sodium beef, chicken, or vegetable broth
500 mL	2 cups water
125 mL	1/2 cup wild rice, rinsed and drained
500 mL	2 cups packed spinach leaves, coarsely chopped
15 mL	1 tablespoon no-salt-added tomato paste
125 mL	1/2 cup seeded and chopped red bell pepper
15 mL	1 tablespoon minced flat-leaf parsley
5 mL	1 teaspoon minced fresh thyme leaves
0.5 mL	1/8 teaspoon freshly ground black pepper

The deep, meaty aroma and woodsy taste of mushrooms and wild rice permeate this soup. Though it may sound like it tastes a bit earthy, it is actually light and elegant. Wild rice is an excellent source of niacin and dietary fiber and contributes significant amounts of protein and iron to your diet.

1. Heat 1 tablespoon (15 mL) of the oil in a large saucepan. Add the mushrooms and onions. Cook over medium-low heat, covered, stirring occasionally, until softened, about 5 minutes.
2. Raise the heat to medium-high. Uncover and cook, stirring occasionally, until the mushrooms and onions are golden, about 5 minutes. Add the garlic and cook for 1 minute.
3. Add the broth, water, and rice and heat to boiling. Cook, covered, until the rice grains burst open exposing the soft inside of each grain, about 55 minutes.
4. Add the spinach and tomato paste and cook, stirring, until the spinach wilts, about 2 minutes.
5. Cook the bell peppers and the remaining 1 teaspoon (5 mL) of oil in a small skillet over medium heat, stirring occasionally, until the peppers are tender, about 5 minutes. Add the parsley, thyme, and black pepper. Spoon on top just before serving.

Per serving: 165 calories, 5 g total fat, 1 g saturated fat, 23 g carbohydrate, 7 g protein, 2 g fiber, 5 mg cholesterol, 451 mg sodium, 29 mg calcium

Barley, Chicken, and Spring Vegetable Soup

Serves 4

PREP TIME: **15 minutes**
COOK TIME: **1 hour**

Studded with colorful spring vegetables and soft, tender, and flavorful beads of barley, this is a luscious, satisfying soup. Barley is an ancient grain high in fiber, magnesium, phosphorus, potassium, and folacin. The spring vegetables add plenty of nutrients and fiber of their own.

500 g	1 pound bone-in chicken breast, skin removed and fat trimmed
2 L	2 quarts water
2	2 cloves garlic, halved
1	1 large carrot
1	1 thick onion slice
1	1 leafy celery top
1	1 bay leaf
125 mL	1/2 cup pearled barley
250 mL	1 cup trimmed asparagus slices (1/4-inch/0.5-cm diagonals)
125 mL	1/2 cup trimmed green bean pieces (1/4 inch/0.5 cm)
125 mL	1/2 cup frozen peas
25 mL	2 tablespoons fresh lemon juice
2 mL	1/2 teaspoon coarse salt
0.5 mL	1/8 teaspoon freshly ground black pepper
50 mL	1/4 cup slivered fresh basil

1. Heat the chicken, water, garlic, carrot, onion, celery, and bay leaf in a large saucepan set over medium-high heat. Bring to a boil, then reduce the heat to low. Skim the foam from the surface, and continue to cook for 45 minutes.
2. Remove the chicken and carrot from the broth and reserve. Pour the broth through a strainer set over a large bowl, and discard the solids. Let stand until the fat comes to the surface of the broth. Discard the fat.
3. Pour 7 cups (1.75 L) of the broth back into the pan. Add the barley and cook, covered, over medium-low heat until tender, 30 to 45 minutes.
4. Cut the chicken into 1/2-inch (1-cm) pieces when it is cool enough to handle. Discard the bones. Slice the carrot into 1/4-inch (0.5-cm) pieces.
5. Stir the chicken, carrots, asparagus, green beans, and peas into the barley and cook, stirring, until the raw vegetables are tender, about 6 minutes. Add the lemon juice, salt, and pepper. Top with the basil.

Per serving: 261 calories, 4 g total fat, 1 g saturated fat, 28 g carbohydrate, 29 g protein, 6 g fiber, 73 mg cholesterol, 459 mg sodium, 45 mg calcium

Roasted Tomato Soup with Toasted Cumin and Brown Rice

Serves 4

PREP TIME: **15 minutes**
COOK TIME: **55 minutes**

Enjoy tomatoes all year long by oven roasting. This simple technique adds extra flavor to the tomatoes, making this soup especially delicious. Tomatoes are an excellent fat-free source of vitamins and minerals, especially vitamins A and C, and potassium.

1 kg	2 pounds tomatoes, trimmed and quartered
1/2	1/2 medium onion, cut into 1/4-inch/0.5 cm wedges
1	1 clove garlic, chopped
15 mL	1 tablespoon extra-virgin olive oil
	Freshly ground black pepper
350 mL	3 cups water, divided
125 mL	1/2 cup long- or medium-grain brown rice
15 mL	1 tablespoon ground cumin
500-750 mL	2 to 3 cups reduced-sodium chicken broth
25 mL	2 tablespoons fresh lime juice
15 mL	1 tablespoon seeded, deveined, and minced jalapeño (wear gloves when handling), or to taste
125 mL	1/2 cup peeled, seeded, and chopped ripe avocado
50 mL	1/4 cup chopped fresh cilantro

1. Preheat the oven to 400°F (200°C). Combine the tomatoes, onions, and garlic on a jelly-roll pan. Drizzle with the oil and pepper and spread in a single layer. Roast, stirring occasionally, until the tomatoes are shriveled and the onions are golden, about 45 minutes.
2. Remove from the oven and transfer to a blender or food processor. Add 1 cup (250 mL) of the water to the pan, scrape any browned bits to loosen, and add them to the blender. Puree until smooth.
3. In a large saucepan, bring the remaining 2 cups (500 mL) of water to a boil over medium-high heat. Add the rice. Cover and cook until tender, about 45 minutes. Drain any excess water.
4. Heat the cumin in a large saucepan over low heat, stirring frequently. Cook until fragrant, about 2 minutes. Add the tomatoes, rice, and broth and heat to a boil. Add the lime juice and jalapeños. Top with the avocado and cilantro.

Per serving: 205 calories, 7 g total fat, 1 g saturated fat, 30 g carbohydrate, 6 g protein, 4 g fiber, 3 mg cholesterol, 117 mg sodium, 46 mg calcium

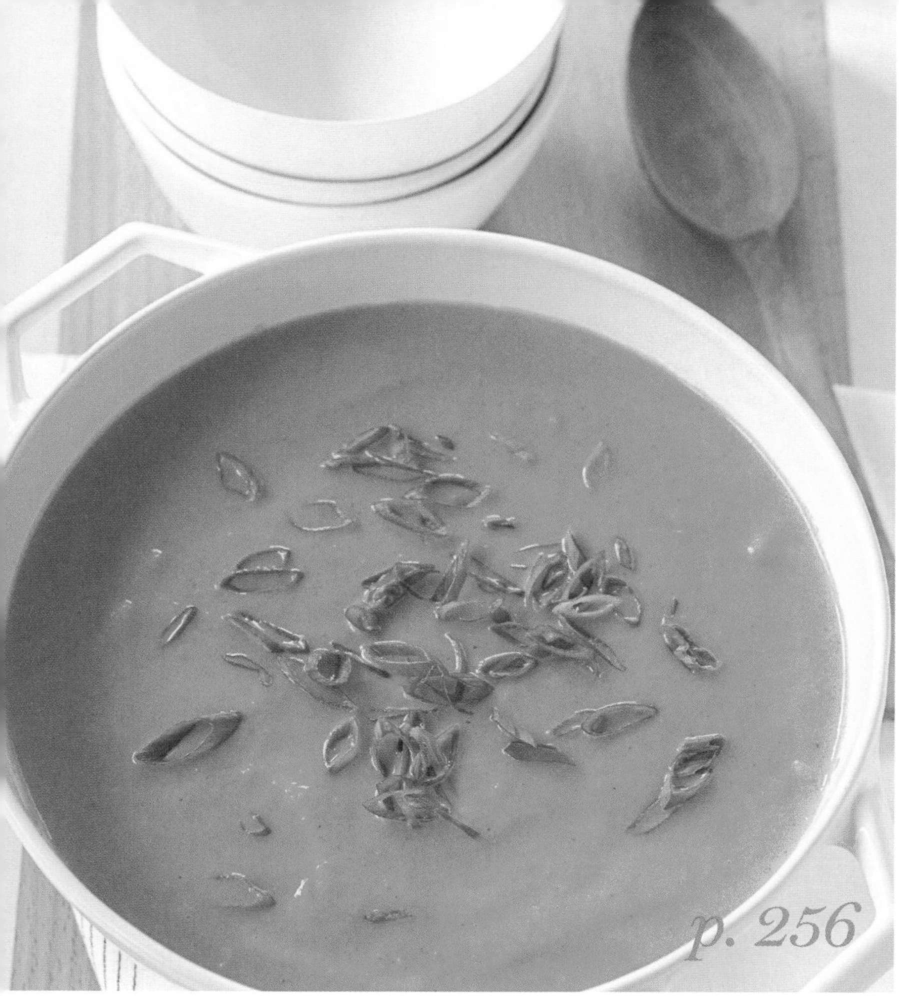
p. 256

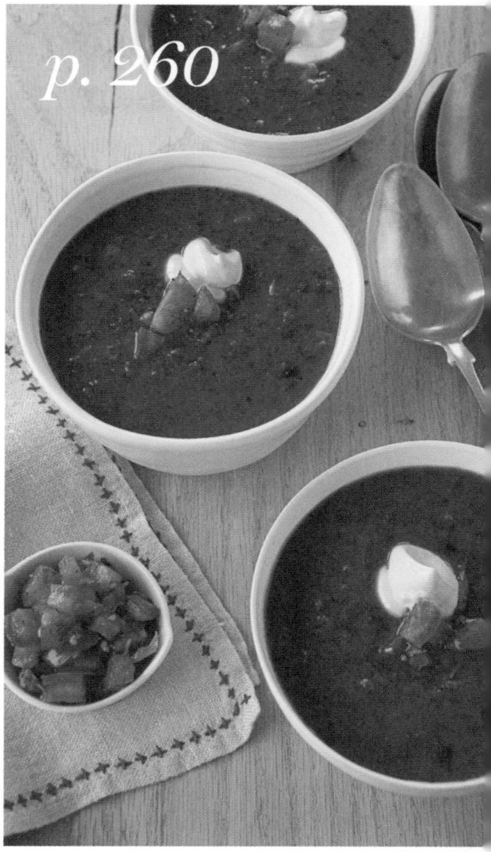
p. 260

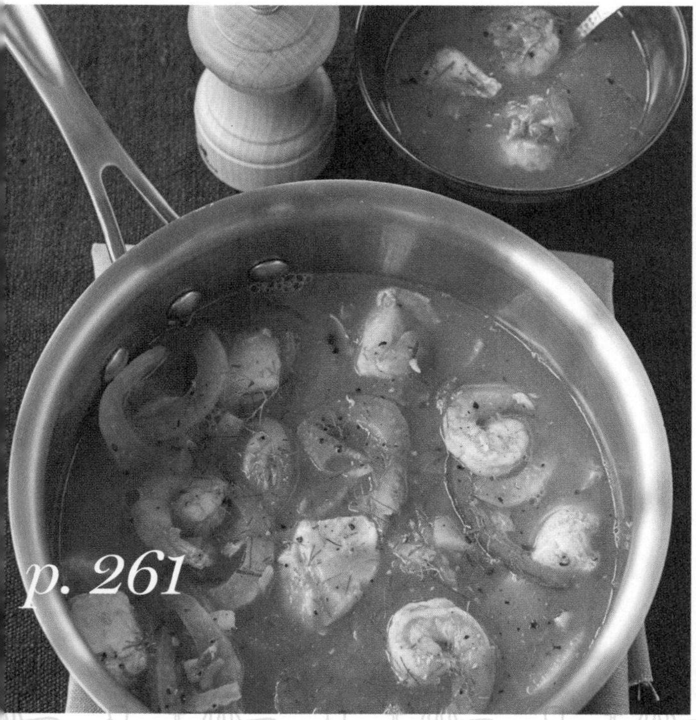
p. 261

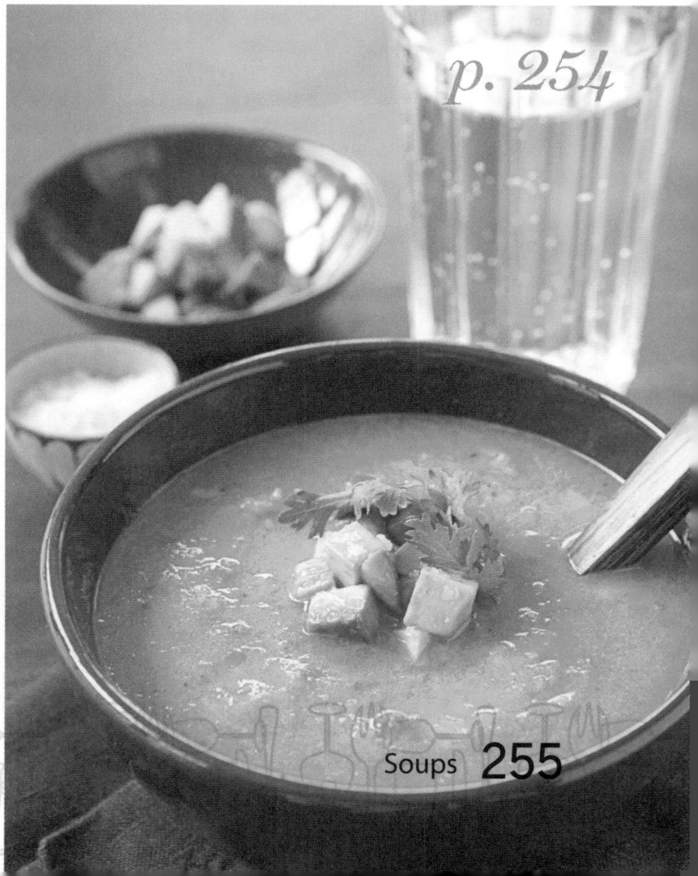
p. 254

Creamy Curried Carrot Soup

Serves 4

PREP TIME: **20 minutes**
COOK TIME: **30 minutes**

Despite the title there is no cream—just milk—in this lusciously smooth, gently spiced soup. Milk adds calcium and vitamin D to your diet, and carrots are an excellent source of antioxidants.

15 mL	1 tablespoon extra-virgin olive oil
125 mL	1/2 cup chopped scallion (white part only)
10 mL	2 teaspoons chopped fresh ginger
10 mL	2 teaspoons Madras curry powder, or to taste
2 mL	1/2 teaspoon ground turmeric
1.5 L	6 cups sliced trimmed carrots (about 1 3/4 pounds/875 g)
500 mL	2 cups reduced-sodium chicken broth
500 mL	2 cups low-fat (1%) milk
2 mL	1/2 teaspoon coarse salt
50 mL	1/4 cup thinly sliced scallion (green part only)

1. Heat the oil in a large saucepan set over medium-high heat, until shimmering. Reduce the heat to low. Stir in the white scallions and cook until tender, about 5 minutes.
2. Add the ginger, curry, and turmeric. Stir until blended. Add the carrots and broth and bring to a boil. Reduce the heat to medium-low. Cook, covered, until the carrots are soft, about 25 minutes. Cool slightly.
3. Puree the soup in a food processor or blender until smooth. Pour back into the saucepan and stir in the milk and salt. Reheat, stirring, over low heat. Sprinkle the top with the green scallions.

Per serving: 180 calories, 5 g total fat, 1 g saturated fat, 27 g carbohydrate, 7 g protein, 6 g fiber, 6 mg cholesterol, 517 mg sodium, 236 mg calcium

Butternut Squash and Apple Soup

Serves 4

PREP TIME: **15 minutes**
COOK TIME: **30 minutes**

Delicate and smooth, this quick-and-easy soup conveniently uses either fresh or frozen squash. The apple juice and grated ginger add a pleasant sweet-and-spicy flavor. Dark orange vegetables, like winter squash, are an excellent source of carotenoids, the building blocks of vitamin A.

15 mL	1 tablespoon extra-virgin olive oil
250 mL	1 cup coarsely chopped leeks (white and light green parts only)
250 mL	1 cup coarsely chopped carrot
5 mL	1 teaspoon chopped garlic
500 mL	2 cups unsweetened apple juice
500 mL	2 cups water
750 g	1 1/2 pounds peeled, seeded, and cubed fresh butternut squash or 2 boxes (12 ounces/340 g each) frozen squash puree
1	1 large apple, peeled, cored, and chopped (1 1/2 cups/375 mL)
15 mL	1 tablespoon chopped fresh ginger
50 mL	1/4 cup fresh lemon juice
125 mL	1/2 teaspoon coarse salt
0.5 mL	1/8 teaspoon ground red pepper, or to taste
125 mL	1/2 cup plain low-fat yogurt

1. Heat the oil in a large saucepan over medium-low heat. Add the leeks and carrots, and cook, stirring, until tender, about 5 minutes. Add the garlic and cook for 1 minute more.
2. Add the apple juice, water, squash, apples, and ginger and heat to a boil. Reduce the heat to low. Cook, covered, until the squash is soft, about 20 minutes. Cool slightly.
3. Puree the soup, in batches, in a food processor or blender. Return to the saucepan and reheat, about 5 minutes. Add the lemon juice, salt, and red pepper.
4. Swirl each serving with 2 tablespoons/25 mL of the yogurt.

Per serving: 279 calories, 4 g total fat, 1 g saturated fat, 60 g carbohydrate, 6 g protein, 5 g fiber, 3 mg cholesterol, 351 mg sodium, 200 mg calcium

Asian-Flavored Chicken, Shiitake, and Bok Choy Soup

Serves 4

PREP TIME: **20 minutes**
COOK TIME: **30 minutes**

750 mL	3 cups water
750 mL	3 cups reduced-sodium chicken broth
250 g	8 ounces boneless, skinless chicken breast, fat trimmed
2	2 trimmed scallions
2	2 cloves garlic, divided
1	1 fresh ginger slice (1 1/4-inches/3-cm thick)
1	1 sprig cilantro
5 mL	1 teaspoon reduced-sodium soy sauce
4	4 medium shiitake mushrooms, stems discarded and thinly sliced
2	2 small heads baby bok choy, trimmed and sliced (1/4 inch/0.5 cm), about 2 cups/500 mL
15 mL	1 tablespoon chopped fresh cilantro
2 mL	1/2 teaspoon fresh grated ginger
2 mL	1/2 teaspoon toasted sesame oil
2 mL	1/2 teaspoon toasted sesame seeds

Steaming aromatic broth with bits of earthy-tasting shiitake, tender lean chicken, and crunchy bok choy make this soup especially appealing. Soup is considered a healthy, low-calorie way to help fill you longer and control overeating. Research shows that when diners sip a bowl of soup before a full-course meal, they consumer fewer calories.

1. Add the water, broth, and chicken to a soup pot set over medium-high heat. Slice the white part of the scallions and add to the pot (reserve the green part of the scallions). With the side of a knife, bruise one of the garlic cloves and add it to the pot. Stir in the ginger slice and the cilantro sprig and bring to a boil. Reduce the heat to low. Cook, covered, for 20 minutes.
2. Lift the chicken from the broth and set aside. Strain the broth over a large bowl. Discard the solids and return the broth to the pot. Slice the reserved green part of the scallions and add to the pot. Grate or crush the remaining garlic clove and add it to the pot. Stir in the mushrooms, bok choy, chopped cilantro, and grated ginger. Cook over low heat for 10 minutes. Add the oil.
3. Cut the chicken into thin crosswise slices. Distribute evenly among four soup bowls. Ladle the broth mixture over the chicken, distributing the vegetables evenly. Top with the sesame seeds.

Per serving: 100 calories, 2 g total fat, 0 g saturated fat, 4 g carbohydrate, 15 g protein, 1 g fiber, 36 mg cholesterol, 191 mg sodium, 54 mg calcium

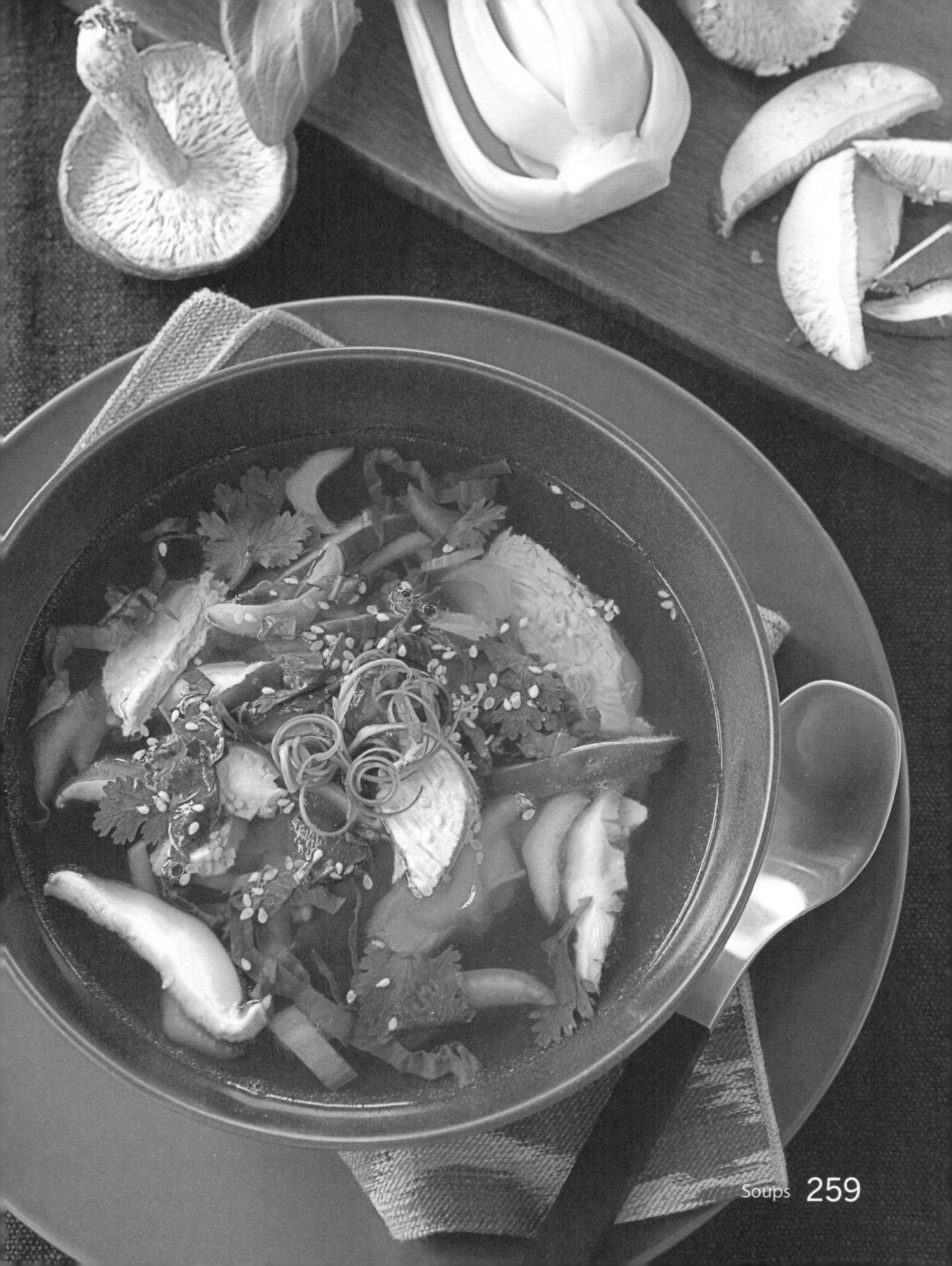

Black Bean Soup with Chipotle Chiles

Serves 4

PREP TIME: **20 minutes**
COOK TIME: **20 minutes**

The rich taste of black beans comes through in this fragrant soup embellished with the complex smokiness of fiery-hot chipotle chiles. Don't worry...the heat of the chiles is tempered by a cooling spoonful of nonfat sour cream in each bowl of soup. Black beans are an excellent low-fat source of protein.

15 mL	1 tablespoon extra-virgin olive oil
1	1 medium onion, chopped
1	1 medium red bell pepper, seeded and chopped
1	1 medium green bell pepper, seeded and chopped
2	2 cloves garlic, chopped
15 mL	1 tablespoon ground cumin
5 mL	1 teaspoon dried oregano
2	2 cans (14.5 ounces/540 mL each) black beans, rinsed and drained
1 L	4 cups reduced-sodium chicken or vegetable broth
10 mL	2 teaspoons finely chopped chipotle chiles in adobo sauce
125 mL	1/2 cup chopped fresh tomato
15 mL	1 tablespoon fresh lime juice
15 mL	1 tablespoon minced fresh cilantro
1 mL	1/4 teaspoon coarse salt
125 mL	1/2 cup nonfat sour cream

1. Heat the oil in large soup pot over medium heat. Add the onions and peppers. Reduce the heat to medium-low and cook, stirring, until golden, about 10 minutes.
2. Stir in the garlic, cumin, and oregano. Cook for 1 minute. Add the beans, broth, and chiles and heat to a boil. Reduce the heat to low. Cook, stirring occasionally, for 20 minutes. Cool slightly.
3. Transfer about half of the mixture into a blender or food processor and puree. Stir back into the remaining soup in the pot.
4. In a small bowl, combine the tomatoes, lime juice, cilantro, and salt. Add 2 tablespoons (25 mL) of the sour cream to each serving and top with the tomato mixture.

Per serving: 249 calories, 5 g total fat, 1 g saturated fat, 37 g carbohydrate, 13 g protein, 9 g fiber, 3 mg cholesterol, 540 mg sodium, 144 mg calcium

Two-Fish Soup with Fennel and Roasted Tomatoes

Serves 4

PREP TIME: **20 minutes**
COOK TIME: **1 hour**

1.25 L	5 cups packed cored and quartered plum tomatoes (1 1/2 pounds/750 g)
1	1 clove garlic, thinly sliced
25 mL	2 tablespoons extra-virgin olive oil, divided
625 mL	2 1/2 cups water
250 mL	1 cup trimmed and sliced (2 × 1/4-inch/5 × 0.5-cm pieces) fennel bulbs
125 mL	1/2 cup red onion slivers (2 × 1/4 inch/5 × 0.5-cm lengthwise pieces)
500 mL	2 cups dry white wine
2 mL	1/2 teaspoon fennel seeds
250 g	8 ounces large shrimp (about 12 pieces)
375 g	12 ounces thick, boneless, skinless fish (swordfish, cod, sea bass, halibut, grouper), cut into 1/2-inch/1-cm pieces
50 mL	1/4 cup finely chopped fennel tops

Laced with the delicate sweet taste of cooked fennel and slow-roasted tomatoes, this versatile soup is especially easy on the cook. Use whatever fish looks good in your market. Both the fish and the shrimp—the most popular of all seafood—are naturally low in fat and calories and are a good source of iron, potassium, and niacin.

1. Preheat the oven to 400°F (200°C).
2. Spread the tomatoes in a 9 × 13-inch (22 × 33-cm) roasting pan. Add the garlic and drizzle with 1 tablespoon (15 mL) of the oil. Roast, stirring every 15 minutes, until the tomato skins are shriveled and the edges begin to brown, about 45 minutes.
3. Add the water to the pan and stir to loosen browned bits from the bottom of the pan. Puree in a blender or food processor. Set aside.
4. Heat the remaining 1 tablespoon (15 mL) of oil in a 10-inch (25-cm) sauté pan or 4 quart (4 L) shallow saucepan over medium heat. Add the fennel bulbs and onions. Reduce the heat to low. Cook, stirring, until the vegetables are tender, about 8 minutes.
5. Add the wine and fennel seeds, then cover and heat to a boil. Boil, uncovered, over medium heat for 2 minutes. Add the tomatoes and heat to boiling. Reduce the heat to low and cook for 10 minutes.
6. Add the shrimp and fish to the pan and cook, covered, until the fish is tender, 3 to 5 minutes. Sprinkle with the fennel tops.

Per serving: 319 calories, 10 g total fat, 2 g saturated fat, 13 g carbohydrate, 30 g protein, 3 g fiber, 121 mg cholesterol, 178 mg sodium, 90 mg calcium

Curried Chicken Breasts with Butternut Squash, Green Beans, and Tomatoes

Serves 4

PREP TIME: **15 minutes**
COOK TIME: **30 minutes**

Fragrant with curry, cumin, and ginger, this luscious chicken dish is simmered in tomato sauce with chunks of potatoes and butternut squash and makes a great quick-and-easy dinner. Tomatoes are a good source of potassium, beta-carotene, and vitamin C, and Indian spices have been shown to have anti-inflammatory properties.

5 mL	1 teaspoon extra-virgin olive oil
125 mL	1/2 cup slivered onions
10 mL	2 teaspoons mild curry powder
5 mL	1 teaspoon ground cumin
625 g	1 1/4 pounds boneless, skinless chicken breasts, cut into 1-inch/2.5-cm pieces
1	1 can (28 ounces/796 mL) diced tomatoes (with juice)
125 mL	1/2 cup light coconut milk
500 mL	2 cups peeled, seeded, and cubed (1/4 inch/0.5 cm) butternut squash
5 mL	1 teaspoon grated fresh ginger
1 mL	1/4 teaspoon coarse salt
0.5 mL	1/8 teaspoon freshly ground black pepper
250 mL	1 cup frozen green peas
250 mL	1 cup trimmed green beans pieces (1 inch/2.5 cm)
500 mL	2 cups hot cooked brown Basmati rice
50 mL	1/4 cup finely chopped fresh cilantro

1. Heat the oil in a deep sauté pan set over medium heat, until shimmering. Add the onions and cook, stirring, until softened, about 3 minutes. Add the curry powder and cumin and stir to blend. Add the chicken and lightly brown, about 3 minutes. Remove the chicken pieces to a plate and set aside.
2. Add the tomatoes (with juice), coconut milk, squash, ginger, salt, and pepper to the onions and bring to a gentle boil over medium-low heat. Continue to cook, uncovered, until the sauce is slightly thickened, about 10 minutes.
3. Add the chicken and any accumulated juices, the peas, and green beans to the tomatoes. Cook, covered, until the chicken and beans are cooked through, about 5 minutes.
4. Serve over the rice and sprinkle with the cilantro.

Per serving: 393 calories, 7 g total fat, 3 g saturated fat, 50 g carbohydrate, 32 g protein, 8 g fiber, 73 mg cholesterol, 736 mg sodium, 105 mg calcium

Pan-Seared Chicken Thighs with Chimichurri Sauce

Serves 4

PREP TIME: **10 minutes**
COOK TIME: **15 minutes**

Chimichurri, a spicy fresh herb, garlic, and olive oil mixture is popular in Argentina, where it is served over meats. Here, it is used as both a marinade and a sauce over quick-seared boneless and skinless chicken thighs. The dark thigh meat of the chicken, while not as lean as the breast, is a great match for this deliciously tangy sauce.

250 mL	1 cup lightly packed cilantro leaves plus tender stems
125 mL	1/2 cup lightly packed parsley leaves plus tender stems
50 mL	1/4 cup fresh lemon juice
25 mL	2 tablespoons extra-virgin olive oil
25 mL	2 tablespoons water
5 mL	1 teaspoon ground cumin
1 mL	1/4 teaspoon coarse salt
0.5 mL	1/8 teaspoon ground red pepper
4	4 boneless, skinless chicken thighs, fat trimmed, patted dry, and halved
1	1 clove garlic, minced

1. Combine the cilantro, parsley, lemon juice, oil, water, cumin, salt, and pepper in a food processor or blender, and pulse until the herbs are finely chopped.
2. Place the chicken in a large bowl. Add 1 tablespoon (15 mL) of the sauce and toss to coat. Stir the garlic into the remaining sauce and transfer to a small serving bowl. Set aside.
3. Heat a large nonstick skillet over medium heat until hot enough that a drop of water sizzles. Coat the pan lightly with nonstick cooking spray. Add the chicken without crowding, cooking it in two batches, if necessary. Pan-sear the chicken, adjusting the heat to maintain a steady sizzle until the meat is browned and cooked through, about 5 minutes per side. With all the chicken thighs in the skillet, add any remaining marinade. Cook, turning the chicken, for about 3 minutes.
4. Transfer to a serving plate and serve the sauce on the side.

Per serving: 158 calories, 10 g total fat, 2 g saturated fat, 3 g carbohydrate, 14 g protein, 1 g fiber, 57 mg cholesterol, 212 mg sodium, 29 mg calcium

Braised Chicken Breasts with Garlic, Lentils, and Asparagus

Serves 4

PREP TIME: **30 minutes**
COOK TIME: **30 minutes**

In this luscious and earthy dish, a richly flavored garlic sauce coats pieces of gently braised chicken. Fiber- and protein-packed lentils, flavored with orange zest, complement the chicken both in flavor and texture. Fear not: Cooking whole garlic cloves mellows the flavor.

4	4 boneless, skinless chicken breasts (about 5 ounces/150 g each), fat trimmed
15 mL	1 tablespoon chopped fresh thyme leaves, divided
5 mL	1 teaspoon minced orange zest, divided
2 mL	1/2 teaspoon freshly ground black pepper, divided
15 mL	1 tablespoon extra-virgin olive oil
10	10 cloves garlic, trimmed and bruised with the side of a knife
625 mL	2 1/2 cups reduced-sodium low-fat chicken broth, divided
150 mL	2/3 cup brown lentils
375 mL	1 1/2 cups trimmed asparagus pieces (1 inch/2.5 cm)

1. In a large bowl, season the chicken with 1 teaspoon (5 mL) of the thyme, 1/2 teaspoon (2 mL) of the orange zest, and 1/4 teaspoon (1 mL) of the pepper.
2. Heat the oil in a deep 10-inch (25-cm) skillet or sauté pan over medium heat, until it shimmers. Reduce the heat to medium-low. Add the chicken and garlic, and cook for 3 minutes. Turn the chicken and cook for an additional 2 minutes. Add 1/2 cup (125 mL) of the broth. Reduce the heat to low. Cover and cook until the chicken is cooked through and the garlic is soft, about 10 minutes. Transfer the chicken to a plate and cover with foil.
3. Transfer the braising liquid and garlic to a blender or food processor and puree. Pour into a small saucepan and keep warm.
4. In the same pan, bring the remaining 2 cups (500 mL) of broth to a boil. Stir in the lentils and cook, covered, over medium-low heat until almost tender; continue to boil, uncovered, over medium heat to evaporate the excess liquid.
5. Stir the asparagus, the remaining 1/2 teaspoon (2 mL) of orange zest, and the remaining 1/4 teaspoon (1 mL) of pepper into the lentils. Arrange the chicken on top. Cook, covered, until asparagus is crisp-tender and chicken is heated, about 3 minutes. Pour the garlic sauce over the chicken and sprinkle with the remaining 2 teaspoons (10 mL) of thyme before serving.

Per serving: 419 calories, 10 g total fat, 2 g saturated fat, 27 g carbohydrate, 55 g protein, 6 g fiber, 136 mg cholesterol, 536 mg sodium, 79 mg calcium

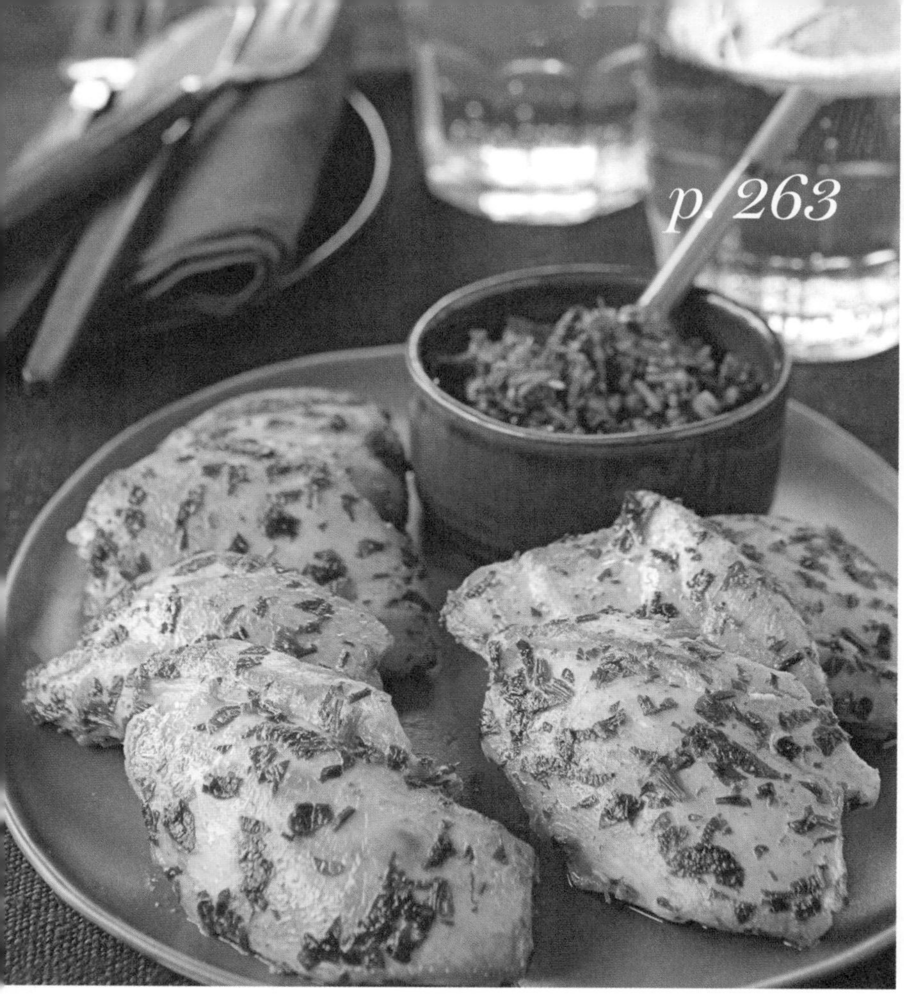
p. 263

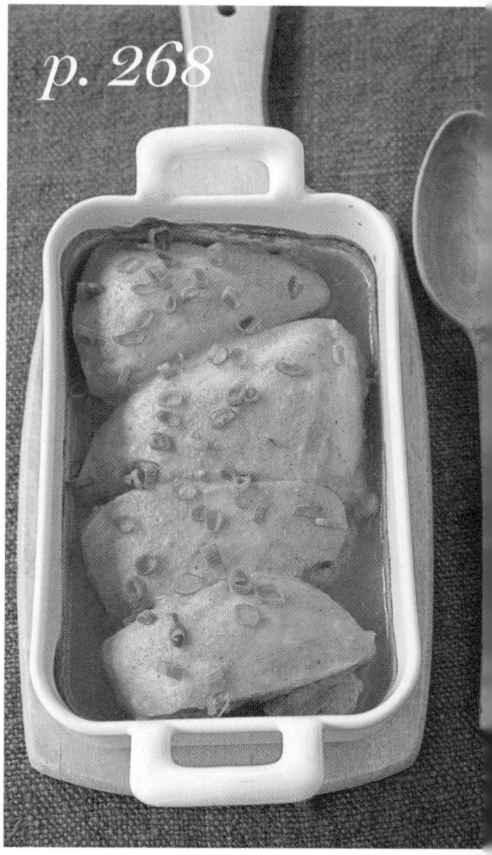
p. 268

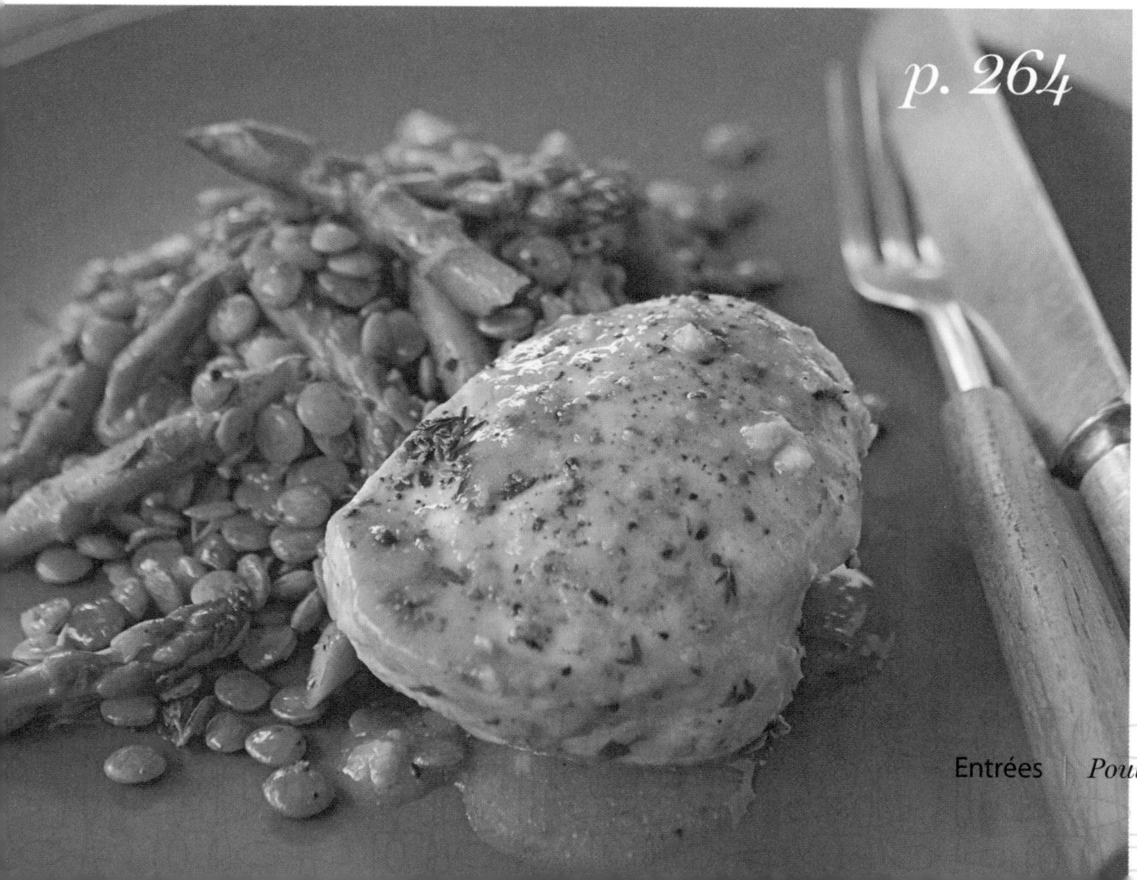
p. 264

Hazelnut-Crusted Turkey Cutlets with Parmesan and Rosemary

Serves 4

PREP TIME: **15 minutes**
COOK TIME: **15 minutes**

Hazelnuts, Parmesan, and rosemary dress up these turkey cutlets, making them crunchy on the outside and moist and tender on the inside. Turkey breast cutlets are a great low-fat source of protein. Hazelnuts, although fairly caloric, add fiber, protein, and good fats to your diet.

125 mL	1/2 cup roasted, peeled, and finely chopped hazelnuts
125 mL	1/2 cup plain breadcrumbs
25 mL	2 tablespoons freshly grated Parmesan
2	2 egg whites
10 mL	2 teaspoons snipped fresh rosemary leaves or 1 teaspoon/5 mL chopped dried
0.5 mL	1/8 teaspoon freshly ground black pepper
8	8 turkey breast cutlets (1/4 inch/0.5 cm thick), about 1 1/2 pounds/ 750 g
25 mL	2 tablespoons extra-virgin olive oil
1	1 sprig of rosemary

1. Combine the nuts, breadcrumbs, and Parmesan in a shallow bowl. In another shallow bowl, whisk together the egg whites, rosemary leaves, and pepper until frothy. Dip the turkey in the egg whites, let the excess drip off, then roll in the nut mixture, pressing to coat.
2. Heat a large nonstick skillet over medium heat until hot enough that a drop of water sizzles. Add the oil and tilt the pan to coat. Add the cutlets, in batches, if necessary, and cook until lightly browned, about 3 minutes. Turn and cook until the turkey is cooked through, about 2 minutes longer.
3. Arrange on a platter and top with the rosemary sprig.

Per serving: 414 calories, 18 g total fat, 3 g saturated fat, 13 g carbohydrate, 49 g protein, 2 g fiber, 60 mg cholesterol, 421 mg sodium, 88 mg calcium

Herb-Roasted Turkey Breast

Serves 8–10

PREP TIME: **30 minutes**
COOK TIME: **2 hours 15 minutes**

The secret to moist, tender turkey meat is not added fat, but to turn the breast as it roasts. This technique allows the meat to self-baste. Turkey breast is an excellent source of protein and is relatively low in total fat. Enjoy the flavor of Thanksgiving anytime of year.

3	3 cloves garlic, divided
25 mL	2 tablespoons minced flat-leaf parsley
10 mL	2 teaspoons dried rosemary, crumbled
2 mL	1/2 teaspoon coarsely ground black pepper
2 mL	1/2 teaspoon grated lemon zest
1	1 bone-in whole turkey breast (6 to 7 pounds/3 to 3.5 kg)
1	1 large onion, cut in thin wedges (1/8 inch/0.25 cm)
1	1 rib celery (with leaves), cut into 1-inch/2.5-cm lengths
1	1 carrot, peeled and diagonally sliced (1/2 inch/1 cm)
1	1 parsnip, peeled, trimmed, and diagonally sliced (1/2 inch/1 cm)
1	1 bay leaf
2	2 cans (14 ounces/398 mL each) fat-free reduced-sodium chicken broth

1. Position an oven rack in the lower third of the oven and preheat the oven to 400°F (200°C).
2. Mince 2 of the garlic cloves and place them in a small bowl. Add the parsley, rosemary, pepper, and lemon zest and stir until well-blended.
3. Rinse the turkey breast with cold water, drain, and pat dry with paper towels. Gently separate the skin from the turkey on either side of the breast bone to make pockets. Rub the herb mixture under the skin and onto the meat.
4. Spread the onions, celery, carrots, and parsnips in the bottom of a medium-size roasting pan. Add the garlic and the bay leaf to the pan. Place the turkey, skin side down, on top of the vegetables. Add the broth and cover the turkey breast loosely with foil.
5. Roast the turkey for 1 hour, basting with the pan juices every 20 minutes. Remove the pan from the oven. Lower the temperature to 350° F (180°C) and remove the foil. Turn the turkey skin side up. Roast, uncovered, basting every 20 minutes, until the temperature on a meat thermometer registers 170°F (80°C), about 1 1/2 hours. Transfer the turkey breast to a cutting board. Place a strainer over a medium saucepan and strain the broth, discarding the vegetables and the bay leaf. Boil over high heat until reduced by half. Serve broth on the side.

Per serving: 254 calories, 1 g total fat, 0 g saturated fat, 7 g carbohydrate, 51 g protein, 2 g fiber, 123 mg cholesterol, 344 mg sodium, 53 mg calcium

Tandoori Chicken

Serves 4

PREP TIME: **15 minutes**
COOK TIME: **20 minutes**

Oven-roasted chicken breasts emerge spicy and moist from a highly seasoned Indian-inspired yogurt marinade. Researchers continue to study the positive impact that compounds in spices like turmeric, ginger, and chiles have on our health.

250 mL	1 cup plain low-fat yogurt
50 mL	1/4 cup chopped scallion (white part only)
15 mL	1 tablespoon chopped fresh ginger
1	1 jalapeño, seeded, deveined, and chopped (wear gloves when handling)
15 mL	1 tablespoon paprika
15 mL	1 tablespoon curry powder
2 mL	1/2 teaspoon ground turmeric
1	1 clove garlic, crushed
4	4 boneless, skinless chicken breasts (5 ounces/150 g each), fat trimmed
25 mL	2 tablespoons thinly sliced scallion (green part only)

1. Puree the yogurt, white scallions, ginger, jalapeños, paprika, curry, turmeric, and garlic in a blender or food processor. Transfer to a medium bowl. Add the chicken and toss to coat. Cover and refrigerate for 30 minutes.
2. Preheat the oven to 450°F (230°C). Arrange the chicken in a roasting pan and spoon half of the marinade over the chicken. Discard the remaining marinade.
3. Roast the chicken until the juices run clear when pierced with knife, about 7 minutes. Sprinkle with the green scallions.

Per serving: 248 calories, 5 g total fat, 2 g saturated fat, 12 g carbohydrate, 36 g protein, 1 g fiber, 98 mg cholesterol, 257 mg sodium, 175 mg calcium

Lamb Stew with Artichoke Hearts and New Potatoes

Serves 4

PREP TIME: **15 minutes**
COOK TIME: **1 hour 10 minutes**

15 mL	1 tablespoon extra-virgin olive oil
125 mL	1/2 cup chopped onion
50 mL	1/4 cup chopped celery
50 mL	1/4 cup diced carrot
1	1 clove garlic, finely chopped
375 g	12 ounces lamb sirloin cut into 3/4-inch/1.5-cm cubes
2 mL	1/2 teaspoon dried oregano
2 mL	1/2 teaspoon salt
0.5 mL	1/8 teaspoon freshly ground black pepper
1	1 can (14.5 ounces/396 mL) diced tomatoes (with juice)
1	1 strip (1/2 × 2 inches/ 1 cm × 5 cm) orange zest
4	4 small unpeeled, new potatoes, quartered
1	1 box (8 ounces/226 g) frozen artichoke hearts
250 mL	1 cup frozen green peas

Tender morsels of lamb, chunks of potatoes, tender green peas, and delicate artichoke hearts make a luscious, easy stew that is perfect anytime, but it's truly remarkable in the spring, when lamb is at its most succulent. Artichokes and potatoes cooked with the skins on are excellent sources of vitamins and fiber.

1. Heat the oil in large deep skillet or sauté pan set over medium-high heat, until shimmering. Add the onions, celery, carrots, and garlic. Cook, stirring continually, over low heat until the vegetables are tender but not browned, about 10 minutes.
2. Raise the heat to high. Add the lamb, oregano, salt, and pepper and sear until brown on all sides, about 5 minutes.
3. Add the tomatoes (with juice) and orange zest, stirring and scraping up any browned bits in the bottom of the pan, and heat to boiling. Reduce the heat to low and cook, covered, until the meat is fork-tender and the juices have thickened, about 45 minutes.
4. Add the potatoes and artichokes and cook, covered, until the vegetables are tender, about 10 minutes. Add the peas and cook for 5 minutes longer.

Per serving: 278 calories, 8 g total fat, 2 g saturated fat, 27 g carbohydrate, 23 g protein, 8 g fiber, 54 mg cholesterol, 596 mg sodium, 76 mg calcium

Marinated Lamb Kebabs with Zucchini, Tomatoes, and Red Onions

Serves 4

PREP TIME: **30 minutes**
COOK TIME: **10–12 minutes**

125 mL	1/2 cup fresh lime juice
15 mL	1 tablespoon finely chopped fresh cilantro
15 mL	1 tablespoon chopped fresh mint
10 mL	2 teaspoons ground cumin
5 mL	1 teaspoon seeded, deveined, and finely chopped jalapeño (wear gloves when handling)
2 mL	1/2 teaspoon coarse salt
0.5 mL	1/8 teaspoon freshly ground black pepper
500 g	1 pound boneless lamb sirloin, cut into 20 (about 2 × 1-inch/5 cm × 2.5 cm) pieces
8	8 pieces zucchini (1 inch/2.5 cm)
8	8 red onion wedges (1/2 inch/1 cm)
16	16 cherry tomatoes

The fresh, clean flavors of lime juice, cilantro, and cumin give this marinade a distinctively Southwestern flavor. Using half of the marinade for the meat and the other half for the vegetables gives these kebabs a superb flavor boost. Lamb is generally less marbled with saturated fat than beef, making it a great lower-fat choice for kebabs.

1. Whisk together the lime juice, cilantro, mint, cumin, jalapeños, salt, and pepper in a medium bowl until blended. Transfer half of the mixture to another medium bowl.
2. Place the meat in one bowl and the zucchini, onions, and tomatoes in the other bowl. Toss to coat and let stand at room temperature for about 10 minutes.
3. Preheat a grill or broiler to medium. Thread the meat and vegetables onto 4 metal skewers, distributing evenly. Brush with any remaining marinade.
4. Grill the kebabs for about 12 minutes (or broil for about 8 minutes), or until the meat reaches the desired doneness, turning often so that the meat and vegetables cook evenly. Arrange on a platter and serve.

Per serving: 284 calories, 7 g total fat, 2 g saturated fat, 29 g carbohydrate, 29 g protein, 8 g fiber, 73 mg cholesterol, 400 mg sodium, 102 mg calcium

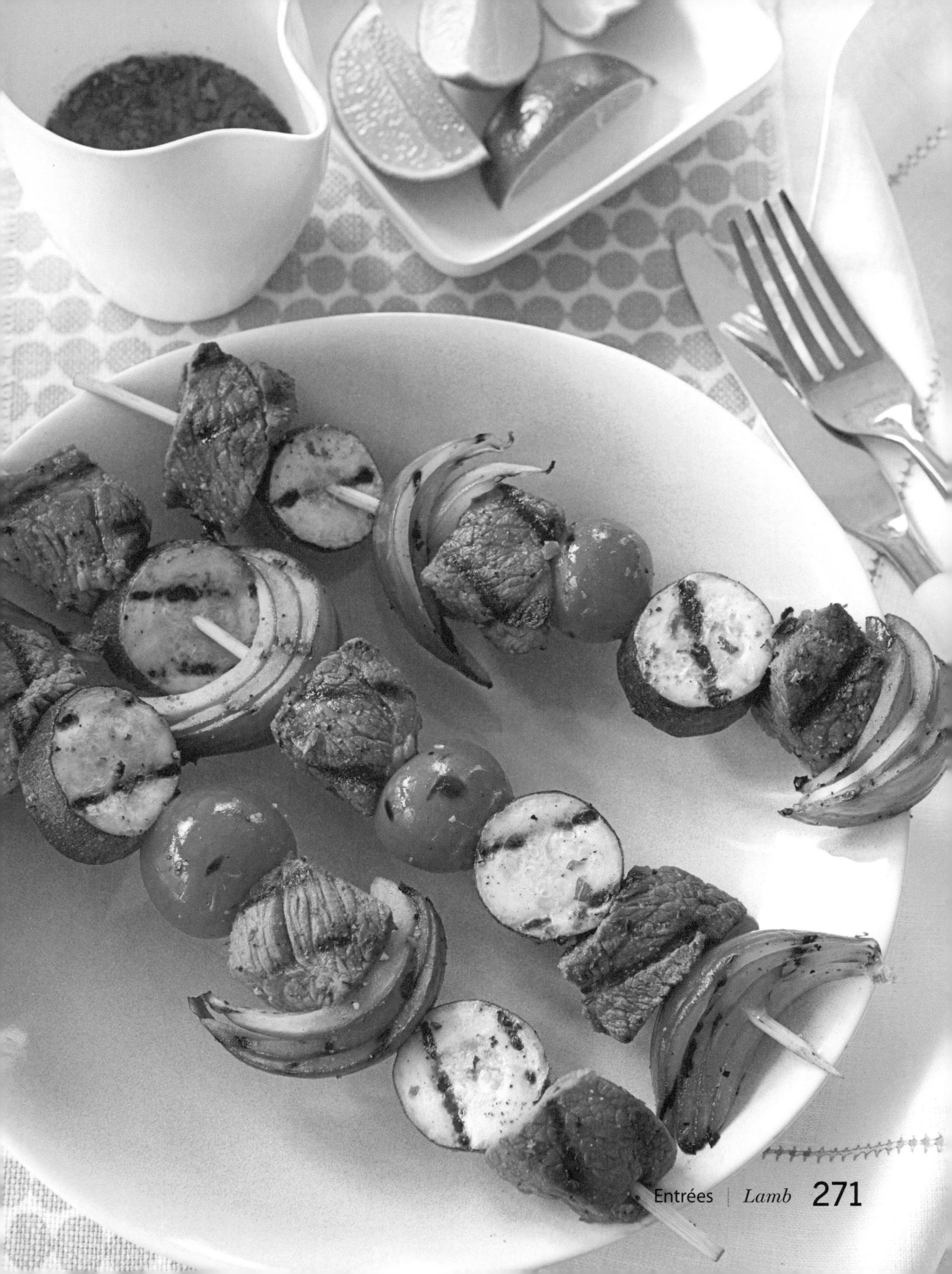

Rosemary-Crusted Pork Tenderloin with Roasted Tomatoes and White Beans

Serves 4

PREP TIME: **20 minutes**
COOK TIME: **55 minutes**

15 mL	1 tablespoon chopped fresh rosemary or 1 teaspoon/5 mL dried
1	1 clove garlic, chopped
1 mL	1/4 teaspoon coarse salt
1 mL	1/4 teaspoon coarsely ground black pepper
625 g	1 1/4 pounds pork tenderloin, patted dry
375 mL	1 1/2 cups cherry or grape tomatoes
2	2 cans (15 ounces/540 mL each) cannellini beans, rinsed and drained
15 mL	1 tablespoon pitted and coarsely chopped Kalamata olives
15 mL	1 tablespoon extra-virgin olive oil, divided

Fragrant rosemary and pungent fresh garlic mashed together with coarsely ground black pepper and coarse salt permeate the pork and flavor the accompanying beans. You don't need to shy away from pork—lean tenderloin is a great choice for the heart-healthy kitchen.

1. Preheat the oven to 400°F (200°C).
2. Place the rosemary and garlic on a cutting board and finely chop them together. Place in a small bowl and mash the salt and pepper into the mixture with the back of a spoon. Spread the paste on the surface of the pork and let stand at room temperature for about 30 minutes.
3. Heat a large nonstick skillet over medium-high heat, and coat with nonstick cooking spray. Add the pork and sear on all sides until lightly browned, about 20 seconds per side. Place it in a 9 × 13-inch (22 × 33-cm) baking pan and scatter the cherry tomatoes around it. Roast until the pork registers 145°F (65°C) on a meat thermometer, about 25 minutes.
4. Remove the pork to a cutting board and loosely cover with foil. Add the beans and olives to the baking dish with the roasted tomatoes. Drizzle with the oil and cover with foil. Roast until heated through, 8 to 10 minutes.
5. Cut the pork in diagonal slices (1/2 inch/1 cm). Remove the beans from the oven and remove the foil. Arrange the pork slices down the center of the pan, overlapping them as needed.

Per serving: 353 calories, 7 g total fat, 2 g saturated fat, 30 g carbohydrate, 41 g protein, 9 g fiber, 92 mg cholesterol, 589 mg sodium, 100 mg calcium

Pork Tenderloin Medallions with Lemon and Honey Mustard Sauce

Serves 4

PREP TIME: **25 minutes**
COOK TIME: **10 minutes**

625 g	1 1/4 pounds pork tenderloin
15 mL	1 tablespoon minced fresh thyme leaves
5 mL	1 teaspoon grated lemon zest
0.5 mL	1/8 teaspoon freshly ground black pepper
5 mL	1 tablespoon olive oil
25 mL	2 tablespoons minced shallots
125 mL	1/2 cup reduced-sodium low-fat chicken broth
25 mL	2 tablespoons fresh lemon juice
5 mL	1 teaspoon honey mustard, or to taste

This tender sauté of pork tenderloin pounded into thin medallions and glazed with a piquant sauce of lemon, honey, and mustard is especially quick and easy to prepare. Pork is an excellent source of thiamin, an important B vitamin, as well as niacin, phosphorus, and potassium.

1. Slice the pork into 12 medallions, each about 3/4-inch/1.5-cm thick. Layer a few at a time between sheets of plastic wrap and pound with a meat pounder or the bottom of a small heavy skillet until they are about 1/4-inch/0.5-cm thick.
2. Combine the thyme, lemon zest, and pepper in a cup and sprinkle it evenly over the pork, pressing it into the surface with your fingertips.
3. Heat the oil in a medium skillet or sauté pan set over medium-high heat until hot enough that a drop of water sizzles. Add the pork, a few slices at a time, and cook for 3 minutes. Turn and cook the other side for 2 minutes longer. Remove to a plate.
4. Reduce the heat to medium-low, add the shallots to the pan and cook, stirring, until tender, about 3 minutes.
5. Add the broth and raise the heat to high. Boil, stirring to loosen any browned bits from the pan, until the liquid is reduced by half. Add the lemon juice and honey mustard, stirring until blended. Return the pork to the pan turning it in the sauce just to heat through.

Per serving: 196 calories, 7 g total fat, 1 g saturated fat, 2 g carbohydrate, 30 g protein, 0 g fiber, 92 mg cholesterol, 143 mg sodium, 14 mg calcium

Grilled Flank Steak and Sweet Potatoes with Dried Tomato, Caper, and Parsley Sauce

Serves 4

PREP TIME: **53 minutes**
COOK TIME: **20 minutes**

Fire up the grill for this new twist on the meat-and-potatoes theme. Bright green parsley pureed with olive oil and vinegar makes a zippy sauce to spoon over thin slices of perfectly cooked flank steak and wedges of bright orange grilled sweet potatoes. Both parsley and sweet potatoes are flush with beta-carotene and vitamin C.

625 g	1 1/4 pounds flank steak, fat trimmed
80 mL	1/3 cup plus 3 tablespoons red-wine vinegar, divided
1 mL	1/4 teaspoon freshly ground black pepper
4	4 small sweet potatoes (preferably Garnet) unpeeled, scrubbed, and quartered lengthwise
5 mL	1 teaspoon extra-virgin olive oil
4	4 sun-dried tomato halves
175 mL	3/4 cup lightly packed Italian parsley with tender stems
50 mL	1/4 cup lightly packed mint leaves
1	1 clove garlic, coarsely chopped
25 mL	2 tablespoons olive oil
25 mL	2 tablespoons water
15 mL	1 tablespoon capers, rinsed and patted dry

1. Place the meat on a platter and sprinkle it with 3 tablespoons (45 mL) of the vinegar and the pepper. Turn to evenly coat and let stand at room temperature for 20 to 30 minutes.
2. Place the sweet potatoes in a large bowl. Drizzle with the extra-virgin olive oil, and toss to coat. Set aside.
3. Place the tomatoes in small bowl and add hot water to cover. Let stand for 10 minutes.
4. Chop the parsley, mint, and garlic in a food processor. Add the remaining 1/3 cup (75 mL) of vinegar, the oil, and water. Pulse just to combine. Transfer to small serving bowl.
5. Drain the tomatoes and cut into 1/4-inch (0.5-cm) pieces. Mix into the parsley sauce, along with the capers. Set aside.
6. Preheat a grill to medium. Place the sweet potatoes and steak on the grill. Cook the sweet potatoes until tender, turning often, 15 to 20 minutes. Grill the steak until it reaches the desired doneness, 6 to 8 minutes per side for medium-rare.
7. Remove the steak to a cutting board and let stand for 5 minutes. Cut across the grain in thin slices and arrange on a platter. Place the sweet potatoes around the edges. Spoon the sauce over the top and serve.

Per serving: 336 calories, 16 g total fat, 4 g saturated fat, 13 g carbohydrate, 32 g protein, 3 g fiber, 47 mg cholesterol, 225 mg sodium, 78 mg calcium

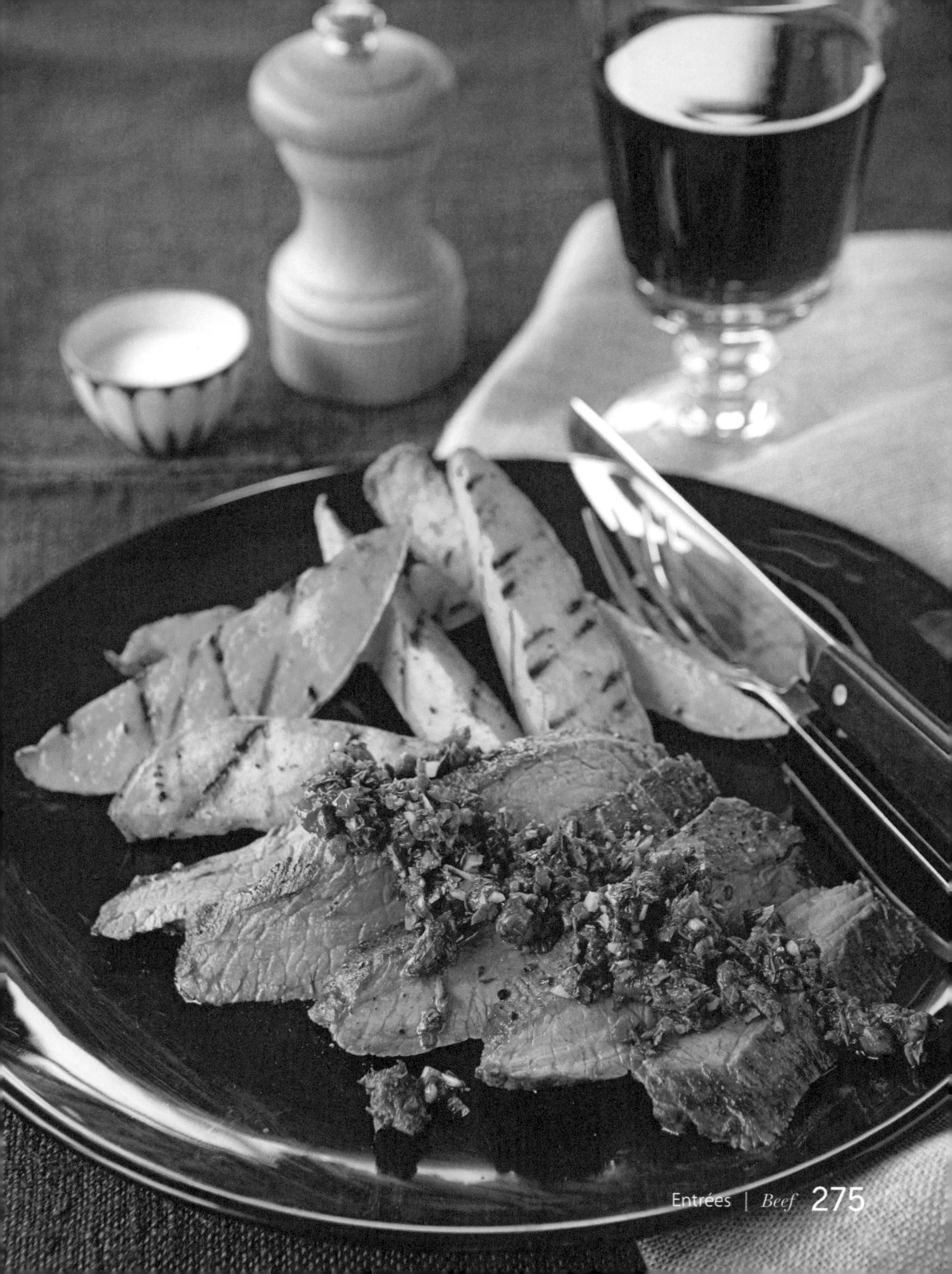

Zinfandel Beef Stew with Roasted Vegetables

Serves 4

Tender chunks of beef are lapped with a rich sauce of pureed vegetables, red wine, and broth. Additional vegetables are oven-roasted to perfect doneness and then folded into the finished stew. Lean cuts of beef such as round are the best choices for a heart-healthy diet.

PREP TIME: **30 minutes**
COOK TIME: **2 hours**

625 g	1 1/4 pounds beef round, patted dry and cut into 1-inch/2.5-cm cubes
2 mL	1/2 teaspoon coarse salt
2 mL	1/2 teaspoon freshly ground black pepper
45 mL	3 tablespoons extra-virgin olive oil, divided
125 mL	1/2 cup chopped onion
125 mL	1/2 cup chopped carrot
125 mL	1/2 cup chopped celery
250 mL	1 cup Zinfandel or other hearty red wine
1	1 bay leaf
1	1 can (15 ounces/540 mL) reduced-sodium low-fat beef broth
1	1 can (14.5 ounces/396 mL) diced tomatoes
2	2 leeks, roots and tops trimmed, washed, cut into 1-inch/2.5-cm pieces
2	2 small carrots, cut into 1/2-inch/1-cm lengths
2	2 Yukon gold potatoes, unpeeled, cut into 1/2-inch/1-cm cubes
1	1 parsnip, trimmed and cut into 1/2-inch/1-cm pieces
5 mL	1 teaspoon chopped fresh thyme leaves
15 mL	1 tablespoon minced flat-leaf parsley

1. Sprinkle the meat with the salt and 1/4 teaspoon (1 mL) of the pepper. Heat a large Dutch oven over medium-high heat and add 2 tablespoons (25 mL) of the oil. When the oil is hot, gradually add the meat and brown it on all sides, turning as needed, about 8 minutes. Add the onions, chopped carrots, and celery and cook, stirring, until tender, about 5 minutes.

2. Add the wine and bay leaf and bring to boil. Cook until reduced by half, about 5 minutes. Add the broth and tomatoes (with juice). Bring to a boil, and cook, covered, over medium-low heat until the meat is tender, about 1 1/2 hours.

3. With a slotted spoon, remove the meat to a large bowl. Remove and discard the bay leaf. Cool the liquid and vegetables, then puree in a blender or food processor until smooth. Return the sauce and meat to the Dutch oven and keep warm over low heat.

4. Preheat the oven to 400°F (200°C). Spread the leeks, the 1/2-inch (1-cm) carrots, the potatoes, and parsnips in a 9 × 13-inch (22 × 33-cm) baking dish. Drizzle with the remaining 1 tablespoon (15 mL) of oil, and add the remaining (5 mL) thyme and the remaining 1/4 teaspoon (1 mL) of pepper. Bake for 25 minutes. Turn with a spatula and bake until golden and tender, about 20 minutes longer.

5. Fold the roasted vegetables into the stew and sprinkle with the parsley. Serve in warm bowls.

Per serving: 497 calories, 18 g total fat, 4 g saturated fat, 36 g carbohydrate, 38 g protein, 6 g fiber, 82 mg cholesterol, 717 mg sodium, 133 mg calcium

Orange and Soy-Glazed Beef Stir-Fry with Green Beans, Mini Bell Peppers, and Peanuts

Serves 4

PREP TIME: **20 minutes**
COOK TIME: **16 minutes**

A quick flash in the pan with a little heart-healthy oil is all it takes to create a colorful and vegetable-filled tasty beef stir-fry. Peanuts add extra crunch and are a good source of protein, niacin, phosphorus, and potassium.

375 g	12 ounces shoulder or round steak, well-trimmed and cut into 1/2-inch/1-cm) cubes
25 mL	2 tablespoons reduced-sodium soy sauce, divided
25 mL	2 tablespoons orange marmalade, divided
3	3 cloves garlic, minced, divided
1 mL	1/4 teaspoon crushed red pepper
15 mL	1 tablespoon extra-virgin olive oil
250 g	8 ounces green beans, trimmed and cut into 1 1/2-inch/3.5-cm lengths
250 g	8 ounces mini multicolored bell peppers or 1 red bell pepper, seeded and cut into strips (1/4-inch/0.5-cm wide)
15 mL	1 tablespoon minced fresh ginger
50 mL	1/4 cup water
25 mL	2 tablespoons thinly sliced scallion
50 mL	1/4 cup chopped unsalted dry-roasted peanuts

1. Combine the beef, 1 tablespoon (15 mL) of the soy sauce, 1 tablespoon (15 mL) of the marmalade, 1 of the garlic cloves, and the crushed red pepper in a large bowl. Stir to blend; set aside.
2. In a small bowl, combine the remaining 1 tablespoon (15 mL) of soy sauce, the remaining 1 tablespoon (15 mL) of marmalade, and another garlic clove. Set aside.
3. Heat a wok or large skillet over high heat until hot. Carefully add the oil and the beef mixture. Stir-fry until no longer pink, about 5 minutes. Transfer to a plate and set aside.
4. Add the beans, bell peppers, ginger, and remaining garlic to the wok and stir-fry for 1 minute. Add the water, cover, and steam the vegetables until crisp-tender, about 4 minutes.
5. Return the beef to the wok. Add the reserved soy sauce mixture and stir until heated. Sprinkle with the scallions and nuts.

Per serving: 260 calories, 12 g total fat, 2 g saturated fat, 17 g carbohydrate, 23 g protein, 4 g fiber, 47 mg cholesterol, 341 mg sodium, 70 mg calcium

Entrées | SEAFOOD

Pan-Seared Shrimp with Lemon Orzo Primavera

Serves 4

PREP TIME: **30 minutes**
COOK TIME: **25 minutes**

625 mL	2 1/2 cups water
250 mL	1 cup coarsely chopped carrot
250 mL	1 cup trimmed asparagus slices
250 mL	1 cup frozen petite peas
250 mL	1 cup whole-wheat or white orzo pasta
375 g	12 ounces large shelled and deveined shrimp
15 mL	1 tablespoon extra-virgin olive oil
5 mL	1 teaspoon lemon zest, divided
2 mL	1/2 teaspoon fresh thyme or 1/4 teaspoon/ 1 mL dried
	Pinch of red pepper flakes
50 mL	1/4 cup fresh lemon juice, divided
50 mL	1/4 cup chopped red bell pepper
25 mL	2 tablespoons finely chopped parsley

Orzo, a tiny, oval-shaped pasta that cooks like rice, tossed with colorful crisp-cooked vegetables is a perfect canvas for lemony seared shrimp. Shrimp is low in fat and calories, but higher in cholesterol, therefore it should be enjoyed in moderation.

1. Bring the water to a boil in a medium saucepan set over medium-high heat. Add the carrots, asparagus, and peas. Boil for 3 minutes. Remove the vegetables with a slotted spoon to a medium bowl.
2. Add the orzo to the water and bring back to a boil. Reduce the heat to low and cook, covered, until the water is absorbed and the orzo is just cooked, about 15 minutes.
3. Meanwhile, combine the shrimp in a medium bowl with the oil, 1/2 teaspoon (2 mL) of the lemon zest, 1/2 teaspoon (2 mL) of the fresh thyme or 1/4 teaspoon (1 mL) of the dried thyme, and the pepper flakes.
4. Heat a 12-inch (30-cm) skillet over medium-high heat until hot enough that a drop of water sizzles. Add the shrimp and sear until browned and cooked through, about 2 minutes per side. Reduce the heat to medium-low. Add 3 tablespoons (45 mL) of the lemon juice and stir with a flat-edged spatula to deglaze the pan and coat the shrimp.
5. Fold the vegetables, red bell peppers, parsley, the remaining 1 tablespoon (15 mL) of lemon juice, and the remaining 1/2 teaspoon (2 mL) of lemon zest into the orzo and spoon into a deep serving dish. Top with the shrimp and drizzle with the pan juices.

Per serving: 382 calories, 6 g total fat, 1 g saturated fat, 54 g carbohydrate, 28 g protein, 5 g fiber, 129 mg cholesterol, 192 mg sodium, 71 mg calcium

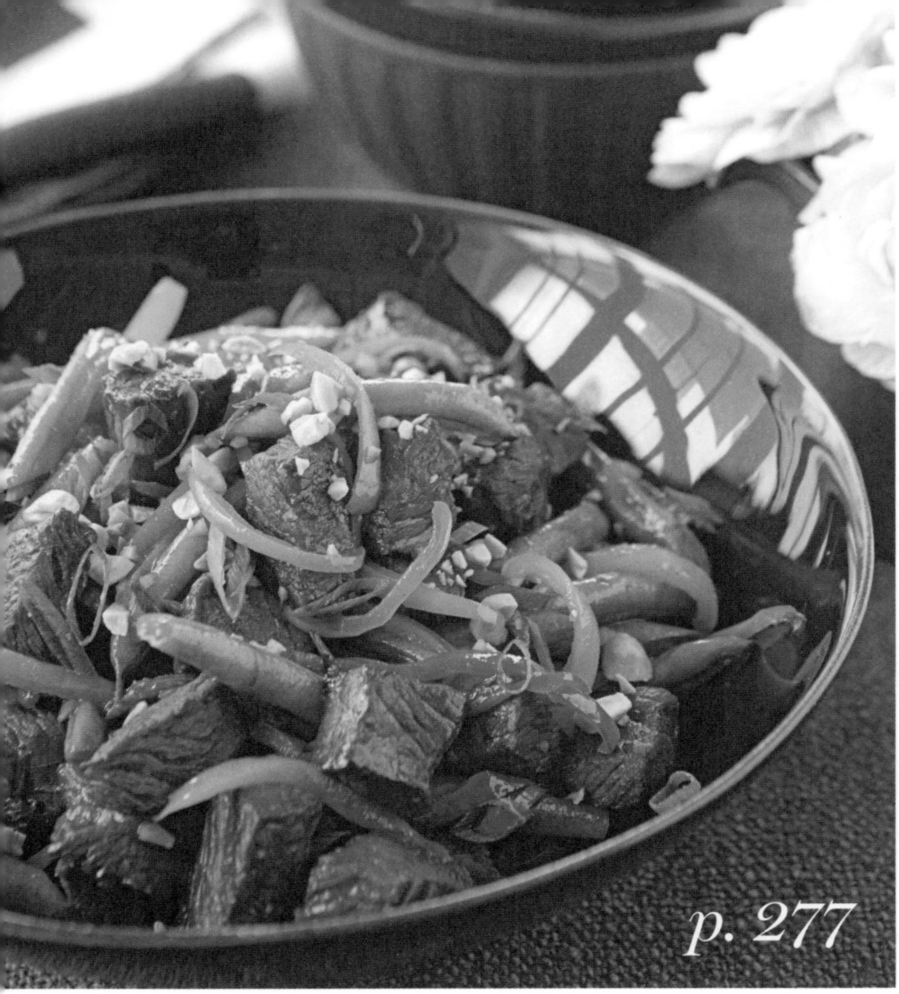
p. 277

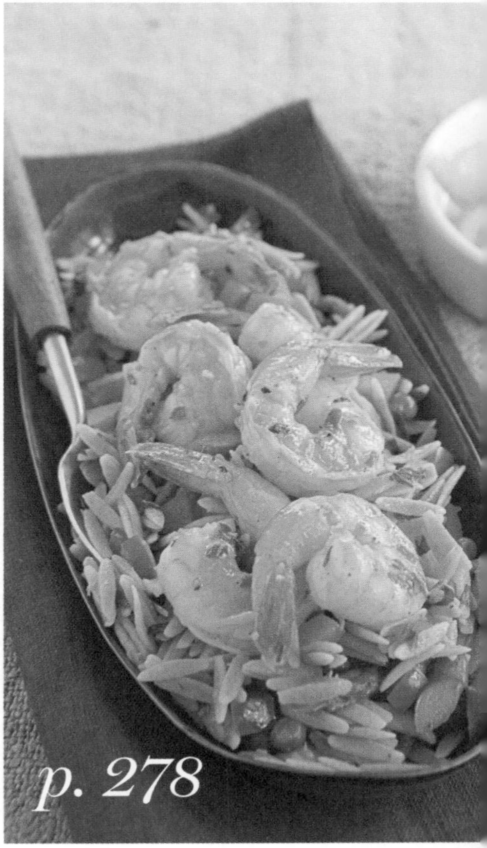
p. 278

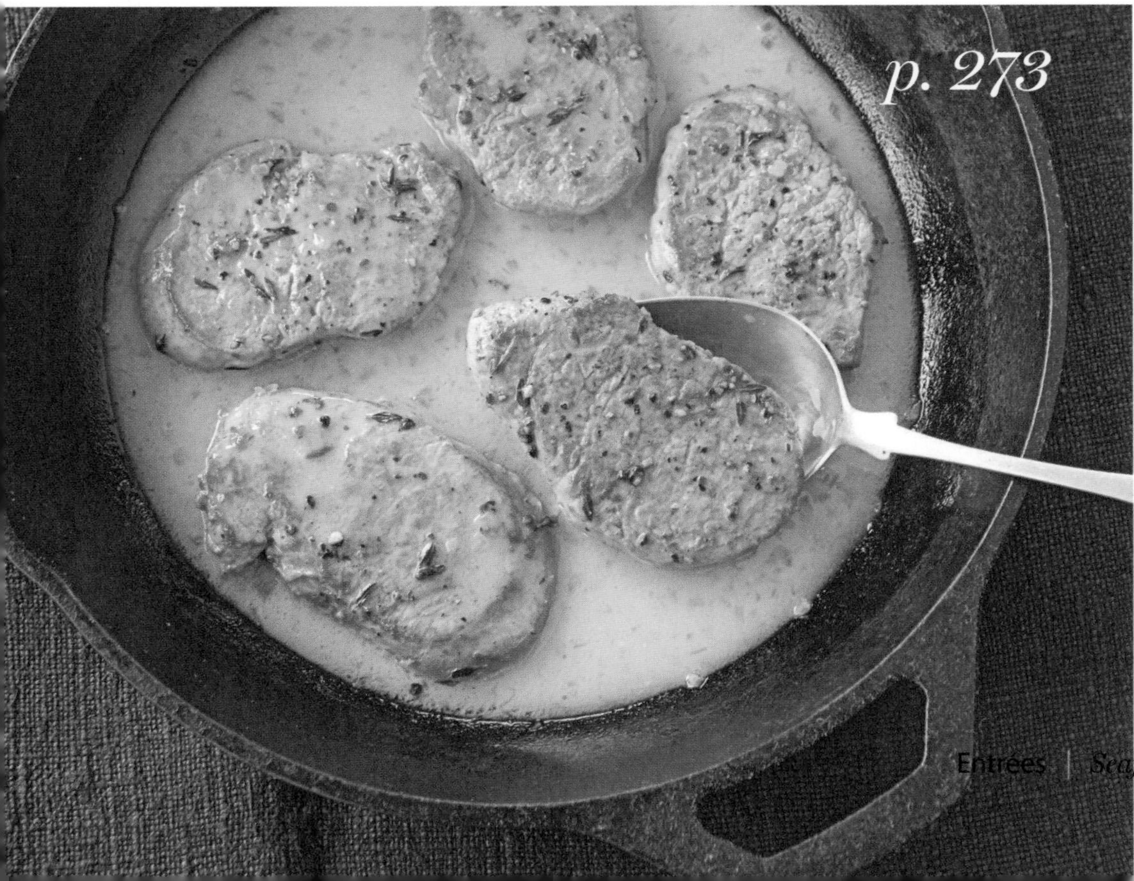
p. 273

Orange-Glazed Roasted Salmon with Tricolor Bell Peppers

Serves 4

Served on a colorful medley of roasted bell peppers, this salmon is glazed with a tangy mixture of orange, honey, and soy sauce. Salmon is an excellent source of omega-3 fatty acids and bell peppers are high in vitamin C and beta-carotene, but red peppers are highest in both nutrients.

PREP TIME: **15 minutes**
COOK TIME: **50 minutes**

1	1 small red bell pepper, seeded, trimmed, and cut into 1/2-inch/1-cm strips
1	1 small yellow bell pepper, seeded, trimmed, and cut into 1/2-inch/1-cm strips
1	1 small green bell pepper, seeded, trimmed, and cut into 1/2-inch/1-cm strips
1	1 medium onion, cut into thin wedges (1/4 inch/0.5 cm)
15 mL	1 tablespoon extra-virgin olive oil
15 mL	1 tablespoon thawed frozen orange juice concentrate
15 mL	1 tablespoon honey
5 mL	1 teaspoon reduced-sodium soy sauce
4	4 boneless, skinless salmon fillets (about 5 ounces/150 g each)

1. Preheat the oven to 400°F (200°F).
2. Spread the red, yellow, and green peppers and onions in a 9 × 13-inch (22 × 33-cm) baking dish and drizzle with the oil. Roast, stirring once or twice, until the peppers are tender and beginning to brown, about 35 minutes.
3. Meanwhile stir the orange juice concentrate, honey, and soy sauce together in small bowl. Set aside.
4. Remove the baking dish from the oven and increase the temperature to 450°F (230°C). Arrange the fish in a single layer, redistributing the vegetables around the fish. Spoon the orange juice mixture over the fish. Roast until the center of the thickest part of the fish is opaque, 10 to 15 minutes, depending on the thickness.
5. To serve, place the vegetables on four plates and top each with a salmon fillet.

Per serving: 279 calories, 13 g total fat, 2 g saturated fat, 12 g carbohydrate, 29 g protein, 2 g fiber, 78 mg cholesterol, 110 mg sodium, 33 mg calcium

Broiled Fish Steaks with Tomato, Peach, and Orange Salsa

Serves 4

PREP TIME: **20 minutes**
COOK TIME: **5 minutes**

4	4 fish steaks (about 5 ounces/150 g each)
5 mL	1 teaspoon extra-virgin olive oil
	Freshly ground black pepper, to taste
375 mL	1 1/2 cups coarsely chopped plum tomatoes
250 mL	1 cup coarsely chopped peeled ripe peaches or nectarines
1	1 seedless orange, peel and white pith removed, sectioned and coarsely chopped
25 mL	2 tablespoons chopped fresh cilantro
25 mL	2 tablespoons fresh lime juice
5 mL	1 teaspoon seeded, deveined, and finely chopped jalapeño (wear gloves when handling), or to taste
2 mL	1/2 teaspoon coarse salt

Seasonally fresh, juicy peaches and tomatoes are summer personified in this sprightly salsa zipped up with jalapeños and lime juice. Serve it on any fish fillet that looks good in the market, especially those high in heart-healthy fat such as swordfish, salmon, bluefish, and mackerel. Try this on the grill too!

1. Place an oven rack so the fish will be about 5 inches (13 cm) from the broiler. Preheat the broiler.
2. Brush the surface of the fish lightly with the oil and sprinkle generously with pepper. Set aside.
3. In a small bowl, gently fold together the tomatoes, peaches or nectarines, orange sections, cilantro, lime juice, jalapeños, and salt until blended. Set aside.
4. Broil the fish, turning with a wide spatula until the center of the thickest part of the fish is opaque, about 5 minutes per side, depending on the thickness.
5. To serve, top each portion with a spoonful of the tomato salsa. Serve any remaining salsa on the side.

Per serving: 228 calories, 5 g total fat, 1 g saturated fat, 15 g carbohydrate, 31 g protein, 3 g fiber, 45 mg cholesterol, 370 mg sodium, 85 mg calcium

Oven-Fried Fish Fillets with Chunky Low-Fat Tartar Sauce

Serves 4

PREP TIME: **30 minutes**
COOK TIME: **20 minutes**

There is nothing like crunchy breaded fish fillets, especially when the guilt-free crust is crisped in a hot oven instead of in a vat of bubbling oil. Enjoy each bite with a dip in the equally guilt-free tangy tartar sauce. Lean fish is an excellent source of low-fat protein and a good choice for a heart-healthy diet.

125 mL	1/2 cup low-fat mayonnaise
25 mL	2 tablespoons minced fresh dill, divided
15 mL	1 tablespoon minced seedless or Kirby cucumber
15 mL	1 tablespoon minced dill pickles, patted dry
15 mL	1 tablespoon minced celery
5 mL	1 teaspoon apple-cider vinegar
4	4 fish fillets (about 5 ounces/150 g each)
	Freshly ground black pepper, to taste
1	1 egg white
25 mL	2 tablespoons water
375 mL	1 1/2 cups panko crumbs
	Olive oil

1. In a small bowl, combine the mayonnaise, 1 tablespoon (5 mL) of the dill, the cucumbers, pickles, celery, and vinegar. Refrigerate until ready to serve.
2. Preheat the oven to 450°F (230°C).
3. Sprinkle the fish with pepper and the remaining dill. Whisk the egg white and water together in a shallow bowl until frothy. Place the panko crumbs in a second shallow bowl. Dip the fish in the egg white to coat, and then dip in the crumbs, pressing to coat evenly.
4. Drizzle oil down the center of a jelly-roll pan and place it in the oven until hot, about 5 minutes. Remove the pan, carefully place the fish on it, and return to the oven for 5 minutes. Using a wide spatula, turn the fish over and bake the other side until the fish is crusty and the center of the thickest part of the fish is opaque, 8 to 10 minutes, depending on the thickness. Serve with the chilled tartar sauce.

Per serving: 399 calories, 11 g total fat, 2 g saturated fat, 39 g carbohydrate, 34 g protein, 0 g fiber, 71 mg cholesterol, 589 mg sodium, 35 mg calcium

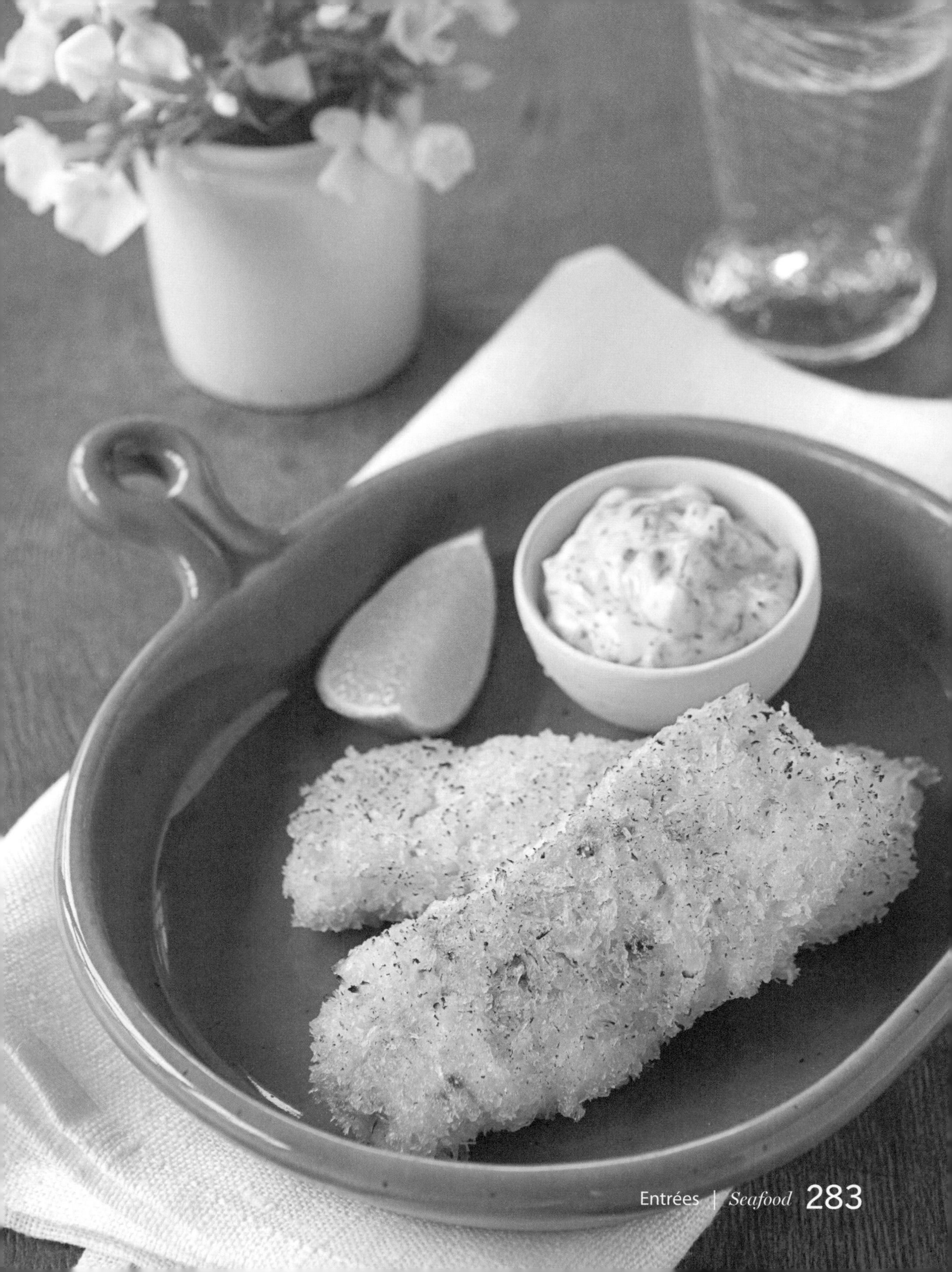

Salmon and Asparagus Farfalle with Walnut-Feta Sauce

Serves 4

PREP TIME: **40 minutes**
COOK TIME: **28 minutes**

Moist chunks of pink salmon, bright green asparagus, and ruffled butterfly pasta are coated with a smooth, creamy sauce of olive oil, feta cheese, and chopped walnuts. Walnuts and olive oil are both high in mono- and polyunsaturated fats (the good fats), and salmon is a good source of omega-3 fatty acids.

250 g	8 ounces boneless salmon fillet
50 mL	1/4 cup extra-virgin olive oil
50 mL	1/4 cup chopped walnuts
1	1 clove garlic, minced or crushed
375 g	12 ounces farfalle or butterfly-shaped pasta
375 g	12 ounces asparagus, trimmed and cut into 1/2-inch/1-cm diagonals
125 mL	1/2 cups crumbled mild goat's milk feta cheese (about 2 ounces/60 g), divided
25 mL	2 tablespoons finely slivered fresh basil leaves

1. Heat a 10-inch (25-cm) nonstick skillet over medium-low heat until hot enough that a drop of water sizzles. Add the salmon and cook on one side for 5 minutes. Turn with a wide spatula and cook until the center of the thickest part of the fish is opaque, about 3 to 5 minutes, depending on the thickness. When cool enough to handle, remove and discard the salmon skin and flake the fish apart into 1/2-inch (1-cm) pieces. Set aside.
2. Wipe out the pan and add the oil, walnuts, and garlic. Heat over medium-low heat, until the garlic sizzles and turns golden, about 2 minutes. (Do not leave the pan unattended; walnuts burn quickly.) Remove from heat.
3. Bring a large pot of water to a boil. Add the pasta and cook, stirring occasionally, until just cooked, 10 to 12 minutes. Add the asparagus and cook until tender, about 2 minutes. Drain, reserving 1/2 cup (125 mL) of the cooking water. Return the pasta to the pot.
4. Reduce the heat to medium-low. Add the reserved cooking water, the walnut mixture, salmon, and 1/4 cup (50 mL) of the feta cheese. Toss gently until heated through and blended, about 2 minutes. Spoon into serving bowls and sprinkle the remaining 1/4 cup (50 mL) of feta cheese and the basil on top.

Per serving: 623 calories, 27 g total fat, 5 g saturated fat, 69 g carbohydrate, 29 g protein, 5 g fiber, 38 mg cholesterol, 83 mg sodium, 76 mg calcium

Cornmeal-Crusted Trout Almondine on Smothered Greens with Lemon

Serves 4

PREP TIME: **20 minutes**
COOK TIME: **30 minutes**

A crunchy golden crust and sliced almonds jazz up this delicious oven-browned trout, making a delicious meal served on a bed of greens smothered with garlic and lemon. Trout is an excellent source of heart-healthy omega-3 fats.

1	1 egg white
25 mL	2 tablespoons water
250 mL	1 cup yellow cornmeal
5 mL	1 teaspoon paprika
2	2 brook or rainbow trout (about 10 ounces/300 g each), gutted and scaled
	Olive oil
50 mL	1/4 cup slivered almonds
1	1 bag (16 ounces/454 g) collards, kale, and Swiss chard mix or 2 bunches (about 1 pound /454 g each) greens, stemmed and torn into pieces
1	1 strip lemon zest (1/2 × 2 inches/1 cm × 5 cm), slivered
1	1 clove garlic, minced or crushed
4	4 lemon wedges

1. Whisk the egg white together with the water in a shallow bowl until frothy. Combine the cornmeal and paprika in another shallow bowl. Dip the fish in the egg white; let the excess drip off. Roll the fish in the cornmeal, pressing to coat evenly. Set aside.
2. Preheat the oven to 450°F (230°C). Drizzle oil down the center of a jelly-roll pan and place in the oven until hot, about 5 minutes. Remove the pan, carefully place the fish on it, and return it to the oven for 5 minutes. Using a wide spatula, turn the fish over and bake until the fish is crusty and the fish is opaque, 10 minutes.
3. Spread the almonds in an 8-inch (20-cm) skillet over medium-high heat, and cook until golden, about 5 minutes. (Do not leave the pan unattended; almonds burn quickly.) Set aside.
4. Rinse greens in a large bowl of water, drain, and place in a large, wide saucepan. Cook, covered, over medium-high heat until wilted, about 2 minutes. Reduce the heat and cook until tender. Add the lemon zest and garlic. Increase the heat to boil off any liquid in the pan.
5. To serve, spread the greens on a platter and top with the trout. Sprinkle with the almonds, and add the lemon wedges.

Per serving (1/2 trout): 412 calories, 9 g total fat, 1 g saturated fat, 4
1 g carbohydrate, 40 g protein, 6 g fiber, 84 mg cholesterol, 131 mg sodium, 287 mg calcium

Sautéed Salmon Fillets with Tomatoes, Zucchini, and Green Olives

Serves 4

PREP TIME: **10 minutes**
COOK TIME: **15 minutes**

In this quick-and-easy one-skillet meal, tomatoes and zucchini are jazzed up with basil to make a garden-fresh pan sauce for salmon fillets. Salmon is high in unsaturated fats and omega-3 heart-healthy fatty acids, niacin, phosphorus, and potassium.

15 mL	1 tablespoon extra-virgin olive oil
4	4 boneless, skinless salmon fillets (about 5 ounces/150 g each)
1	1 can (14.5 ounces/396 mL) no-salt-added diced tomatoes (with juice)
500 mL	2 cups coarsely chopped trimmed zucchini
25 mL	2 tablespoons chopped fresh basil
25 mL	2 tablespoons pitted and chopped green olives
1	1 clove garlic, minced or crushed
0.5 mL	1/8 teaspoon freshly ground black pepper

1. Heat a large nonstick skillet over high heat. Add the oil and tilt the pan to coat evenly. When the oil is shimmering, place the salmon in the pan and cook for 2 minutes. Turn with a wide spatula and cook for another 2 minutes. Remove to a plate, and set aside.
2. Add the tomatoes (with juice), zucchini, basil, olives, garlic, and pepper to the skillet. Heat to a boil and cook, stirring, over medium heat, until slightly reduced, about 3 minutes.
3. Return the salmon to the skillet. Spoon the sauce over the salmon and cook, uncovered, until the center of the thickest part of the fish is opaque, about 5 minutes, depending on the thickness.

Per serving: 277 calories, 14 g total fat, 2 g saturated fat, 7 g carbohydrate, 30 g protein, 1 g fiber, 78 mg cholesterol, 137 mg sodium, 47 mg calcium

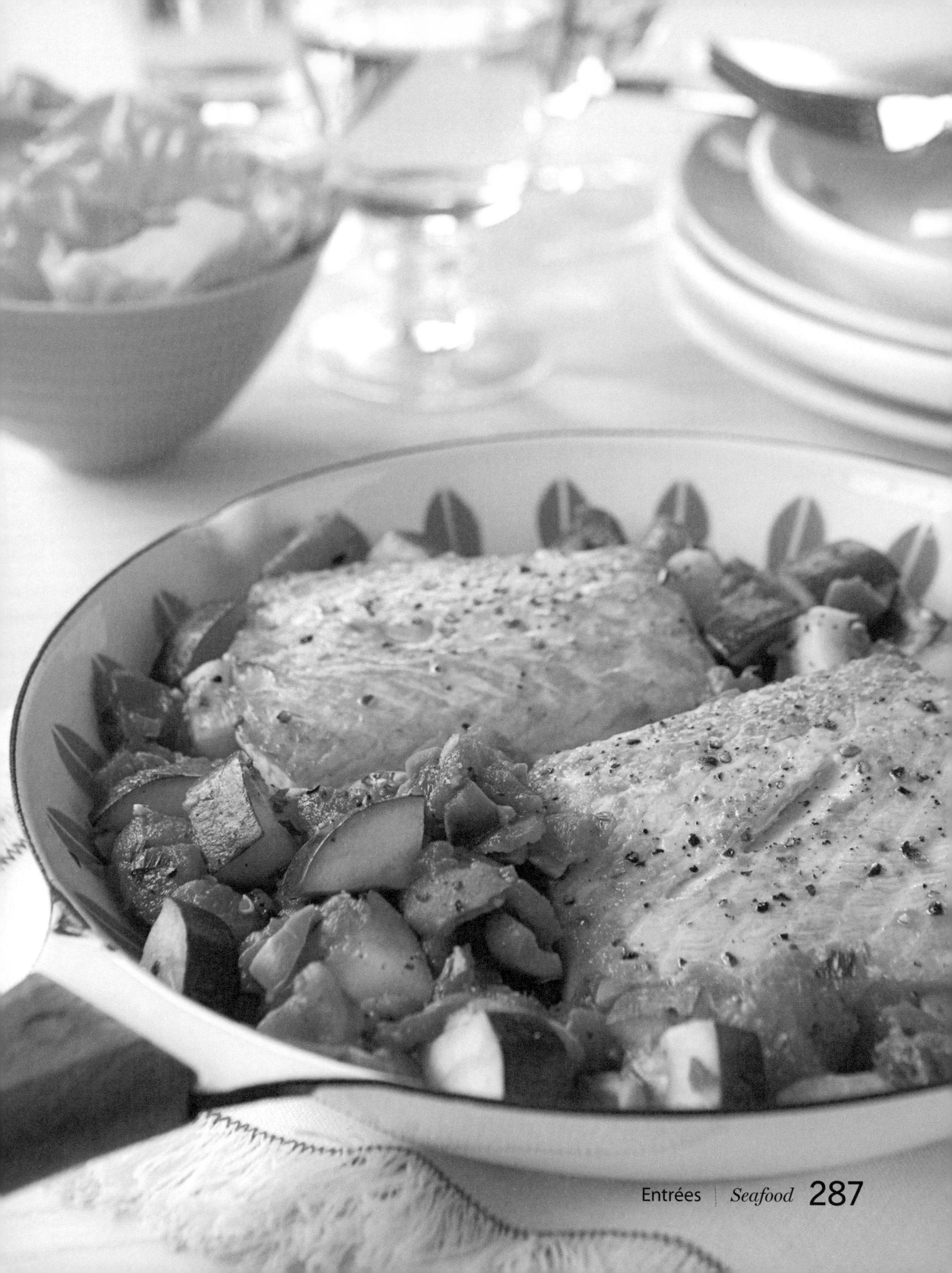

Oven-Roasted Mackerel with Cherry Tomatoes, Potatoes, and Smoked Paprika

Serves 4

PREP TIME: **15 minutes**
COOK TIME: **40 minutes**

Crisp, oven-browned potatoes and seared tomatoes offset the richness of mackerel in this simple and convenient one-pan meal. Mackerel is among the fish highest in omega-3 fatty acids, which are widely known for their heart-healthy advantages.

500 g	1 pound small Yukon Gold or red-skinned potatoes, unpeeled, cut into 1/2-inch/1-cm wedges
375 mL	1 1/2 cups small cherry tomatoes
1/2	1/2 medium onion, cut into thin slices
1	1 clove garlic, thinly sliced
15 mL	1 tablespoon extra-virgin olive oil
7 mL	1 1/2 teaspoons smoked paprika, divided
1 mL	1/4 teaspoon freshly ground black pepper, divided
4	4 boneless, skinless mackerel fillets (4 ounces/125 g each)
15 mL	1 tablespoon chopped flat-leaf parsley
1	1 lemon, cut into wedges

1. Preheat the oven to 400°F (200°C).
2. Toss the potatoes, tomatoes, onions, garlic, and oil in a large shallow baking dish or roasting pan. Spread in single layer and sprinkle with 1 teaspoon (5 mL) of the paprika and 1/8 teaspoon (0.5 mL) of the pepper. Roast the vegetables, turning once, until lightly browned, about 30 minutes.
3. Remove the pan from the oven and increase the temperature to 450°F (230°C). Arrange the fish in a single layer, redistributing the vegetables on top of and around the fish. Sprinkle with the remaining 1/2 teaspoon (2 mL) of paprika and the remaining 1/8 teaspoon (2 mL) of pepper. Roast until the center of the thickest part of the fish is opaque, about 10 minutes, depending on the thickness.
4. Sprinkle with the parsley and serve with the lemon wedges.

Per serving: 366 calories, 20 g total fat, 4 g saturated fat, 23 g carbohydrate, 24 g protein, 3 g fiber, 79 mg cholesterol, 114 mg sodium, 41 mg calcium

Whole-Grain Pasta Primavera with Ricotta

Serves 4

PREP TIME: **40 minutes**
COOK TIME: **20 minutes**

Bright-tasting multicolored vegetables, cut in strips to match the shape of the pasta are tossed with spaghetti and a creamy sauce of low-fat ricotta. The technique of cooking vegetables in pasta cooking water omits the need for oil and keeps fat and calories at a minimum.

500 g	1 pound plum tomatoes, halved
50 mL	1/4 cup slivered fresh basil leaves, divided
2 mL	1/2 teaspoon coarse salt
0.5 mL	1/8 teaspoon freshly ground black pepper
1	1 large carrot, cut into 2 × 1/4 inch/5 × 0.5 cm sticks
8	8 pieces of thin asparagus, cut into 2-inch/5-cm lengths
1	1 small green zucchini, cut into 2 × 1/4 inch/5 × 0.5 cm sticks (about 1 cup/250 mL)
1	1 small yellow zucchini, cut into 2 × 1/4 inch/5 × 0.5 cm sticks (about 1 cup/250 mL)
125 mL	1/2 cup frozen peas
250 g	8 ounces whole-wheat spaghetti
125 mL	1/2 cup low-fat ricotta cheese
125 mL	1/2 cup thinly slivered red onion
25 mL	2 tablespoons freshly grated Parmesan cheese

1. Scoop the pulp and seeds from the tomatoes into a strainer set over a large bowl. Cut the tomato flesh into strips (1/4-inch/0.5-cm wide). Press the pulp and seeds into the strainer to extract the tomato juices. Add the tomato flesh, 2 tablespoons (25 mL) of the basil, the salt, and pepper to the juices in the bowl. Discard the pulp and seeds.
2. Bring a large pot of water to boiling. Add the carrots and boil for 3 minutes. Add the asparagus, green and yellow zucchini, and peas to the water and boil for 2 minutes. Remove the vegetables with a slotted spoon and add to the tomatoes.
3. Add the spaghetti to the boiling water and cook, uncovered, stirring occasionally, until al dente or firm to the bite, 10 to 12 minutes. Drain, reserving 1/2 cup (125 mL) of the cooking water. Return the pasta to the pot. Reduce the heat to low.
4. Stir the ricotta and 1/4 cup (50 mL) of the reserved cooking water together in a small bowl until blended. Add to the pasta, along with the vegetable mixture and red onions. Stir until blended and heated through, about 3 minutes.
5. Transfer to a serving bowl, sprinkle with the remaining 2 tablespoons (25 mL) of basil and sprinkle with the Parmesan.

Per serving: 325 calories, 6 g total fat, 2 g saturated fat, 53 g carbohydrate, 18 g protein, 13 g fiber, 13 mg cholesterol, 427 mg sodium, 168 mg calcium

Soup Bowl Lasagna with Spinach, Turkey Sausage, and Three Cheeses

Serves 4

PREP TIME: 15 minutes
COOK TIME: 35 minutes

This exciting new take on old-fashioned lasagna contains turkey sausage as a flavorful and less-fatty alternative to ground beef. Fresh spinach, which contains folacin and is an excellent source of vitamin A, is layered between the noodles for extra goodness. Everyone loves a cheesy lasagna, and this version doesn't disappoint.

125 g	4 ounces raw Italian turkey sausage, casings removed, crumbled
1	1 can (28 ounces/796 mL) no-salt-added Italian plum tomatoes (with juice)
1	1 clove garlic, minced or crushed
1	1 bag (10 ounces/283 g) fresh spinach, trimmed
8	8 spinach or whole-wheat lasagna noodles, broken in half
250 mL	1 cup low-fat ricotta cheese
125 mL	1/2 cup shredded part-skim mozzarella cheese (2 ounces/60 g)
0.5 mL	1/8 teaspoon freshly ground black pepper
0.5 mL	1/8 teaspoon freshly ground nutmeg
10 mL	2 teaspoons freshly grated Parmesan

1. Place four shallow ovenproof soup or pasta bowls in the oven set at the lowest temperature.
2. Cook the sausage in a 10-inch (25-cm) skillet over medium heat until browned. Remove to a plate lined with paper towels.
3. Add the tomatoes (with juice) to the skillet and cook, breaking up with the side of a spoon, until slightly thickened, about 5 minutes. Stir in the sausage and garlic; keep warm over low heat.
4. Bring a large pot of water to a boil. Add the spinach and cook until wilted, about 20 seconds. Remove the spinach: drain and cool. Squeeze out all the moisture and chop roughly. Add the noodles to the boiling water and cook, stirring occasionally, until al dente or firm to the bite, about 12 minutes. Drain the noodles.
5. Meanwhile, heat the ricotta in a small saucepan over low heat, stirring, until warm. Stir in the mozzarella and remove from the heat. Stir in the pepper and nutmeg.
6. Line up the warmed soup bowls. Spoon half of the tomato sauce into the bowls, dividing evenly. Top with two noodles, side by side. Add a layer of spinach on top of the noodles. Spread the ricotta mixture on the spinach. Add a second layer of noodles and top with remaining sauce. Sprinkle with 1/2 teaspoon (2 mL) of the Parmesan.

Per serving: 417 calories, 12 g total fat, 6 g saturated fat, 48 g carbohydrate, 28 g protein, 10 g fiber, 49 mg cholesterol, 472 mg sodium, 365 mg calcium

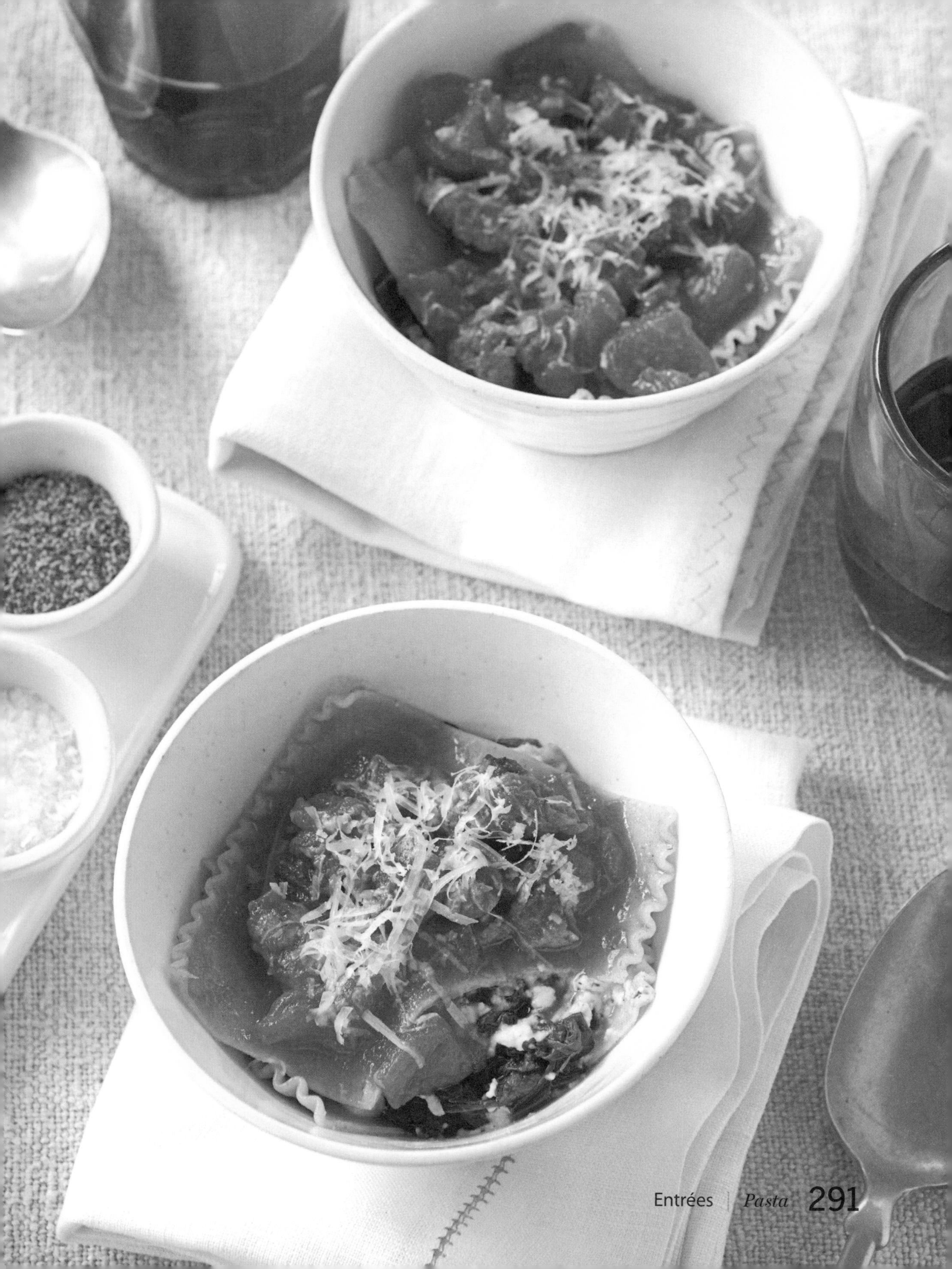

Cheesy Curly Macaroni with Broccoli and Cherry Tomatoes

Serves 6

PREP TIME: **25 minutes**
COOK TIME: **16 minutes**

15 mL	1 tablespoon extra-virgin olive oil
375 mL	1 1/2 cups coarsely chopped broccoli florets
50 mL	1/4 cup chopped onion
250 mL	1 cup sweet 100s or other bite-size cherry tomatoes
1	1 clove garlic, minced
300 g	10 ounces curly macaroni, fusilli, or elbow noodles
250 mL	1 cup low-fat ricotta cheese
25 mL	2 tablespoons grated Parmesan cheese
	Pinch of crushed red pepper
125 mL	1/2 cup coarsely shredded cheddar cheese (2 ounces/60 g)

The creamy topping on this red and green vegetable-studded macaroni and cheese is broiled, instead of baked, allowing the pasta mixture to stay moist and velvety with low-fat ricotta cheese. The low-fat version of ricotta tastes great, has a pleasant texture, and is an excellent source of protein.

1. Heat the oil in a 10-inch (25-cm) skillet or sauté pan over medium-low heat until the garlic begins to sizzle. Add the broccoli and onions and cook, stirring, until tender, about 5 minutes. Add the tomatoes and garlic and cook 1 minute longer. Remove from the heat and let stand.

2. Heat a large pot of water to boiling. Add the pasta and cook, stirring occasionally, until al dente or firm to the bite, 10 to 12 minutes. Drain, reserving 1/2 cup (125 mL) of the cooking water. Leave the pasta in the colander.

3. Whisk the ricotta and 1/4 cup (50 mL) of the reserved cooking water in the pasta pot over medium heat until smooth. Add the vegetables, Parmesan, and crushed red pepper. Stir to blend. Toss in the pasta and combine to evenly distribute the sauce and vegetables. Add the remaining 1/4 cup (50 mL) of cooking water, if the pasta seems too dry. Heat through, stirring, for 3 minutes.

4. Coat a 9 × 13-inch (22 × 330-cm) oval gratin pan that can safely go under the broiler with nonstick cooking spray. Adjust the oven rack so that the top of the dish will be 2 to 3 inches (5 to 7.5 cm) from the broiler. Preheat the broiler.

5. Spread the pasta mixture into the prepared pan. Sprinkle with the cheddar cheese. Broil until the top is golden and the cheese is melted, about 5 minutes.

Per serving: 317 calories, 10 g total fat, 5 g saturated fat, 41 g carbohydrate, 15 g protein, 2 g fiber, 25 mg cholesterol, 161 mg sodium, 232 mg calcium

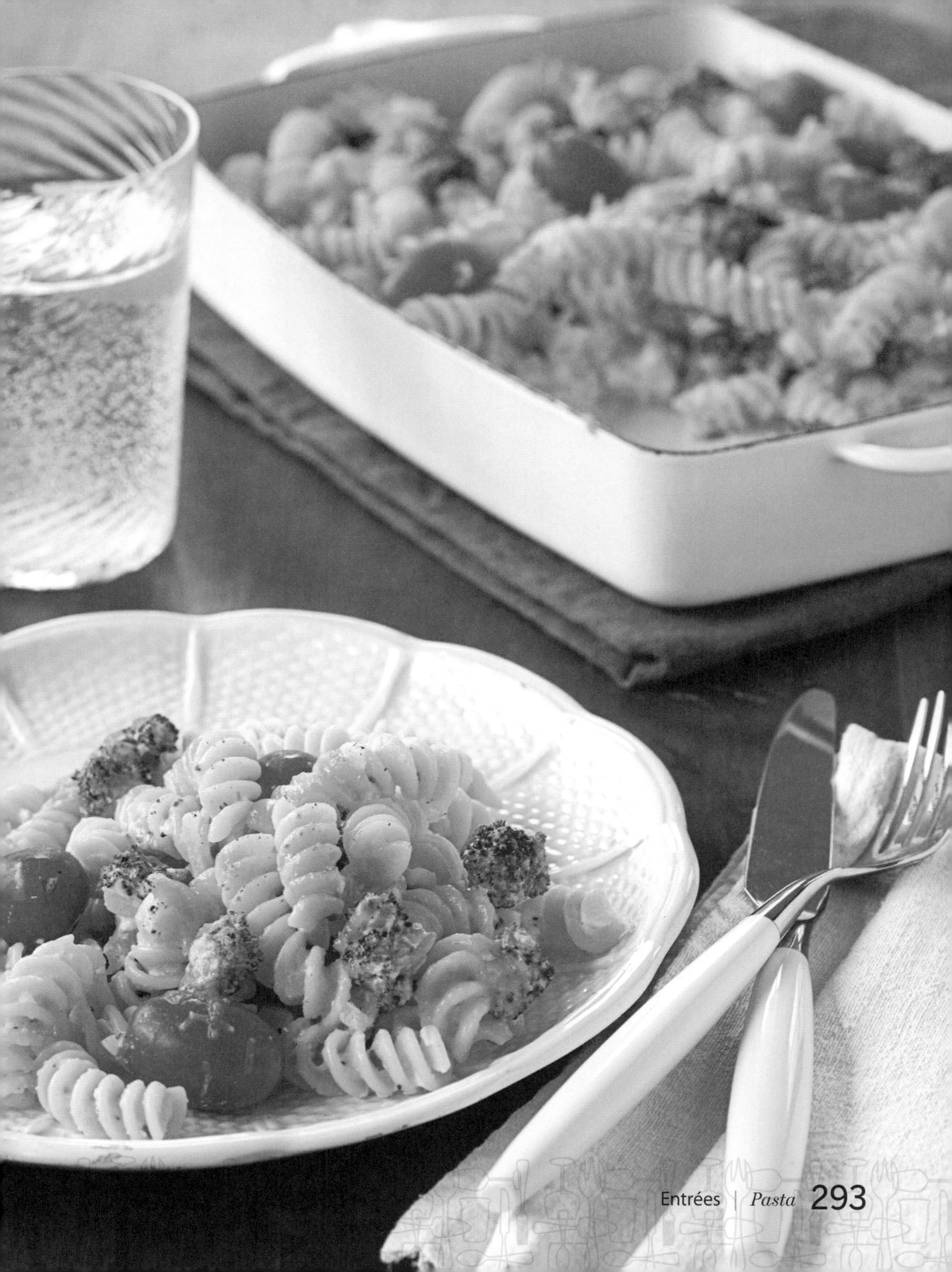

Fusilli with Pinto Beans, Kalamata Olives, Tomatoes, and Broccolini

Serves 4

PREP TIME: **13 minutes**
COOK TIME: **30 minutes**

Pasta and beans with a zesty sauce of tomatoes and crushed red pepper makes a comforting meal. A bit of black olive in every bite adds a pleasant salty hit, and the mild broccolini helps to balance the flavor. Beans are an excellent low-fat source of fiber, folacin, and potassium.

25 mL	2 tablespoons extra-virgin olive oil
2	2 cloves garlic, minced or grated
1	1 can (28 ounces/796 mL) Italian plum tomatoes (with juice)
0.5 mL	1/8 teaspoon red pepper flakes
1	1 can (14.5 ounces/540 mL) pinto beans, rinsed and drained
15 mL	1 tablespoon pitted and coarsely chopped Kalamata olives
250 g	8 ounces fusilli or spiral pasta
500 mL	2 cups broccolini pieces (1 inch/2.5 cm)
20 mL	1 tablespoon plus 1 teaspoon grated Romano cheese

1. Heat the oil and garlic in a 10-inch (25-cm) deep skillet or sauté pan over medium-low heat until the garlic begins to sizzle.
2. Add the tomatoes (with juice) and red pepper flakes. Cook, breaking up with the side of a spoon or potato masher, until the sauce is thickened, about 15 minutes. Add the beans and olives and keep warm over low heat.
3. Bring a large pot of water to a boil and add the pasta. Cook, stirring, until almost al dente or firm to the bite, about 12 minutes.
4. Add the broccolini and cook until tender and the pasta is ready, about 2 minutes. Drain, reserving 1/2 cup (125 mL) of the cooking water. Return the pasta to the pot.
5. Add the tomato sauce and stir to blend. Add the reserved cooking water, if the pasta seems too dry. Spoon into a serving bowl and sprinkle with the Romano.

Per serving: 404 calories, 10 g total fat, 2 g saturated fat, 63 g carbohydrate, 14 g protein, 7 g fiber, 3 mg cholesterol, 786 mg sodium, 102 mg calcium

Barley Risotto with Mushrooms and Spinach

Serves 4–6

PREP TIME: **20 minutes**
COOK TIME: **1 hour**

An ample portion of flavorful mushrooms turns mild-tasting barley into a delicious, creamy, and comforting one-pot meal. While all mushrooms have virtually no fat or calories, some species continue to be studied for their antiviral and antitumor qualities.

15 mL	1 tablespoon extra-virgin olive oil
125 mL	1/2 cup chopped onion
500 g	1 pound coarsely chopped button and/or cremini mushrooms
25 mL	2 tablespoons minced flat-leaf parsley
15 mL	1 tablespoon minced garlic
250 mL	1 cup pearl barley
1 to 1.5 L	4 to 5 cups reduced-sodium low-fat chicken broth, divided
50 mL	1/4 cup chopped dried tomatoes
1	1 bag (5 ounces/142 g) baby spinach
0.5 mL	1/8 teaspoon freshly ground black pepper

1. Heat the oil in a large heavy saucepan over medium heat. Add the onions and cook, stirring, until golden, 3 minutes. Add the mushrooms and cook until tender and golden, about 10 minutes. Add the parsley and garlic and cook for 1 minute longer.
2. Add the barley and 4 cups (1 L) of the broth and bring to a boil. Reduce the heat to medium-low and cook, covered, until most of the liquid is absorbed, about 35 minutes.
3. Add 1/2 cup (125 mL) of the remaining broth and the tomatoes. Cook, stirring frequently, until the barley is tender, adding the remaining 1/2 cup (125 mL) of broth, if necessary, for a creamy texture, about 15 minutes.
4. Stir in the spinach until wilted, about 1 minute. Add the pepper and serve.

Per serving: 263 calories, 5 g total fat, 1 g saturated fat, 48 g carbohydrate, 11 g protein, 10 g fiber, 0 mg cholesterol, 527 mg sodium, 69 mg calcium

Roasted Eggplant, Zucchini, and Red Pepper Parmigiano

Serves 4

PREP TIME: **30 minutes**
COOK TIME: **1 hour 30 minutes**

25 mL	2 tablespoons extra-virgin olive oil
2	2 eggplants (about 1 pound/500 g each), cut into 24 slices (1/2 inch/1 cm)
2	2 medium zucchini, cut into 10 lengthwise slices (1/2 inch/1 cm)
250 mL	1 cup coarsely crumbled multi-grain bread
1	1 can (28 ounces/796 mL) diced tomatoes (with juice)
25 mL	2 tablespoons finely chopped Italian parsley
1	1 clove garlic, minced or grated
	Pinch of crushed red pepper
250 mL	1 cup jarred roasted and peeled red bell peppers, drained, rinsed, and cut into 1-inch/2.5-cm strips
325 mL	1 1/4 cups coarsely shredded part-skim mozzarella cheese (4 ounces/125 g)
15 mL	1 tablespoon freshly grated Parmesan cheese

There is nothing more seductive than a layer of golden eggplant slices sauced with tomatoes and topped with melted cheese. This recipe is enhanced with antioxidant-rich quick-and-easy homemade tomato sauce, roasted red peppers, and crunchy multi-grain bread crumbs. To cut the fat, the eggplant is oven-browned instead of pan-fried.

1. Preheat the oven to 450°F (230°C). Lightly brush two jelly-roll pans with the oil.
2. Place the eggplant and zucchini on the pans and roast for 15 minutes. Remove the zucchini to a plate. Turn the eggplant over and roast for 15 minutes longer.
3. Meanwhile spread the bread in a large skillet and toast over medium-high heat, stirring, until crisp and golden, 7 to 10 minutes. Transfer to a small bowl.
4. Reduce the heat to medium. Add the tomatoes (with juice) to the skillet and cook, stirring, until thickened, about 15 minutes. Stir in the parsley, garlic, and crushed red pepper.
5. Reduce the oven temperature to 400°F (200°C). In a shallow 2 1/2-quart (2.5-L) baking dish, layer half of each of the eggplant, zucchini, roasted red peppers, bread, tomato sauce, and mozzarella. Repeat with the second layer and sprinkle with the Parmesan.
6. Bake until the top is golden, about 20 minutes. Remove from the oven and let stand for 10 minutes before cutting and serving.

Per serving: 312 calories, 15 g total fat, 5 g saturated fat, 33 g carbohydrate, 15 g protein, 12 g fiber, 17 mg cholesterol, 793 mg sodium, 363 mg calcium

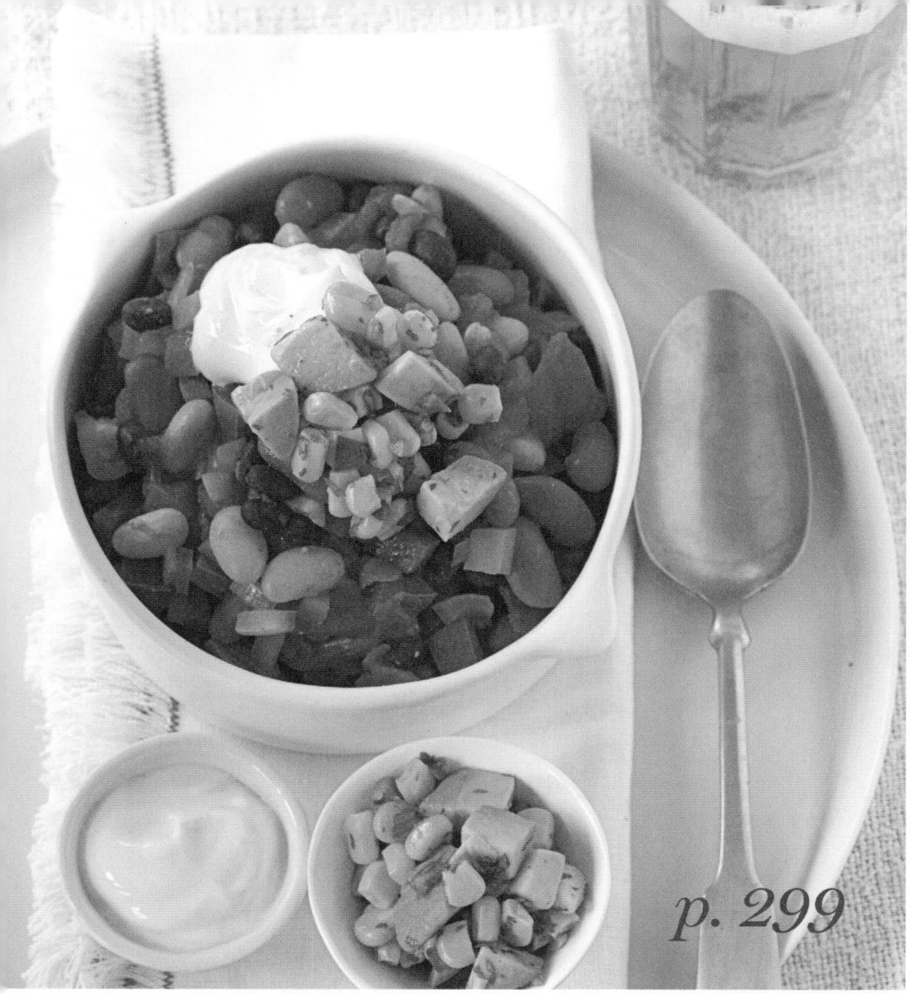
p. 299

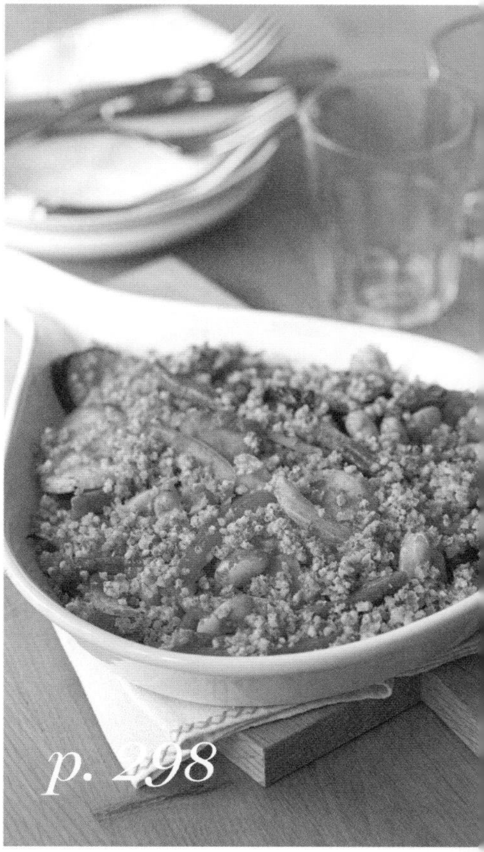
p. 298

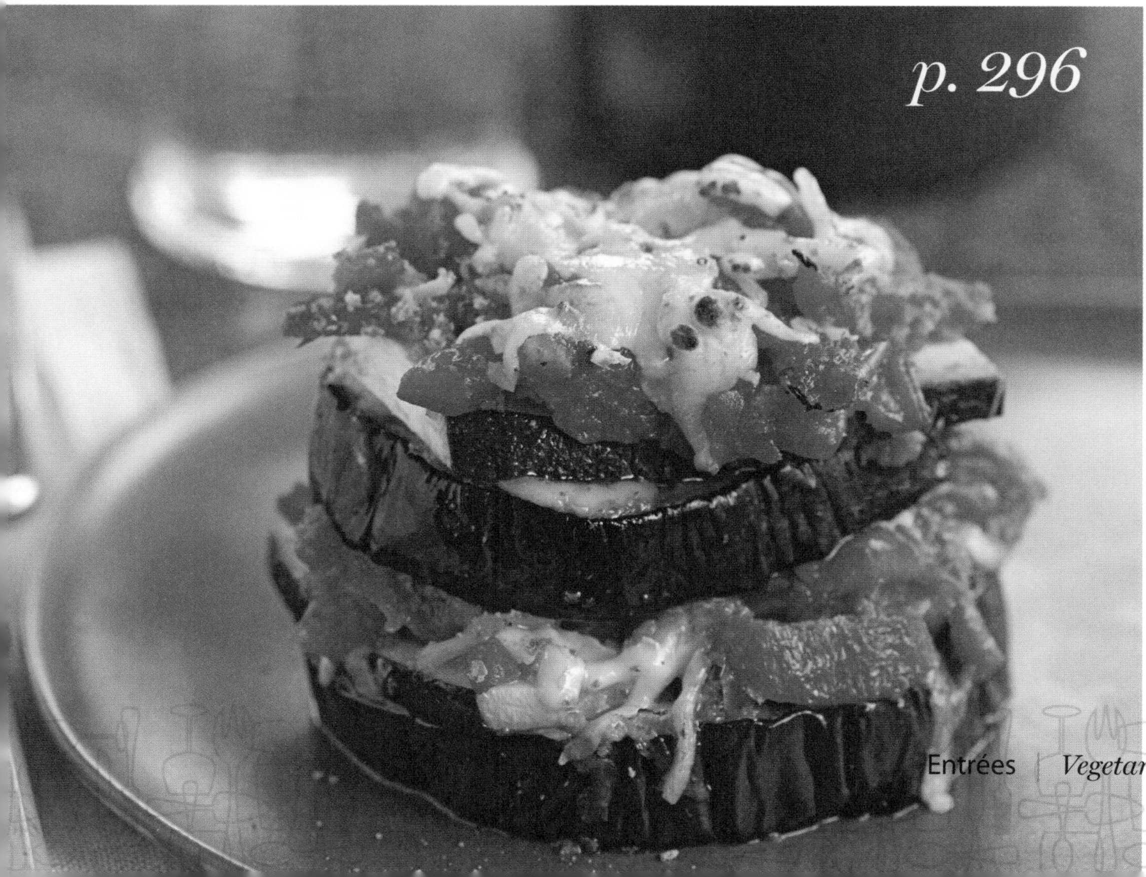
p. 296

White Bean and Roasted Vegetable Casserole with Millet and Crumb Crust

Serves 4

PREP TIME: **40 minutes**
COOK TIME: **1 hour 25 minutes**

A medley of colorful roasted vegetables, cannellini beans, and harissa, a spicy Tunisian hot sauce (if unavailable, substitute Chinese or Thai red chile paste found in most supermarkets), are combined to make this hearty casserole. The dish is topped with a crust of whole-wheat breadcrumbs tossed with cooked millet. Millet, an underconsumed grain, is an excellent source of protein, B vitamins, and minerals.

2	2 red bell peppers, seeded and cut into strips
1	1 large onion, cut into thin wedges (1/4 inch/0.5 cm)
250 mL	1 cup diagonally cut carrots (1/4 inch/0.5 cm)
250 mL	1 cup diagonally cut zucchini (1/4 inch/0.5 cm)
250 mL	1 cup cut yellow squash or zucchini (1/4 inch/0.5 cm)
250 mL	1 cup trimmed and cut green beans (1 inch/2.5 cm)
22 mL	1 tablespoon plus 1 1/2 teaspoons extra-virgin olive oil, divided
10 mL	2 teaspoons ground cumin, divided
1	1 can (28 ounces/796 mL) diced tomatoes
1	1 can (15 ounces/540 mL) cannellini beans, rinsed and drained
10 mL	2 teaspoons *harissa* or 1 1/2 teaspoons (7 mL) Chinese or Thai red chile paste, or to taste
25 mL	2 tablespoons finely chopped fresh cilantro
125 mL	1/2 cup millet
625 mL	2 1/2 cups water
125 mL	1/2 cup whole-wheat breadcrumbs

1. Preheat the oven to 400°F (200°C). Spread the peppers, onions, carrots, zucchini, squash, and green beans on a jelly-roll pan in a single layer. Drizzle with 1 tablespoon (15 mL) of the oil and stir to coat. Sprinkle with 1 teaspoon (5 mL) of the cumin. Roast, until the edges are browned, 40 to 45 minutes.
2. Add the tomatoes (with juice) to a 10-inch (25-cm) skillet and bring to a boil. Boil gently, uncovered, breaking up with the side of a spoon until thickened, about 10 minutes. Stir in the cannellini beans and *harissa* or chile paste. Remove from heat.
3. Heat the millet over medium heat in another 10-inch (25-cm) skillet, stirring, until lightly toasted, about 5 minutes. Add the water and bring to a boil. Reduce the heat and cook, covered, until the millet is tender, 15 to 20 minutes. Drain and cool.
4. Increase heat to medium. Wipe out the skillet and add the breadcrumbs and remaining 1 1/2 teaspoons (7 mL) of oil. Heat, stirring, until lightly toasted, about 3 minutes. Reduce heat to medium-low. Add millet and stir until blended.
5. Reduce the oven temperature to 350°F (180°C). Add the vegetables and the tomato mixture to a 9 × 13-inch (22 × 33-cm) baking dish and blend. Sprinkle the millet mixture evenly on top. Bake until heated through and the topping is crisp, about 25 minutes.

Per serving: 354 calories, 8 g total fat, 1 g saturated fat, 60 g carbohydrate, 13 g protein, 12 g fiber, 0 mg cholesterol, 720 mg sodium, 138 mg calcium

Three-Bean Vegetarian Chili with Tomato, Avocado, and Corn Topping

Serves 6

PREP TIME: **25 minutes**
COOK TIME: **55 minutes**

15 mL	1 tablespoon olive oil
1 each	1 each green bell pepper and onion, chopped
1	1 cup chopped carrot
2	2 cloves garlic, chopped
10 mL	2 teaspoons chile powder
5 mL	1 teaspoon ground cumin
1	1 can (28 ounces/ 796 mL) no-salt plum tomatoes
1 each	1 can (15 ounces/ 540 mL) each white, black, and red kidney beans, rinsed and drained
1	1 can (8 ounces/227 g) tomato sauce
10 mL	2 teaspoons chopped chipotle chiles in adobo
125 mL	1/2 cup corn kernels
1/2	1/2 small avocado, chopped
15 mL	1 tablespoon each fresh lime juice and fresh cilantro
5 mL	1 teaspoon seeded minced jalapeño
125 mL	1/2 cup fat-free sour cream

Fragrant with chile powder and smokey chipotle chiles, this easy one-pot dish uses three colors of beans: black, red kidney, and Great Northern or cannellini white. Beans are supernutritious, contributing low-fat protein, a wide variety of vitamins and minerals, and, of course, heart-healthy dietary fiber.

1. Heat the oil in large heavy saucepan over medium-low heat. Add the peppers, onions, carrots, and garlic. Cook, stirring, until golden, about 10 minutes.
2. Stir in the chile powder and cumin and cook until toasted, about 1 minute. Add the tomatoes (with juice), white (Great Northern or cannellini) beans, black beans, kidney beans, tomato sauce, and chiles,, and heat to boiling. Reduce the heat to low. Cook, covered, stirring occasionally, until the flavors are blended, about 45 minutes. If the chili is too thick, thin with a little water.
3. Stir the corn, avocado, lime juice, cilantro, and jalapeño together in a small bowl.
4. Ladle the chili into bowls and top with the sour cream and the corn mixture.

Per serving: 269 calories, 6 g total fat, 1 g saturated fat, 43 g carbohydrate, 13 g protein, 13 g fiber, 1 mg cholesterol, 621 mg sodium, 138 mg calcium

Roasted Asparagus with Orange Gremolata

Serves 4

PREP TIME: **15 minutes**
COOK TIME: **15 minutes**

A fresh tasting finely chopped mixture of orange zest, garlic and parsley—a great salt substitute—adds a bright taste to tender oven roasted asparagus. Super low in calories, asparagus contains a number of nutrients, especially folate.

1	1 bunch asparagus (1 pound/500 g), trimmed
15 mL	1 tablespoon extra-virgin olive oil
1 mL	1/4 teaspoon freshly ground black pepper
50 mL	1/4 cup loosely packed flat-leaf parsley leaves and tender stems
1	1 strip (2 x 2 inches/ 5 × 5 cm) orange zest
1	1 clove garlic

1. Preheat the oven to 400°F (200°C). Coat a jelly-roll pan or shallow baking dish with nonstick cooking spray.
2. Spread the asparagus in the pan. Drizzle with the oil and sprinkle with the pepper. Roast until the asparagus is tender, about 15 minutes.
3. On a cutting board, finely chop the parsley, orange zest, and garlic together. Sprinkle over the asparagus before serving.

Per serving: 61 calories, 4 g total fat, 1 g saturated fat, 6 g carbohydrate, 3 g protein, 3 g fiber, 0 mg cholesterol, 3 mg sodium, 35 mg calcium

Green Beans with Ground Toasted Almonds

Serves 6

PREP TIME: **15 minutes**
COOK TIME: **5 minutes**

Tender green beans tossed with crunchy flavorful toasted almonds gives this favorite combination a healthy new look. Almonds are considered an important part of a heart-healthy, low-saturated-fat diet. Eaten with their natural skins intact adds extra fiber to their already impressive nutritional profile of vitamin E, protein, riboflavin, iron, and magnesium.

50 mL	1/4 cup whole almonds (skin on)
500 g	1 pound green beans, trimmed
1	1 clove garlic, halved
7 mL	1 1/2 teaspoons extra-virgin olive oil
1 mL	1/4 teaspoon coarse salt

1. Preheat the oven to 350°F (180°C).
2. Spread the almonds in a small pan and bake until toasted, about 10 minutes. Cool. Finely chop in a food processor and set aside.
3. Heat a large pot of water to boiling. Add the beans and cook until tender, 4 to 6 minutes. Drain.
4. Rub the inside of a serving bowl with the cut sides of the garlic, then discard the garlic. Add the beans, oil, and salt to the bowl, tossing to coat. Sprinkle with the almonds and toss to blend.

Per serving: 71 calories, 4 g total fat, 0 g saturated fat, 7 g carbohydrate, 3 g protein, 3 g fiber, 0 mg cholesterol, 102 mg sodium, 31 mg calcium

Oven-Roasted Beets with Herbed Vinegar Dressing

Serves 4

PREP TIME: **10 minutes**
COOK TIME: **1 hour**

4 to 5	4 to 5 beets (1 1/2 pounds/750 g), trimmed
45 mL	3 tablespoons red-wine vinegar
25 mL	2 tablespoons extra-virgin olive oil
1	1 clove garlic, crushed or grated
2 mL	1/2 teaspoon grated orange zest
1 mL	1/4 teaspoon coarse salt
0.5 mL	1/8 teaspoon freshly ground black pepper
15 mL	1 tablespoon chopped chives or green scallion tops
15 mL	1 tablespoon chopped fresh mint

The rich sweetness and earthy flavor of beets is retained when they're oven-roasted and sauced with a warm, tangy, red-wine-vinegar dressing laced with herbs. Beets are a good source of fiber, potassium, iron, and folate, an important B vitamin.

1. Preheat the oven to 400°F (200°C).
2. Wrap each beet tightly in foil. Place on a jelly-roll pan or in a shallow baking pan. Roast until tender when a skewer is inserted into the thickest part, about 55 minutes. Let cool in the foil. Rub the skins off the beets and cut into 1/4-inch (0.5-cm) wedges. Place in a large bowl.
3. In a small bowl, whisk the vinegar, oil, garlic, orange zest, salt, and pepper until blended. Pour over the beets. Sprinkle with the chives or scallions and mint. Stir to blend.

Per serving: 140 calories, 7 g total fat, 1 g saturated fat, 17 g carbohydrate, 3 g protein, 5 g fiber, 0 mg cholesterol, 279 mg sodium, 33 mg calcium

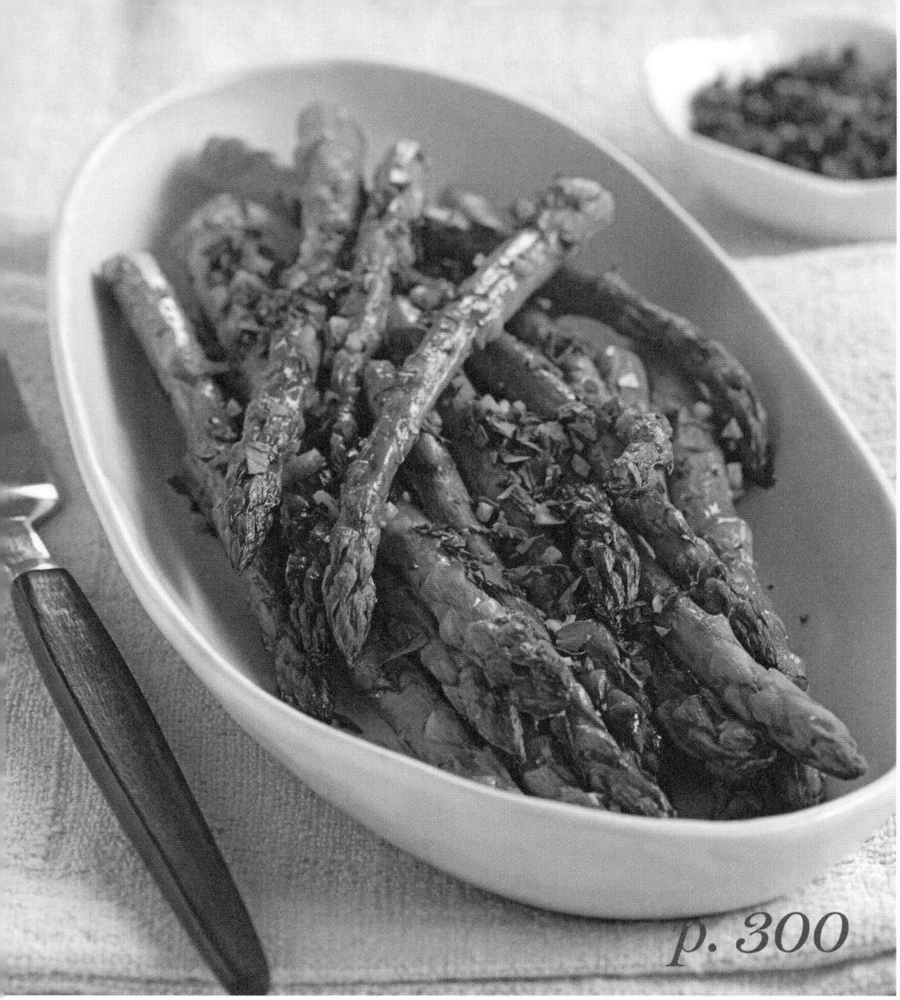
p. 300

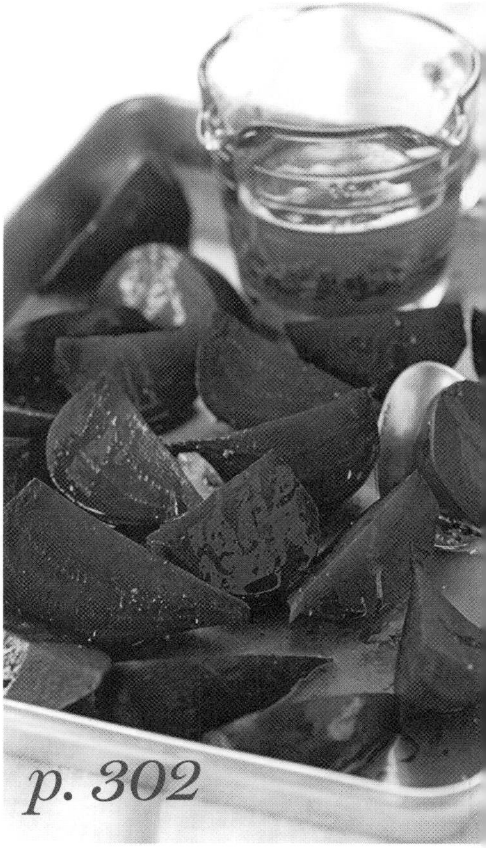
p. 302

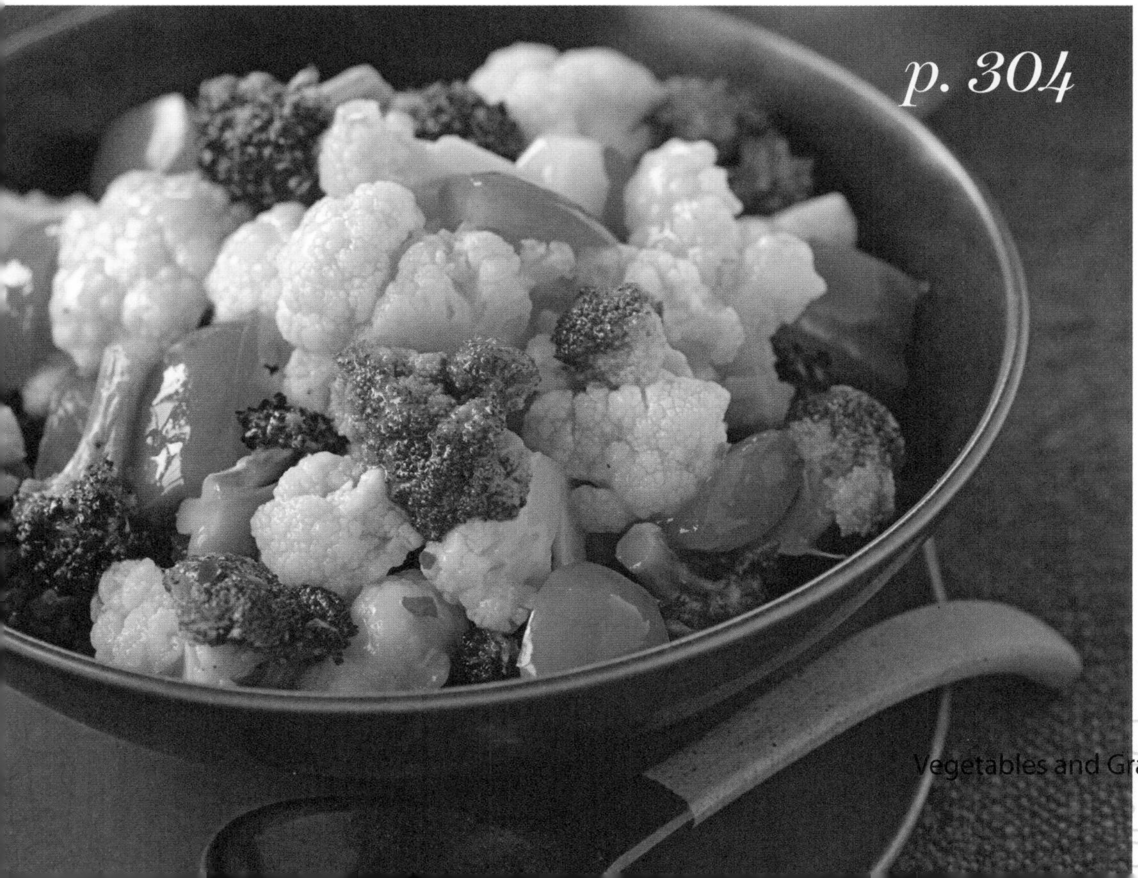
p. 304

Honey-and-Soy-Glazed Broccoli, Cauliflower, and Red Peppers

Serves 4

PREP TIME: **5 minutes**
COOK TIME: **13 minutes**

500 mL	2 cups broccoli florets (1 inch/2.5 cm)
500 mL	2 cups cauliflower florets (1 inch/2.5 cm)
50 mL	1/4 cup water
25 mL	2 tablespoons fresh orange juice
25 ml	2 tablespoons honey
15 mL	1 tablespoon reduced-sodium soy sauce
10 mL	2 teaspoons cornstarch
	Pinch of crushed red pepper (optional)
125 mL	1/2 cup seeded and chopped red bell pepper (1/2-inch/1-cm pieces)

Bags of trimmed florets of broccoli and cauliflower, conveniently available in the produce section of most markets, make this pretty stir-fry a quick-and-easy side dish to serve with meat or fish or over rice. Studies have shown that broccoli and cauliflower, both cruciferous vegetables, are high in compounds called indoles that may protect against certain cancers.

1. Cook the broccoli, cauliflower, and water in a large skillet over medium heat, covered, until tender, 6 to 10 minutes, adding additional water, if needed. Drain the water from the pan.
2. Whisk the orange juice, honey, soy sauce, cornstarch, and red pepper flakes in a small bowl until smooth. Pour over the vegetables.
3. Add the red bell pepper and cook, stirring, until the sauce is thickened and the vegetables are coated, about 3 minutes.

Per serving: 74 calories, 0 g total fat, 0 g saturated fat, 17 g carbohydrate, 3 g protein, 3 g fiber, 0 mg cholesterol, 124 mg sodium, 31 mg calcium

Oven-Roasted Brussels Sprouts with Smoked Ham and Peanuts

Serves 4–6

PREP TIME: **10 minutes**
COOK TIME: **25–30 minutes**

Oven-roasted firm-cooked Brussels sprouts are a revelation in this surprise combo of smoky ham and peanuts. Brussels sprouts, a member of the nutritionally superior cruciferous family of vegetables, are an excellent source of disease-protecting phytochemicals.

500 g	1 pound Brussels sprouts, halved
25 mL	2 tablespoons chopped smoked ham
15 mL	1 tablespoon extra-virgin olive oil
0.5 mL	1/8 teaspoon freshly ground black pepper
25 mL	2 tablespoons chopped dry-roasted unsalted peanuts

1. Preheat the oven to 400°F (200°C).
2. Heat a medium saucepan half-filled with water to boiling. Add the Brussels sprouts and cook for 2 minutes. Drain well.
3. Toss the Brussels sprouts, ham, and oil on a jelly-roll pan. Sprinkle with the pepper. Roast, turning every 10 minutes with a wide spatula, until crisp-tender and lightly browned, about 25 minutes.
4. Sprinkle with the peanuts.

Per serving: 120 calories, 7 g total fat, 1 g saturated fat, 9 g carbohydrate, 5 g protein, 4 g fiber, 4 mg cholesterol, 88 mg sodium, 30 mg calcium

Broccoli Rabe with Sautéed Cremini Mushrooms

Serves 4

PREP TIME: **10 minutes**
COOK TIME: **15 minutes**

Broccoli rabe, braised to temper its mildly bitter taste, and golden slices of mushrooms and garlic combine to make a pleasant and heart-healthy side dish. Look for presliced cremini sold in many produce sections. Mushrooms add a sweet, almost meaty, taste to meals with no added fat or calories.

15 mL	1 tablespoon extra-virgin olive oil
500 mL	2 cups sliced cremini mushrooms (about 5 ounces/150 g)
15 mL	1 tablespoon finely chopped flat-leaf parsley
1	1 clove garlic, crushed
	Pinch of crushed red pepper, or to taste
1	1 bunch broccoli rabe (about 1 pound/500 g), 1 inch/2.5 cm trimmed from stems, cut into 1 1/2-inch/1-cm lengths

1. Heat the oil in a large nonstick skillet set over medium-high heat until hot enough to sizzle a mushroom. Add the mushrooms and cook, stirring, until golden, 4 to 5 minutes.
2. Stir in the parsley, garlic, and red pepper flakes until blended. Remove to a plate and set aside.
3. Rinse the broccoli rabe and lightly shake in a colander, leaving some water clinging to the leaves. Heat the same skillet over medium heat until hot enough that a drop of water sizzles. Add the broccoli rabe and stir until wilted, about 10 minutes. Reduce the heat to medium-low. Cover and cook until tender, 4 to 5 minutes.
4. Stir in the mushrooms and cook, stirring, until reheated, about 1 minute.

Per serving: 76 calories, 4 g total fat, 1 g saturated fat, 7 g carbohydrate, 5 g protein, 1 g fiber, 0 mg cholesterol, 36 mg sodium, 60 mg calcium

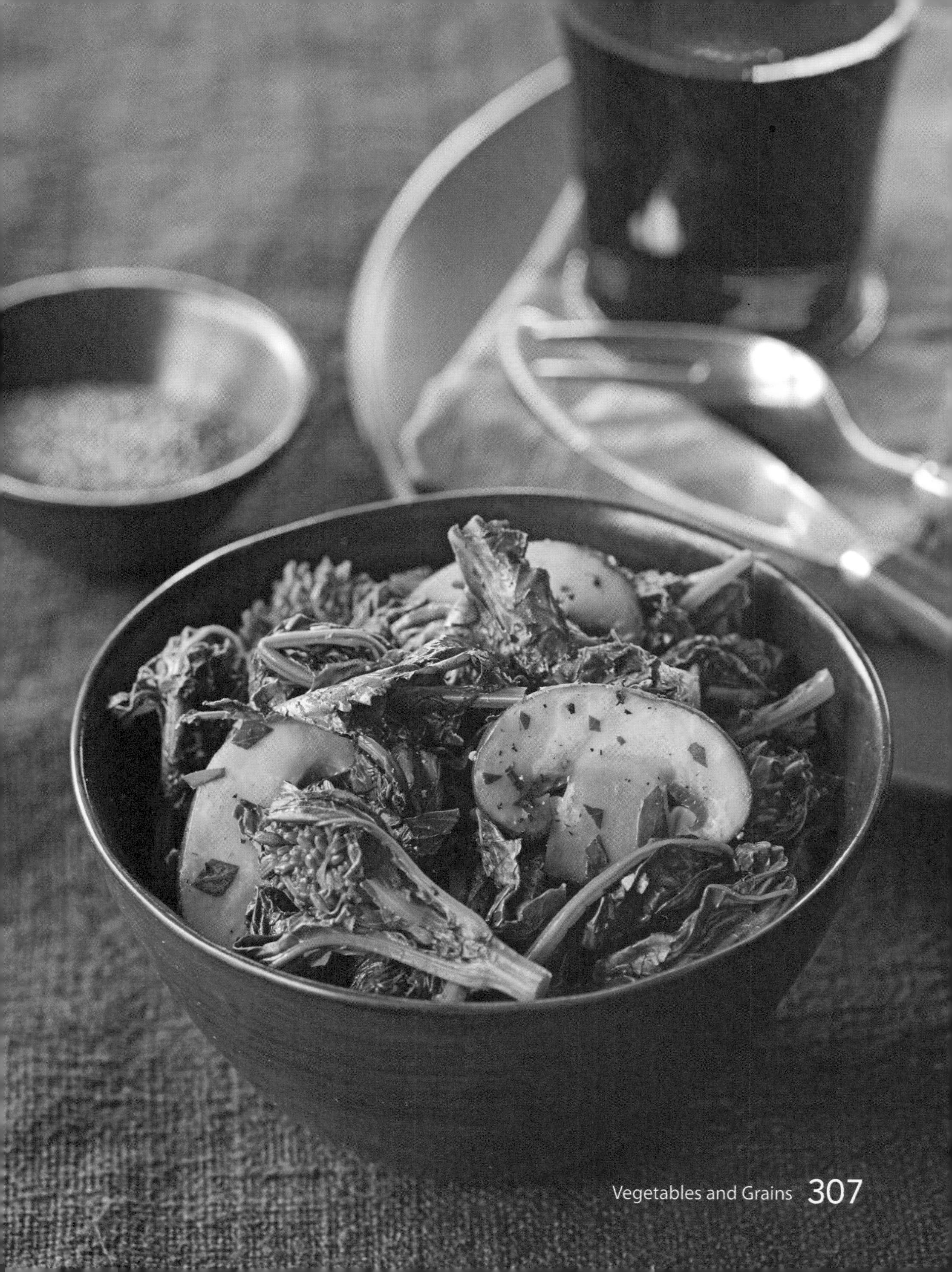

Stir-Fried Cabbage with Tamari and Ginger

Serves 6

PREP TIME: **10 minutes**
COOK TIME: **8–10 minutes**

Quick and easy with two popular tastes: Smooth-tasting tamari and fresh grated ginger. Once all the ingredients are prepped, this vegetable side dish goes together in a matter of minutes.

15 mL	1 tablespoons extra-virgin olive oil or unflavored oil
10 mL	2 teaspoons grated fresh ginger
1	1 small head Savoy cabbage (about 1 pound/500 g), quartered, cored, and cut into 1/4-inch/0.5-cm wide slices
25 mL	2 tablespoons water
10 mL	2 teaspoons reduced-sodium tamari

1. Heat the oil and ginger in a wok or large skillet over medium-low heat until the ginger sizzles, about 1 minute. Immediately add the cabbage and water.
2. Raise the heat to medium-high. Cook, tossing the cabbage with tongs and adjusting the temperature as needed to keep the cabbage sizzling, until crisp-tender, 5 to 6 minutes.
3. Raise the heat to high. Add the tamari and stir-fry until the cabbage is coated, about 1 minute.

Per serving: 42 calories, 2 g total fat, 0 g saturated fat, 5 g carbohydrate, 2 g protein, 2 g fiber, 0 mg cholesterol, 81 mg sodium, 27 mg calcium

Carrots and Sugar Snaps with Tarragon and Orange

Serves 4

PREP TIME: **12 minutes**
COOK TIME: **8 minutes**

Fresh and festive, bright orange carrots and green sugar snap peas are especially delicious seasoned with fresh tarragon and zesty orange. Sugar snap peas, a cross between snow peas and green peas, have plump, edible pods filled with very sweet, tender peas. They are both low in fat and high in fiber.

15 mL	1 tablespoon extra-virgin olive oil
4	4 medium carrots, cut into 1/4-inch/0.5-cm diagonal slices (about 1 1/2 cups/375 mL)
10 mL	2 teaspoons finely chopped orange zest
1	1 clove garlic, crushed
25 mL	2 tablespoons water
250 g	8 ounces stringless sugar snap peas, trimmed
10 mL	2 teaspoons chopped fresh tarragon
	Freshly ground black pepper

1. Heat the oil in a large skillet over medium heat. Add the carrots, orange zest, and garlic. Cook, stirring, until coated, about 1 minute.
2. Add the water and cook, covered, until the carrots are almost crisp-tender, 3 minutes.
3. Stir in the peas and tarragon. Cook, covered, until the carrots and peas are both crisp-tender, 3 to 4 minutes.
4. Sprinkle with the pepper.

Per serving: 81 calories, 4 g total fat, 1 g saturated fat, 10 g carbohydrate, 2 g protein, 3 g fiber, 0 mg cholesterol, 40 mg sodium, 63 mg calcium

Roasted Carrots, Red Onions, and Bell Peppers with Lemon

Serves 4–6

PREP TIME: **15 minutes**
COOK TIME: **45 minutes**

A colorful trio of roasted vegetables gussied up with thin slivers of lemon combine to make an easy and tasty side dish. Carrots contain a spectacular amount of beta-carotene, an antioxidant researchers believe may help reduce the risk of heart disease and some cancers.

500 mL	2 cups carrot slices (1-inch/2.5-cm diagonals)
1	1 medium red onion, cut into 1-inch/2.5-cm wedges (1 3/4 cups/ 425 mL)
1	1 red bell pepper, seeded and cut into 1 × 2-inch/2.5 × 5-cm strips, or 8 whole mini bell peppers
4	4 thin slices lemon, seeded and halved
15 mL	1 tablespoon extra-virgin olive oil
5 mL	1 teaspoon fresh thyme leaves
0.5 mL	1/8 teaspoon freshly ground black pepper

1. Preheat the oven to 400°F (200°C). Coat a jelly-roll pan or a shallow baking dish with nonstick cooking spray.
2. Combine the carrots, onions, bell peppers, lemons, oil, thyme, and black pepper in the pan. Toss to coat and arrange in a single layer.
3. Roast, stirring once or twice, until the carrots are tender and golden, about 45 minutes.

Per serving: 84 calories, 4 g total fat, 1 g saturated fat, 12 g carbohydrate, 1 g protein, 3 g fiber, 0 mg cholesterol, 61 mg sodium, 38 mg calcium

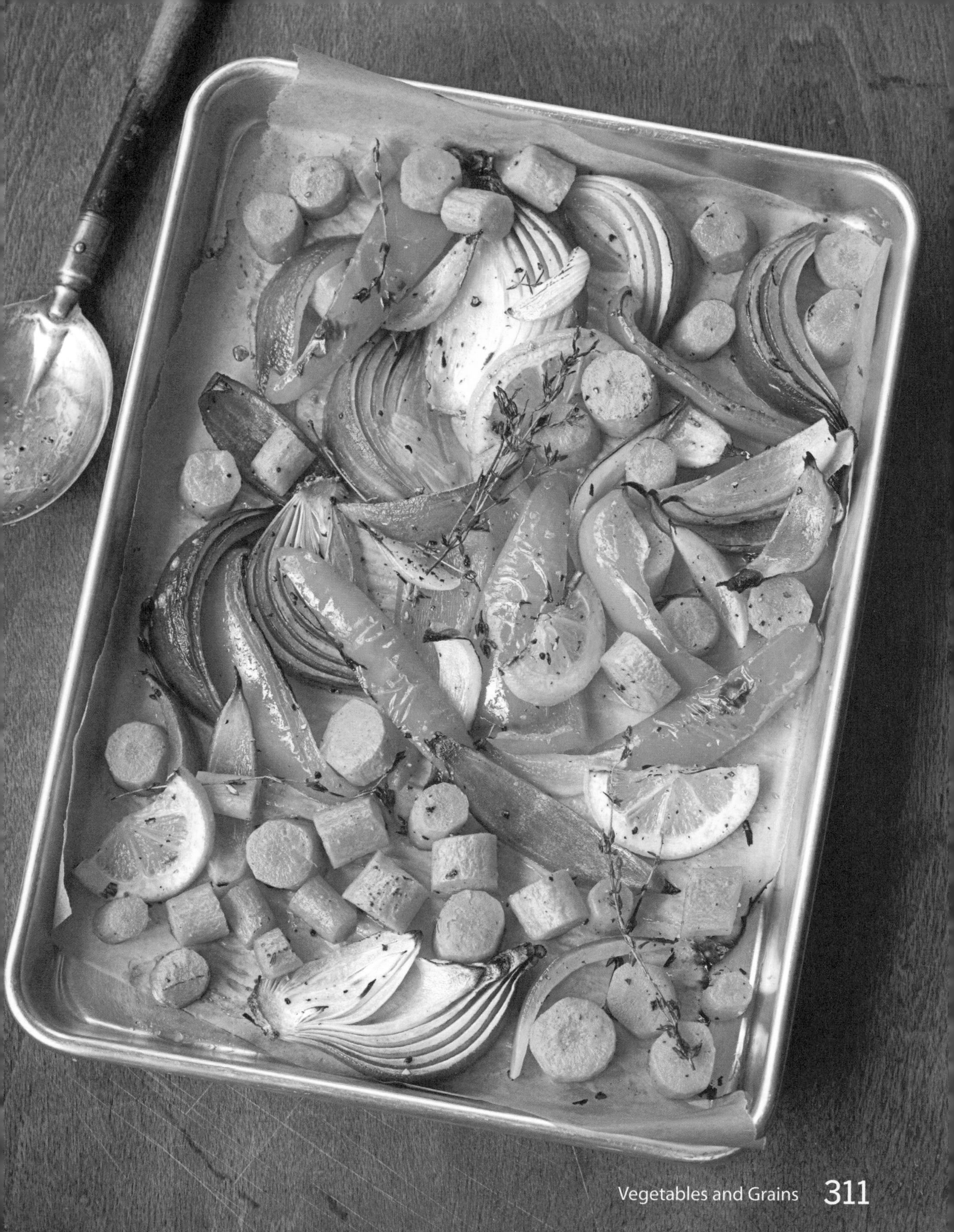

Oven-Roasted Cauliflower with Madras Curry Powder

Serves 4

PREP TIME: **10 minutes**
COOK TIME: **35–40 minutes**

1	1 whole head cauliflower (about 1 1/2 pounds/ 750 g), trimmed
15 mL	1 tablespoon extra-virgin olive oil
5 mL	1 teaspoon Madras curry powder, divided
0.5 mL	1/8 teaspoon freshly ground black pepper
25 mL	2 tablespoons finely chopped fresh cilantro, dill, or mint

Aromatic curry powder stands up to the distinctive taste of oven-roasted cauliflower. A member of the cruciferous family of vegetables, cauliflower is highly touted for its important nutritional contributions to a healthy diet.

1. Preheat the oven to 400°F (200°C). Coat a jelly-roll pan with nonstick cooking spray.
2. Slice through the cauliflower head at 3/4-inch (1.5-cm) the intervals to make thick slices or "steaks." Arrange them on the pan in a single layer. Brush with the oil and sprinkle with 1/2 teaspoon (2 mL) of the curry powder. Roast until the cauliflower begins to brown on the edges, about 20 minutes.
3. Remove the pan from the oven and turn the cauliflower over with a wide spatula. Sprinkle with the remaining 1/2 teaspoon (2 mL) of curry powder and the pepper. Return to the oven and roast until tender and golden, 15 to 20 minutes longer.
4. Sprinkle with the cilantro, dill, or mint.

Per serving: 76 calories, 4 g total fat, 1 g saturated fat, 9 g carbohydrate, 3 g protein, 4 g fiber, 0 mg cholesterol, 52 mg sodium, 40 mg calcium

Braised Mixed Greens with Slow-Cooked Garlic and Dried Currants

Serves 4–6

PREP TIME: **10 minutes**
COOK TIME: **17 minutes**

Leafy greens, now conveniently sold in big bags in produce departments, sweetened with slow-cooked garlic and dried currants make a quick-and-easy skillet braise. Dark, leafy greens are highly touted for their abundance of nutrients, including beta-carotene, vitamin C, folate, iron, calcium, and fiber.

15 mL	1 tablespoon extra-virgin olive oil
3	3 cloves garlic, thinly sliced
1	1 bag (1 pound/500 g) mixed braising greens (collards, kale, turnip greens, and mustard), rinsed and slightly drained
15 mL	1 tablespoon dried currants

1. Heat the oil and garlic in a small skillet over low heat, stirring, until the garlic begins to sizzle. Watch carefully and remove from the heat when the garlic begins to turn golden, about 5 minutes. Set aside.
2. Cook the greens and currants in a large wide pan over medium heat, covered, turning once or twice with tongs, until wilted and tender, about 10 minutes. Raise the heat to high. Cook, uncovered, to evaporate any excess moisture.
3. Add the garlic. Reheat, stirring, for 1 minute.

Per serving: 81 calories, 4 g total fat, 1 g saturated fat, 10 g carbohydrate, 3 g protein, 4 g fiber, 0 mg cholesterol, 24 mg sodium, 178 mg calcium

Velvet Spinach with Sesame

Serves 6

PREP TIME: **10 minutes**
COOK TIME: **5 minutes**

Gentle steam quickly cooks spinach to a velvety texture. Spinach offers an array of nutrients, including vitamins, minerals, beta-carotene, lutein, and zeaxanthin, which are absorbed when the leaves are coated with a fat, like olive oil.

20 mL	1 tablespoon plus 1 teaspoon light olive oil
1	1 clove garlic, crushed
2 mL	1/2 teaspoon dark sesame oil
2	2 bunches (1 1/2 pounds/750 g) leaf spinach, rinsed, long stems trimmed
2 mL	1/2 teaspoon sesame seeds

1. Heat the olive oil and garlic in a small skillet over low heat, stirring, until the garlic begins to sizzle, about 30 seconds. Remove from the heat. Stir in the sesame oil.
2. Steam the spinach in a vegetable steamer insert set over 1 inch (2.5 cm) of boiling water, covered, until wilted, about 2 minutes.
3. Using tongs, remove the spinach to a serving dish. Top with the garlic and sprinkle with the sesame seeds.

Per serving: 60 calories, 4 g total fat, 1 g saturated fat, 5 g carbohydrate, 3 g protein, 3 g fiber, 0 mg cholesterol, 90 mg sodium, 115 mg calcium

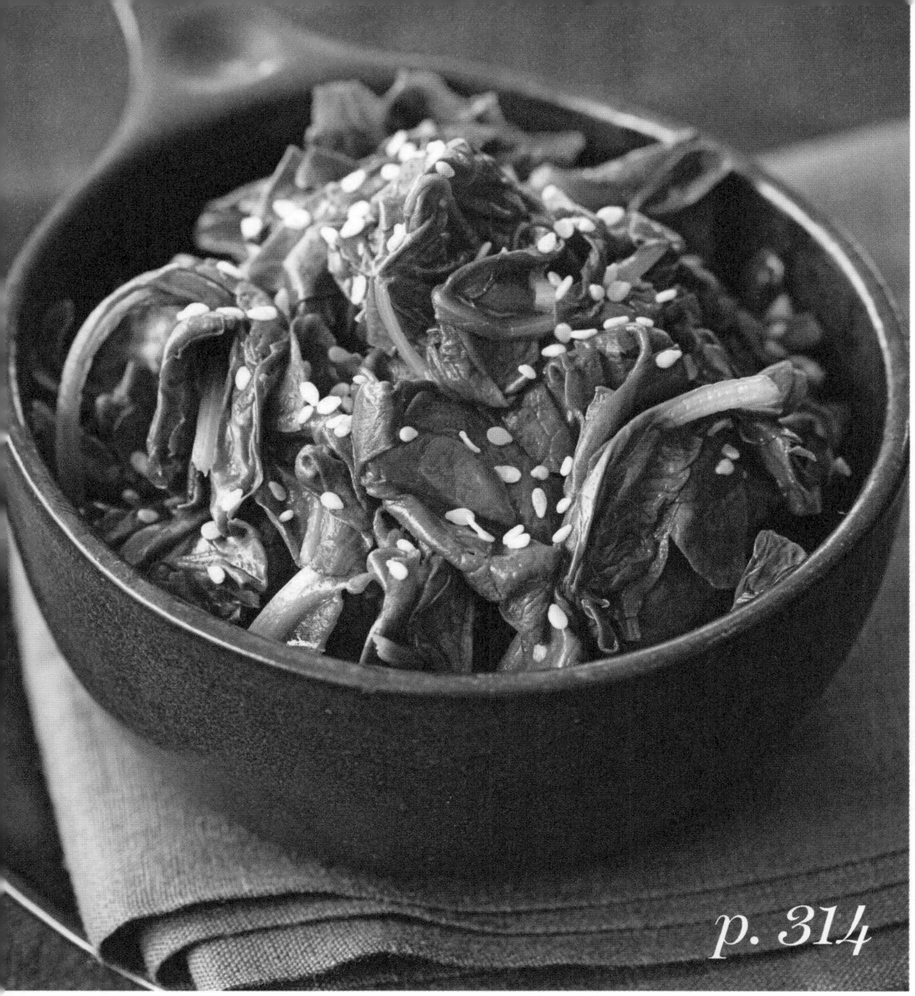
p. 314

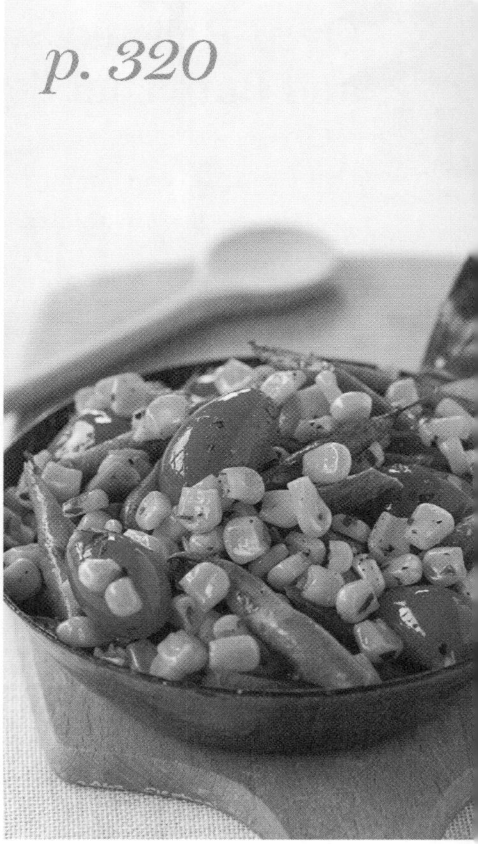
p. 320

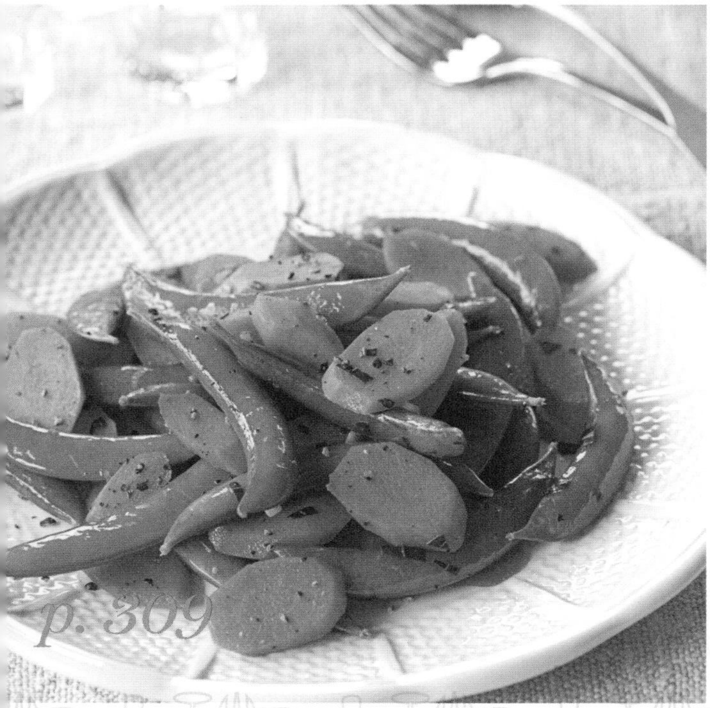
p. 309

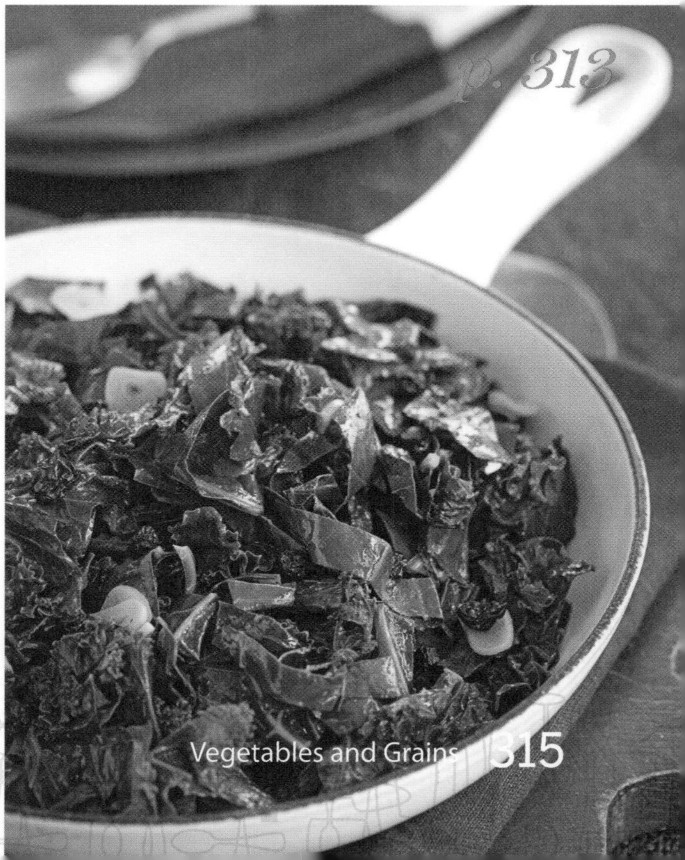
p. 313

Oven-Roasted Sweet Potatoes and Butternut Squash with Pecans

Serves 4–6

PREP TIME: **10 minutes**
COOK TIME: **30 minutes**

The aromatic spice blend typically used for pumpkin pie is used here, along with crunchy pecans, to give roasted sweets and winter squash a delicious twist. Pecans, rich in zinc, thiamin, and fiber, also provide plenty of heart-healthy monounsaturated and polyunsaturated fats.

500 g	1 pound butternut squash, unpeeled, seeds removed, and cut into 1-inch/2.5-cm pieces (4 to 5 cups/1 to 1.25 L)
250 g	8 ounces sweet potato, unpeeled, cut into 1-inch/2.5-cm pieces (1 1/4 cups/300 mL)
15 mL	1 tablespoon extra-virgin olive oil
5 mL	1 teaspoon pumpkin pie spice
1 mL	1/4 teaspoon coarse salt
0.5 mL	1/8 teaspoon freshly ground black pepper
15 mL	1 tablespoon maple syrup
50 mL	1/4 cup chopped pecans

1. Preheat the oven to 400°F (200°C). Coat a jelly-roll pan or shallow baking dish with nonstick cooking spray.
2. Place the squash, potatoes, oil, pumpkin pie spice, salt, and pepper on the pan and toss until coated. Spread in a single layer. Roast, turning once or twice with a wide spatula, until the vegetables are tender and golden, about 30 minutes.
3. Drizzle with the syrup and turn to coat. Sprinkle with the pecans and roast for 5 minutes longer.

Per serving: 193 calories, 9 g total fat, 1 g saturated fat, 29 g carbohydrate, 3 g protein, 5 g fiber, 0 mg cholesterol, 182 mg sodium, 85 mg calcium

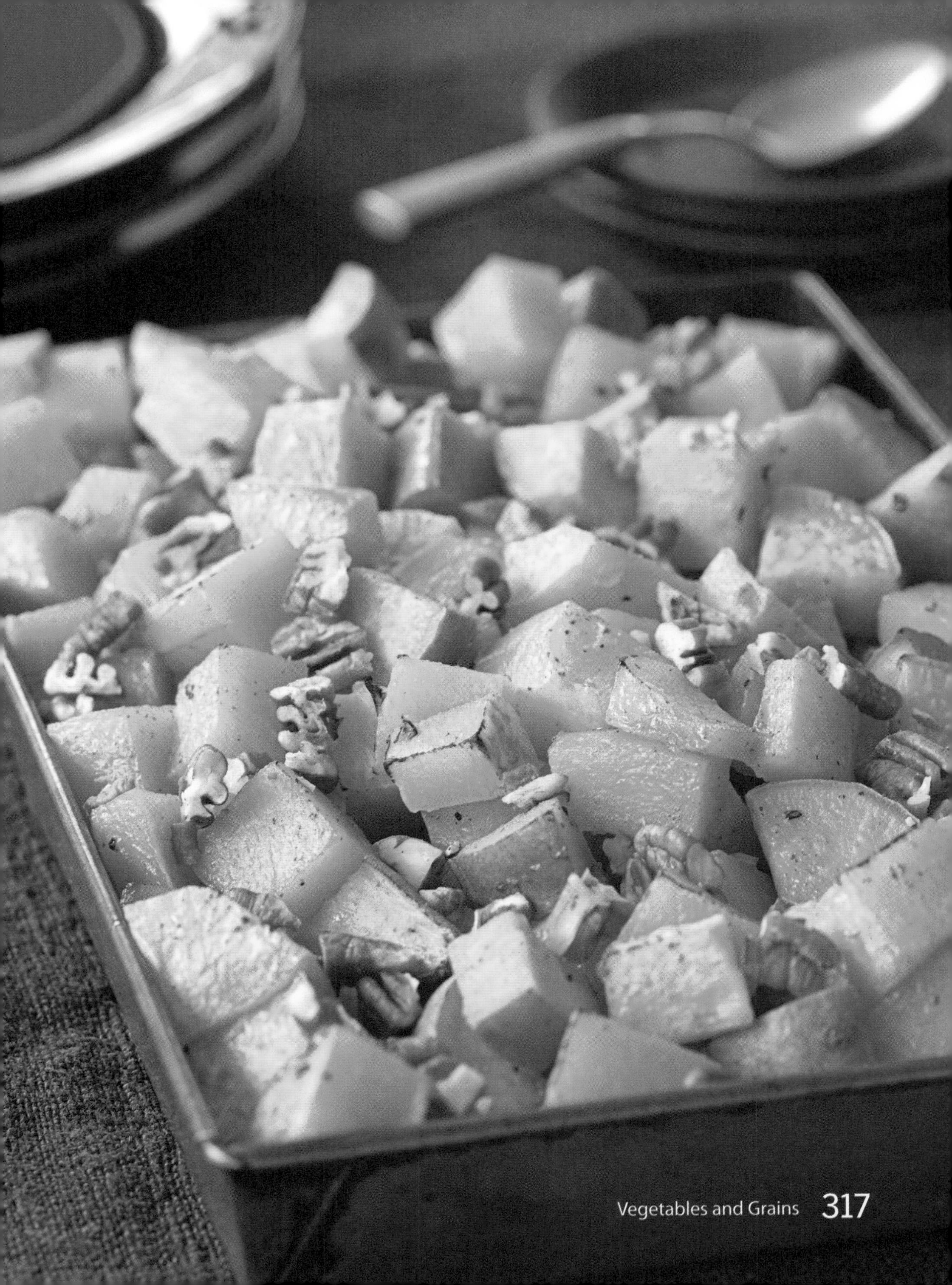

Rough-Mashed Olive Oil and Garlic Potatoes

Serves 5

PREP TIME: **5 minutes**
COOK TIME: **15 minutes**

The secret to mashed potatoes without guilt is this fragrant mélange flavored with herbs, garlic, and fruity olive oil. In addition to carbohydrates, potatoes provide protein, vitamin C, potassium, and iron, while the skins provide lots of fiber.

1 kg	2 pounds Yukon gold potatoes, unpeeled and cubed (1/2 inch/1 cm)
4	4 cloves garlic, bruised with the side of a knife
1	1 bay leaf
1	1 fresh thyme stem (2 inches/5 cm)
2 mL	1/2 teaspoon coarse salt
50 mL	1/4 cup extra-virgin olive oil, divided
0.5 mL	1/8 teaspoon freshly ground black pepper

1. Combine the potatoes, garlic, bay leaf, thyme, and salt in a medium saucepan and add water to cover. Bring to a boil over high heat. Reduce the heat to medium. Cook, covered, until tender, about 15 minutes. Drain, reserving 1/4 cup (50 mL) of the cooking water. Discard the bay leaf and thyme stem.
2. Return the potatoes to the pan and mash with a potato masher or pastry blender, adding 2 tablespoons (25 mL) of the oil and as much of the reserved cooking water as needed to reach the desired consistency.
3. Mound the potatoes on individual serving plates. Make an indention in the surface of each mound and drizzle evenly with the remaining 2 tablespoons (25 mL) of oil. Sprinkle on fresh ground black pepper.

Per serving: 238 calories, 11 g total fat, 2 g saturated fat, 31 g carbohydrate, 4 g protein, 3 g fiber, 0 mg cholesterol, 245 mg sodium, 31 mg calcium

Summer Squash, Edamame, and Leek Sauté with Lemon and Thyme

Serves 6

PREP TIME: **15 minutes**
COOK TIME: **8 minutes**

Edamame, fresh soybeans, are high in protein, fiber, and B vitamins, plus potassium and magnesium—all heart-healthy nutrients. Lemon and thyme brighten the flavors of summer squash and leeks, making this dish a terrific addition to your favorite vegetable recipes.

15 mL	1 tablespoon extra-virgin olive oil
250 mL	1 cup sliced trimmed leeks (1/4-inch/0.5-cm slices)
250 mL	1 cup thawed frozen shelled edamame
250 g	8 ounces small zucchini, halved lengthwise and cut into 1/4-inch/0.5-cm crosswise slices (about 1 cup/250 mL)
250 g	8 ounces small yellow summer squash, halved lengthwise and cut into 1/4-inch/0.5-cm crosswise slices (about 1 cup/250 mL)
10 mL	2 teaspoons chopped fresh thyme leaves
10 mL	2 teaspoons grated lemon zest
0.5 mL	1/8 teaspoon freshly ground black pepper
1	1 clove garlic, crushed

1. Heat the oil in a large nonstick skillet over medium heat until hot enough to sizzle a leek. Add the leeks and cook, stirring, for 1 minute.
2. Add the edamame and cook, stirring, for 1 minute.
3. Add the zucchini, squash, thyme, and lemon zest and cook, stirring, for 1 minute.
4. Reduce the heat to medium-low. Cook, covered, until the squash is crisp-tender, 3 to 4 minutes. Stir in the pepper and garlic. Cook, stirring, for 30 seconds.

Per serving: 70 calories, 4 g total fat, 1 g saturated fat, 7 g carbohydrate, 4 g protein, 2 g fiber, 0 mg cholesterol, 7 mg sodium, 41 mg calcium

Blistered Tomatoes with Corn, Green Beans, and Basil

Serves 4–6

PREP TIME: **15 minutes**
COOK TIME: **10 minutes**

Fresh tomatoes, corn, and green beans accented with fresh basil make a tasty combo packed with the great flavors of summer. Fresh produce is the backbone of healthy eating with the goal set at 8 to 10 servings a day. Here, you get a good start with three vegetables in every spoonful.

15 mL	1 tablespoon extra-virgin olive oil
50 mL	2 cups cherry, sugar plum, grape, or other small tomatoes
250 mL	1 cup sliced trimmed green beans (1/4-inch/0.5-cm diagonals)
500 mL	2 cups corn kernels cut from 2 ears of corn
1	1 clove garlic, crushed
25 mL	2 tablespoons finely chopped fresh basil leaves
0.5 mL	1/8 teaspoon freshly ground black pepper

1. Heat the oil in a medium skillet over medium-high heat until hot. Add the tomatoes and cook, shaking the pan until the tomatoes are blistered and softened, about 5 minutes.
2. Reduce the heat to medium-low. Stir in the beans and cook, covered, until crisp-tender, about 3 minutes.
3. Stir in the corn and garlic. Cook, stirring, for 2 minutes. Stir in the basil and pepper.

Per serving: 108 calories, 4 g total fat, 1 g saturated fat, 15 g carbohydrate, 3 g protein, 3 g fiber, 0 mg cholesterol, 6 mg sodium, 21 mg calcium

Orzo Pilaf with Spinach and Walnuts

Serves 6

PREP TIME: **10 minutes**
COOK TIME: **15 minutes**

Embellished with tender spinach leaves and crunchy walnuts, orzo, a tender rice-shaped pasta, lends itself to being cooked pilaf-style, like rice. Although high in complex carbohydrates, pasta is a good source of protein and is enriched with B vitamins, iron, and selenium. It should be enjoyed in moderation.

50 mL	1/4 cup broken walnuts
550 mL	2 1/4 cups reduced-sodium low-fat chicken broth
250 mL	1 cup orzo
500 mL	2 cups firmly packed washed and dried baby spinach leaves

1. Heat the walnuts in a small skillet over medium-low heat, stirring, until the walnuts are golden, about 5 minutes. Set aside.
2. Heat the broth to boiling in a medium saucepan. Stir in the orzo and cook, covered, until the broth is absorbed and the orzo is al dente or firm to the bite, about 15 minutes.
3. Stir in the spinach and cook until wilted, about 30 seconds. Sprinkle with the walnuts.

Per serving: 186 calories, 4 g total fat, 1 g saturated fat, 30 g carbohydrate, 8 g protein, 2 g fiber, 0 mg cholesterol, 37 mg sodium, 25 mg calcium

Lentils with Dill and Sun-Dried Tomatoes

Serves 6

PREP TIME: **10 minutes**
COOK TIME: **15 minutes**

Little bits of dried tomatoes and chopped dill add a bright taste to meaty-tasting lentils. Tiny disk-shaped lentils have a positive nutritional profile providing fiber and other vitamins, but are particularly rich in the B vitamin folate—1/2 cup (125 mL) of cooked lentils provides almost half the daily requirement.

2	2 cloves garlic, divided
250 mL	1 cup brown lentils, rinsed and sorted
1	1 bay leaf
25 mL	2 tablespoons fresh lemon juice
15 mL	1 tablespoon extra-virgin olive oil
0.5 mL	1/8 teaspoon freshly ground black pepper
75 mL	1/3 cup chopped fresh dill
25 mL	2 tablespoons chopped oil-packed sun-dried tomatoes, rinsed thoroughly and drained

1. Bruise 1 of the garlic cloves with the side of a knife. Cook the garlic, lentils, and bay leaf in plenty of boiling water until the lentils are tender, about 15 minutes. Drain well. Discard the bay leaf and garlic.
2. Crush the remaining clove of garlic. In a serving bowl, whisk together the garlic, lemon juice, oil, and pepper.
3. Fold in the lentils, dill, and tomatoes. Serve warm.

Per serving: 130 calories, 3 g total fat, 0 g saturated fat, 20 g carbohydrate, 7 g protein, 5 g fiber, 0 mg cholesterol, 10 mg sodium, 19 mg calcium

Quinoa Pilaf with Dried Apples and Sliced Almonds

Serves 4

PREP TIME: **10 minutes**
COOK TIME: **15 minutes**

50 mL	1/4 cup sliced almonds (skins on)
250 mL	1 cup quinoa
500 mL	2 cups water
125 mL	1/2 cup chopped dried apples
2 mL	1/2 teaspoon coarse salt

Fluffy with a pleasant crunch and sweet, nutty flavor, the taste of quinoa is a revelation to those who have yet to experience it. Quinoa is a complete protein, which is rare in the plant world. It is relatively low in fat and provides vitamin E, riboflavin, zinc, potassium, iron, magnesium, and fiber.

1. Heat the almonds in a small skillet set over low heat, stirring, until golden, 3 to 5 minutes. Set aside.
2. Rinse the quinoa in a strainer under running water or swish in a bowl of water and strain. Shake dry. Heat in a deep skillet or wide saucepan over medium-low heat, stirring, until the quinoa begins to darken slightly, 7 to 10 minutes.
3. Add the water, apples, and salt and bring to a boil. Reduce the heat to low. Cook, covered, until the liquid is absorbed and the quinoa is fluffy, 12 to 18 minutes.
4. Sprinkle with the almonds.

Per serving: 217 calories, 5 g total fat, 1 g saturated fat, 35 g carbohydrate, 7 g protein, 4 g fiber, 0 mg cholesterol, 361 mg sodium, 35 mg calcium

Wild Rice with Two-Mushroom Sauté and Toasted Hazelnuts

Serves 6

PREP TIME: **20 minutes**
COOK TIME: **55 minutes**

Nutty, tasty, wild rice and rich, earthy mushrooms combine to make a hearty, but elegant, side dish. For ease in preparation, look for peeled and toasted hazelnuts. Hazelnuts contain good heart-healthy fats and more vitamin E than other nuts, while wild rice is higher in protein than other rice and contains niacin and B vitamins.

750 mL	3 cups water
250 mL	1 cup wild rice, rinsed
25 mL	2 tablespoons extra-virgin olive oil
750 mL	3 cups chopped white button mushrooms (8 ounces/250 g)
300 mL	1 1/4 cups chopped (stems discarded) shiitake mushrooms (4 ounces/125 g)
1	1 clove garlic, finely chopped
25 mL	2 tablespoons chopped flat-leaf parsley
5 mL	1 teaspoon chopped fresh thyme
0.5 mL	1/8 teaspoon freshly ground black pepper
25 mL	2 tablespoons chopped peeled toasted hazelnuts

1. Heat the water and rice to boiling in a medium saucepan. Reduce the heat to medium. Cook, covered, stirring occasionally, until the water is absorbed and the rice is tender, about 45 minutes. Let stand, covered, for 10 minutes.
2. Heat the oil in a medium skillet over medium-high heat until hot enough to sizzle a piece of mushroom. Add the button and shiitake mushrooms and cook, stirring, until browned and tender, about 5 minutes.
3. Stir in the garlic and cook for 1 minute. Stir in the parsley, thyme, and pepper.
4. Stir into the rice and sprinkle with the hazelnuts.

Per serving: 166 calories, 7 g total fat, 1 g saturated fat, 23 g carbohydrate, 5 g protein, 2 g fiber, 0 mg cholesterol, 4 mg sodium, 18 mg calcium

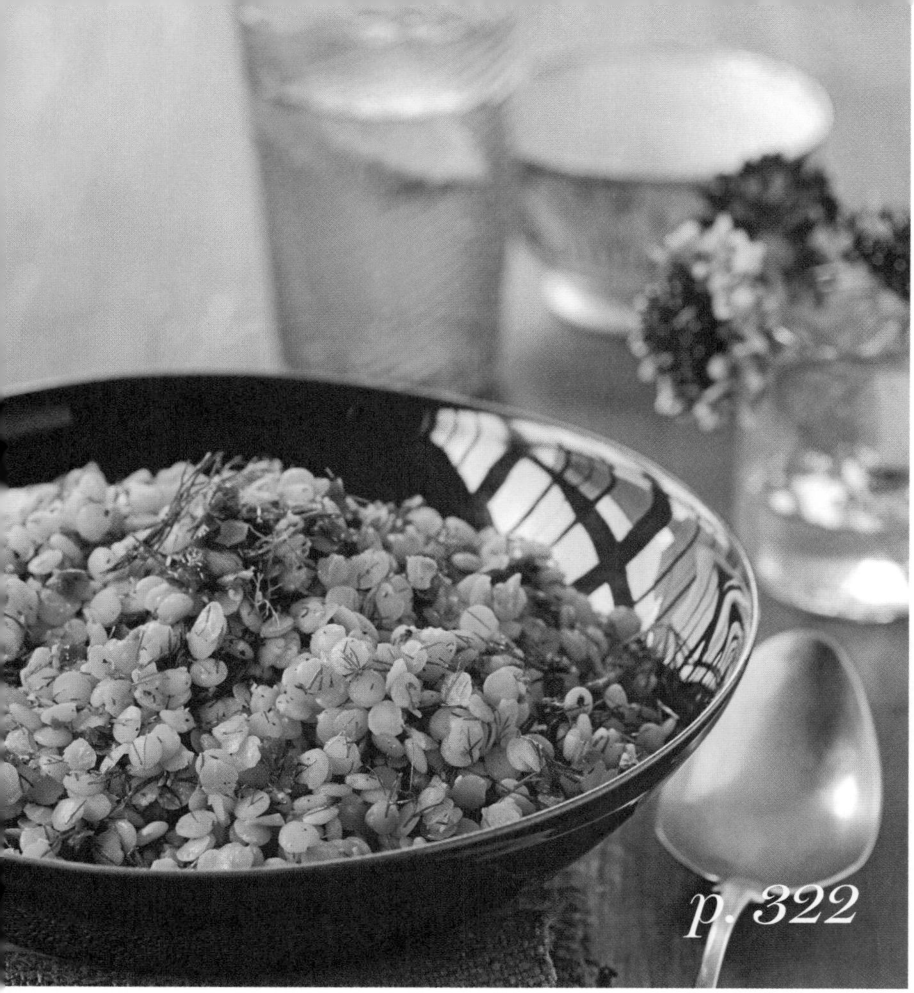
p. 322

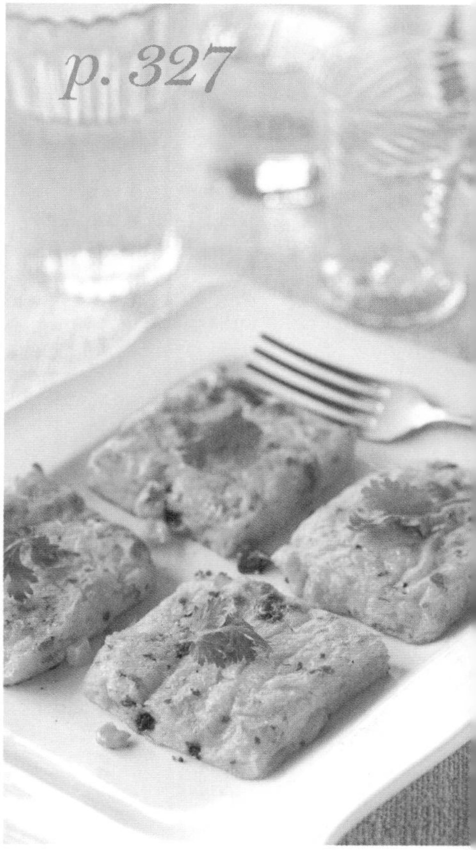
p. 327

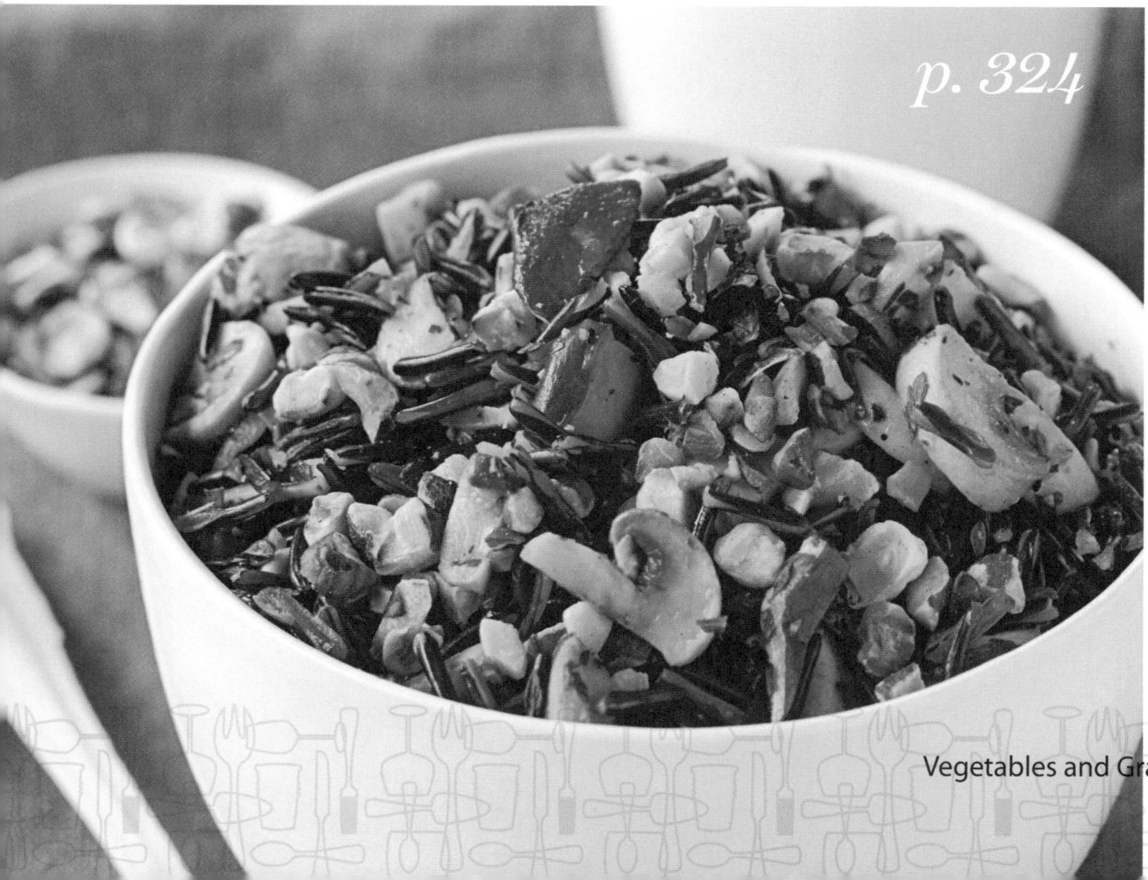
p. 324

Bulgur Pilaf with Dried Cranberries and Pistachios

Serves 6

PREP TIME: **5 minutes**
COOK TIME: **20 minutes**

Garnet gems of dried cranberries and bright green pistachios add sparkle to this easy-on-the-cook bulgur pilaf. Look for cranberries naturally sweetened with unsweetened fruit juice. Dried cranberries are an excellent source of vitamin C, potassium, and fiber.

15 mL	1 tablespoon extra-virgin olive oil
50 mL	1/4 cup chopped onion
250 mL	1 cup medium-grain bulgur
500 mL	2 cups water
25 mL	2 tablespoons chopped dried cranberries
25 mL	2 tablespoons chopped natural pistachios

1. Heat the oil in a 10-inch (25-cm) skillet or sauté pan over medium heat. Cook the onions, stirring, until golden, about 5 minutes.
2. Add the bulgur and cook, stirring, until the bulgur is toasted a shade darker, about 5 minutes.
3. Add the water and cranberries and heat to boiling. Reduce the heat to medium-low. Cook, covered, stirring occasionally, until all the water is absorbed, 10 minutes. Let stand, uncovered and undisturbed, for 5 minutes.
4. Spoon into a serving dish and sprinkle with the pistachios.

Per serving: 125 calories, 4 g total fat, 1 g saturated fat, 21 g carbohydrate, 3 g protein, 5 g fiber, 0 mg cholesterol, 4 mg sodium, 12 mg calcium

Double Corn Polenta Toast with Cilantro

Serves 6

PREP TIME: **15 minutes**
COOK TIME: **35 minutes**

Crispy on the outside and soft and tasty on the inside, double corn polenta toasts are conveniently made from chilled cornmeal mush or polenta. Yellow corn is the most nutritious with the highest numbers for beta-carotene, but all whole-grain cornmeal is high in protein, fiber, and other nutrients.

25 mL	2 tablespoons finely chopped onion
5 mL	1 teaspoon extra-virgin olive oil
375 mL	1 1/2 cups water
125 mL	1/2 cup coarse-ground polenta or yellow cornmeal
125 mL	1/2 cup low-fat (1%) milk
125 mL	1/2 cup fresh or thawed frozen corn kernels
15 mL	1 tablespoon finely chopped fresh cilantro
15 mL	1 tablespoon chopped oil-packed sun-dried tomatoes, well-rinsed and drained
10 mL	2 teaspoons seeded, deveined, and finely chopped jalapeño (wear gloves when handling), or to taste
75 mL	1/3 cup coarsely shredded Manchego or Monterey Jack cheese

1. Coat a 9-inch (22-cm) square metal or glass baking dish with nonstick cooking spray.
2. Cook the onions and oil in a medium saucepan over low heat, stirring, until tender, about 3 minutes.
3. Add the water and cornmeal. Cook, stirring constantly, until boiling. Adjust the heat to maintain a simmer and cook, stirring, until thickened, 6 to 8 minutes.
4. Stir in the milk, corn, cilantro, tomatoes, and jalapeños. Cook, stirring, for 5 minutes.
5. Stir in the cheese and spoon into the pan. Cover with plastic wrap and refrigerate for several hours or until cold and firm. Loosen the sides, turn out of pan, and cut into 12 evenly sized portions.
6. Preheat the oven to 400°F (200°C). Coat a jelly-roll pan with nonstick cooking spray.
7. Place the polenta portions on the pan and bake until lightly browned on the bottoms, about 10 minutes. Turn with a wide spatula and brown the other side, about 10 minutes.

Per serving: 105 calories, 3 g total fat, 2 g saturated fat, 16 g carbohydrate, 4 g protein, 2 g fiber, 7 mg cholesterol, 57 mg sodium, 27 mg calcium

Toasted Almond and Chocolate Soufflé Cake

Serves 10

PREP TIME: **20 minutes**
COOK TIME: **25 minutes**

150 mL	1/2 cup plus 2 tablespoons sugar, divided
75 mL	1/3 cup chopped almonds (skin on)
125 mL	1/2 cup unsweetened cocoa powder
8	8 large egg whites
0.5 mL	1/8 teaspoon salt
25 mL	2 tablespoons sliced almonds (skin on)

Smooth and creamy, dense and chocolaty, this easy-to-make cake is pure chocolate decadence...with zero cholesterol! It is made with a minimum of unsaturated fat and lots of protein-rich egg whites. It gets its intense chocolate flavor from cocoa—the pure, fat-free form of chocolate being touted for its natural nutrients and health-promoting flavanol antioxidants.

1. Preheat the oven to 325°F (160°C). Line the bottom of an 8-inch (20-cm) springform pan with parchment. Coat the parchment and the sides of the pan with nonstick cooking spray. Sprinkle the bottom and sides with 1 tablespoon (15 mL) of the sugar.
2. Spread the chopped almonds in a baking pan and bake until lightly toasted, 7 to 10 minutes. Remove from the oven and let cool. Combine them with 1 tablespoon (15 mL) of the remaining sugar in a food processor and pulse to finely grind. Pour into a large bowl. Add the remaining 1/2 cup (125 mL) of sugar and the cocoa powder. Stir to blend.
3. In a medium bowl, beat the egg whites and salt with an electric mixer until soft peaks form. Fold the egg whites, in three additions, into the cocoa mixture. Spoon into the springform pan and smooth the top. Sprinkle with the sliced almonds.
4. Bake until the cake puffs and a tester inserted in the center comes out smeared but at the edges is clean, about 25 minutes. Cool the cake on a wire rack for 30 minutes (cake will fall). Loosen the sides of the cake with a knife and remove the pan sides. Cool cake completely before serving.

Per serving: 147 calories, 3 g total fat, 0 g saturated fat, 17 g carbohydrate, 15 g protein, 1 g fiber, 0 mg cholesterol, 239 mg sodium, 20 mg calcium

Whole-Grain Scones with Dried Currants and Walnuts

Makes 8

PREP TIME: **20 minutes**
COOK TIME: **19 minutes**

There is nothing more tempting than a warm scone! These are even more inviting because they are made wholesome with heart-healthy ingredients. Low-fat buttermilk and unsaturated vegetable oil add a soft light crumb to the batter and wheat germ and ground flaxseed add multiple nutritional benefits.

425 mL	1 3/4 cups unbleached all-purpose flour
50 mL	1/4 cup wheat germ
50 mL	1/4 cup sugar
15 mL	1 tablespoon ground flaxseed
5 mL	1 teaspoon ground cinnamon
2 mL	1/2 teaspoon salt
125 mL	1/2 cup coarsely chopped walnuts
75 mL	1/3 cup dried currants
175 mL	3/4 cup buttermilk
2 mL	1/2 teaspoon baking soda
75 mL	1/3 cup light olive oil or other unflavored vegetable oil

1. Preheat the oven to 350°F (180°C). Coat a baking sheet with nonstick cooking spray.
2. Combine the flour, wheat germ, sugar, flaxseed, cinnamon, and salt in a large bowl and stir to blend. Add the walnuts and currants and toss to coat.
3. Combine the buttermilk and baking soda in a cup. Add it and the oil to the dry ingredients and stir just until blended. Do not overmix. Gather the dough together, adding a little more buttermilk to moisten dry particles, if needed.
4. Transfer the dough to a lightly floured work surface and shape into a flat 7-inch (17.5-cm) round. Use a wide spatula to transfer the dough to the baking sheet. Cut into 8 wedges, leaving a slight separation between each wedge.
5. Bake for 15 minutes. Increase the oven temperature to 375°F (190°C) and bake until lightly browned, about 8 minutes longer. Serve warm.

Per scone: 237 calories, 12 g total fat, 2 g saturated fat, 29 g carbohydrate, 5 g protein, 2 g fiber, 1 mg cholesterol, 141 mg sodium, 39 mg calcium

Fresh Fruit and Cheese Tartlets

Makes 6

PREP TIME: **1 hour 50 minutes**
COOK TIME: **15 minutes**

These cream-filled, fresh-fruit-topped tarts are dainty, pretty, and a snap to make. The easy-to-handle whole-grain dough is made with healthful trans-fat-free vegetable shortening and is simply pressed into the pans with your fingertips.

125 mL	1/2 cup all-purpose flour
50 mL	1/4 cup whole-wheat pastry flour
25 mL	2 tablespoons trans-fat-free vegetable oil
20 mL	1 tablespoon plus 1 teaspoon sugar, divided
60 -75 mL	4 to 5 tablespoons cold water
125 mL	1/2 cup low-fat cottage cheese
125 mL	1/2 cup low-fat (1/3 less fat) cream cheese (4 ounces/125 g)
5 mL	1 teaspoon grated orange zest
2 mL	1/2 teaspoon vanilla extract
6	6 slices peeled kiwifruit (1/4 inch/0.5 cm thick)
250 mL	1 cup blueberries

1. Combine the all-purpose flour, pastry flour, oil, and 1 teaspoon (5 mL) of the sugar in a large bowl and toss with a fork to blend. Gradually add the water, 1 tablespoon (15 mL) at a time, to form the dough. Gather into a ball, flatten into a disk, wrap in foil, and refrigerate for 20 minutes.
2. Preheat the oven to 350°F (180°C). Coat six 3- to 3 1/2-inch (7.5- to 8.5-cm) tartlet pans with nonstick cooking spray. Divide the dough into six even pieces and shape into balls. Roll each into a 4- to 5-inch (10- to 12.5-cm) circle.
3. Carefully lift each round of dough and place in the tartlet pans, pressing the dough along the bottom and up the sides of each pan. Patch any tears with your fingertips. Poke holes in the dough with a fork to keep the shells from shrinking. Place the tart pans on a baking sheet and bake until the edges are lightly browned, about 15 minutes. Remove from the oven and cool on a wire rack.
4. Meanwhile, combine the cottage cheese, cream cheese, the remaining 1 tablespoon (15 mL) of sugar, the orange zest, and vanilla in a food processor and process until light and fluffy. Divide among the tart shells and smooth the tops. Place a kiwi slice in the center of each tartlet and surround with the blueberries. Carefully remove the tartlets from the pans to serve.

Per tartlet: 174 calories, 8 g total fat, 3 g saturated fat, 22 g carbohydrate, 5 g protein, 2 g fiber, 12 mg cholesterol, 159 mg sodium, 77 mg calcium

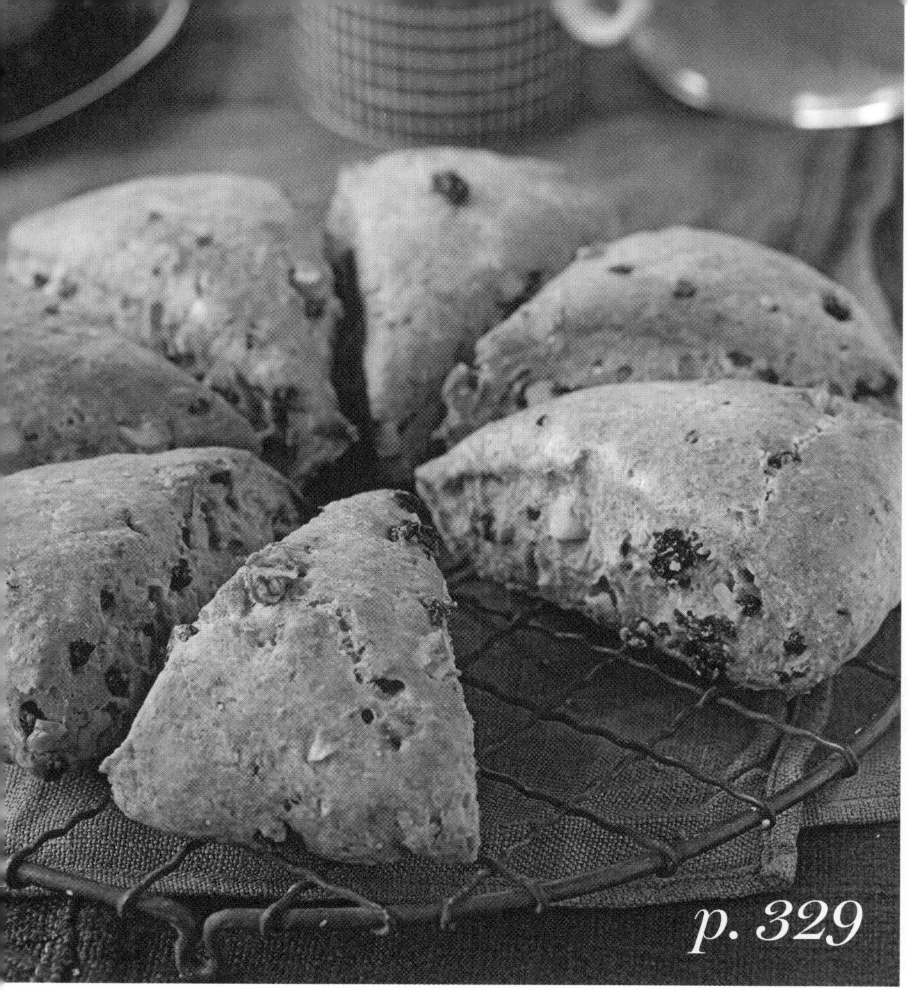
p. 329

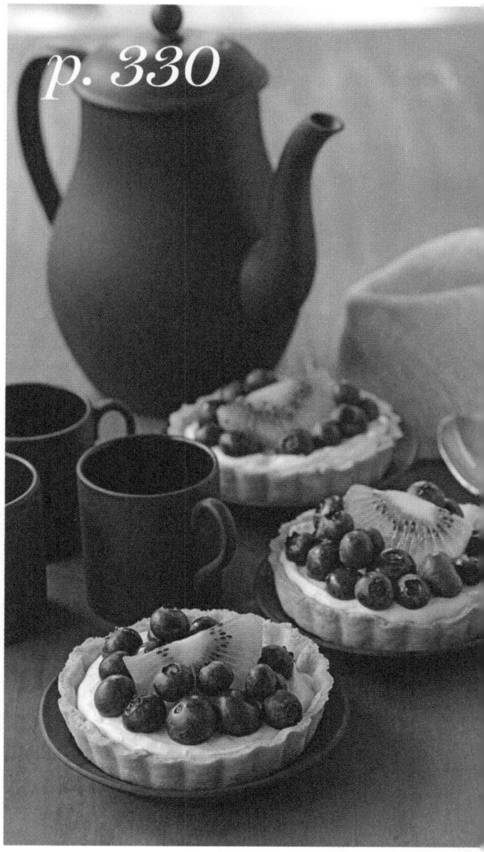
p. 330

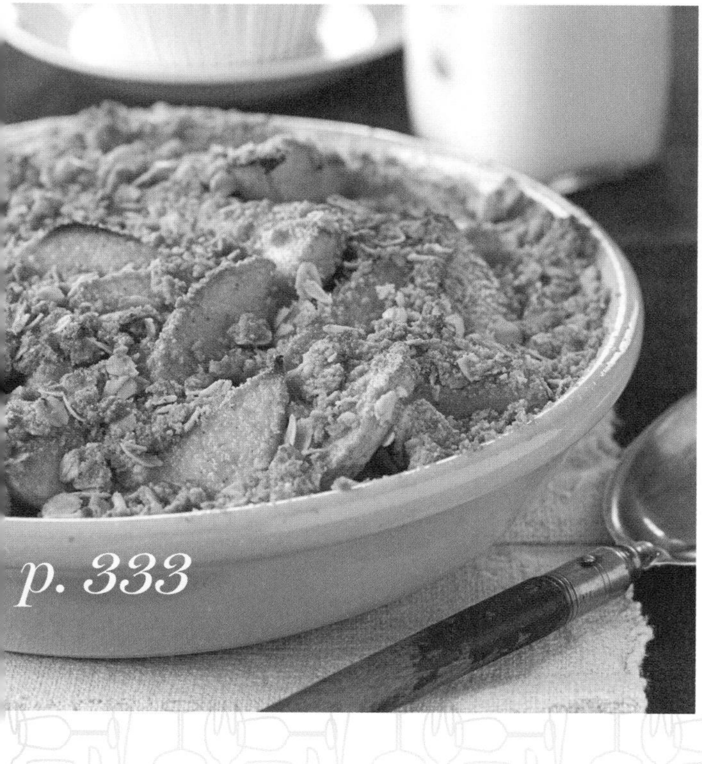
p. 333

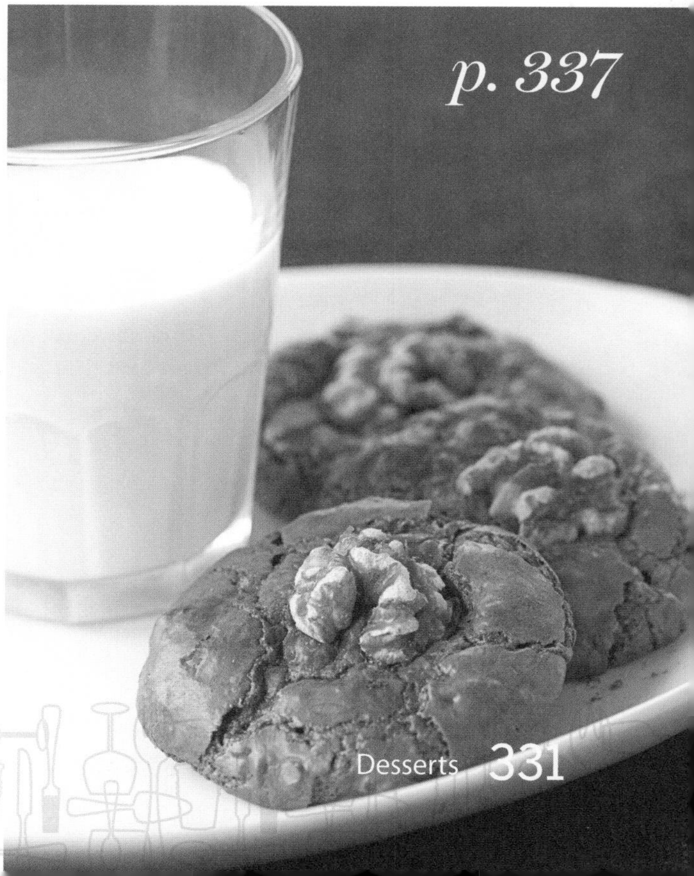
p. 337

Pistachio and Chocolate Chip Biscotti

Makes 16

PREP TIME: **15 minutes**
COOK TIME: **30 minutes**

2	2 large eggs
75 mL	1/3 cup sugar
125 mL	1/2 cup unbleached all-purpose flour
50 mL	1/4 cup whole-wheat pastry flour
2 mL	1/2 teaspoon ground cinnamon
2 mL	1/2 teaspoon baking powder
50 mL	1/4 cup toasted, peeled, and coarsely chopped natural pistachios
50 mL	1/4 cup semi-sweet mini chocolate chips

Crunchy and luscious, these chocolate chip biscotti are perfect with a cup of coffee or tea. Look for semi-sweet mini chips or, even better, dark chocolate chunks that can be chopped into smaller pieces. The darker the chocolate, the less fat and the more heart-healthy antioxidants it provides.

1. Preheat the oven to 350°F (180°C). Coat a baking sheet with nonstick cooking spray.
2. With an electric mixer, beat the eggs and sugar in a large bowl until the sugar is dissolved and the mixture is light and fluffy.
3. Combine the all-purpose flour, pastry flour, cinnamon, baking powder, and pistachios in a food processor and pulse until the nuts are chopped. Fold into the eggs along with the chocolate chips to make a stiff batter.
4. Spoon the batter onto the baking sheet making two 11 × 2 inch (28 × 5 cm) logs, leaving about 3 inches (7.5 cm) between. Bake for 20 minutes. Remove from the oven and reduce the temperature to 325°F (160°C).
5. Use two spatulas to slide the logs to a cutting board. Cut into diagonal slices (1-inch/2.5-cm wide). Place the slices, cut sides down, on the baking sheet and return to the oven. Bake until golden, 10 to 12 minutes. Cool on a wire rack.

Per biscotti: 73 calories, 2 g total fat, 1 g saturated fat, 11 g carbohydrate, 2 g protein, 1 g fiber, 27 mg cholesterol, 26 mg sodium, 10 mg calcium

Apple Streusel Pie

Serves 8

PREP TIME: **25 minutes**
COOK TIME: **50 minutes**

175 mL	3/4 cup all-purpose flour
50 mL	1/4 cup whole-wheat pastry flour
25 mL	2 tablespoons packed light brown sugar, divided
0.5 mL	1/8 teaspoon salt
50 mL	1/4 cup trans-fat-free vegetable shortening
75 mL	1/4 cup plus 1 tablespoon cold water
1 to 1.5 L	4 to 5 cups peeled and cored baking apple slices (1/8 inch/0.25 cm)
25 mL	2 tablespoons fresh lemon juice
5 mL	1 teaspoon ground cinnamon

STREUSEL TOPPING

125 mL	1/2 cup quick-cooking (not instant) oatmeal
50 mL	1/4 cup all-purpose flour
50 mL	1/4 cup whole-wheat pastry flour
50 mL	1/4 cup packed light brown sugar
2 mL	1/2 teaspoon ground cinnamon
45 mL	3 tablespoons cold butter, cut into small pieces

Everybody loves a slice of pie. This one is special with its buttery streusel topping over cinnamon-laced apples tucked into a crispy crust. It only sounds sinful. The crisp crust uses heart-healthy trans-fat-free vegetable shortening and fiber-rich whole-wheat flour. With this dish, you can love your pie and eat it, too.

1. Combine the all-purpose flour, pastry flour, 1 tablespoon (15 mL) of the brown sugar, and the salt in a food processor. Pulse once to blend. Add the shortening and pulse just until the mixture is crumbly. Add the water, 1 tablespoon (15 mL) at a time, pulsing with each addition, only until the dough pulls away from the sides of the bowl. Gather the dough into a ball, wrap it in foil, and refrigerate for 20 minutes.
2. Preheat the oven to 375°F (190°C).
3. Prepare the streusel topping. Combine the oatmeal, all-purpose flour, pastry flour, brown sugar, and cinnamon in the bowl of a food processor and pulse once to blend. Add the butter and pulse until crumbly, 4 to 5 times. Do not overblend or the oatmeal will be too finely chopped.
4. Toss the apples in a large bowl with the lemon juice, the remaining 1 tablespoon (15 mL) of brown sugar, and the cinnamon. Set aside.
5. Roll the dough into a round shape large enough to fit into a 9-inch (22-cm) pie plate. Carefully transfer to the pie plate, turning the edges under and crimping to form an edge. Spread the apple mixture in the crust and top with the streusel.
6. Bake until the streusel is browned and the apples are tender, about 50 minutes.

Per serving: 222 calories, 11 g total fat, 5 g saturated fat, 29 g carbohydrate, 3 g protein, 1 g fiber, 11 mg cholesterol, 50 mg sodium, 18 mg calcium

Three-Berry Oatmeal and Almond Crisp

Serves 8

PREP TIME: **20 minutes**
COOK TIME: **35 minutes**

A crunchy oatmeal and almond topping crowns this bubbly berry crisp. Crisps are easy to make with almost any fruit on the bottom, but when it comes to nutrients, colorful berries are the tops. Make double the amount of topping and freeze it for a repeat performance another day.

375 mL	1 1/2 cups strawberries, hulled and cut into 1/2-inch/1-cm pieces
250 mL	1 cup blueberries, rinsed and drained
250 mL	1 cup raspberries, rinsed and drained
15 mL	1 tablespoon all-purpose flour
45 mL	3 tablespoons packed light brown sugar, divided
5 mL	1 teaspoon grated lemon zest
125 mL	1/2 cup quick-cooking (not instant) oatmeal
25 mL	2 tablespoons whole-wheat pastry flour
25 mL	2 tablespoons light olive oil or unflavored vegetable oil
25 mL	2 tablespoons sliced almonds (skin on)
125 mL	1/2 cup low-fat vanilla yogurt

1. Preheat the oven to 350°F (180°C).
2. Combine the strawberries, blueberries, and raspberries in a 9-inch (22-cm) pie plate.
3. Combine the all-purpose flour, 1 tablespoon (15 mL) of the brown sugar, and the lemon zest, in a small bowl and stir to blend. Sprinkle on top of the berries and lift gently with a spoon to coat evenly.
4. In a medium bowl, combine the oatmeal, pastry flour, the remaining 2 tablespoons (25 mL) of brown sugar, the oil, and almonds. Blend with a fork or your fingertips. Squeeze the mixture in your hand to make small "pebbles" and drop evenly on top of the berries.
5. Bake until the top is browned and the fruit is bubbly, about 35 minutes. Top each serving with 1 tablespoon (15 mL) of the yogurt.

Per serving: 127 calories, 5 g total fat, 1 g saturated fat, 19 g carbohydrate, 3 g protein, 4 g fiber, 1 mg cholesterol, 12 mg sodium, 51 mg calcium

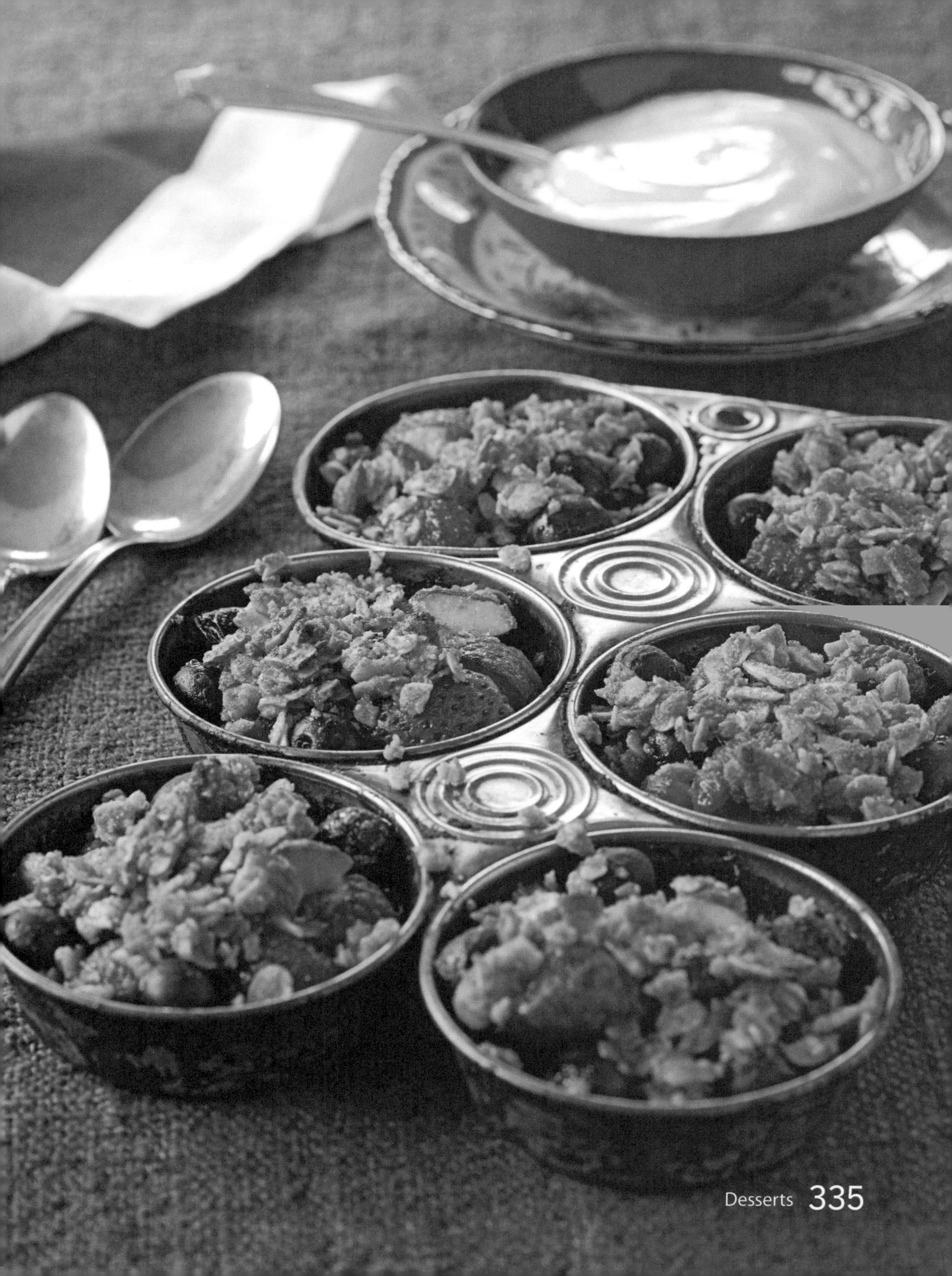

Fresh Pineapple-Mango Sorbet

Serves 6

PREP TIME: **10 minutes**
FREEZE TIME: **30 minutes in ice cream maker; about 3 hours in freezer**

Cool, refreshing, and bursting with the natural sweetness of two luscious tropical fruits, this is a sorbet to savor. This requires some freezing time, so plan ahead. If you have an ice-cream maker, just follow the manufacturer's directions—it will be ready quicker. Either way, the natural sweetness of the fruits will sing to your palate.

250 mL	1 cup fresh pineapple chunks
250 mL	1 cup peeled and seeded mango chunks
250 mL	1 cup naturally sweetened apple juice
15 mL	1 tablespoon fresh lime juice

1. Puree the pineapples, mangoes, apple juice, and lime juice in a food processor until smooth.
2. Pour the mixture into a large glass loaf pan or other nonreactive pan and freeze until the edges begin to set, 1 to 1 1/2 hours. Stir the firm edges into the soft center and freeze until solid, 1 to 2 hours longer. Break into chunks with the side of a spoon and transfer to a food processor. Process until smooth, then spoon into a plastic container and freeze until firm, about 45 minutes.

Per serving: 54 calories, 0 g total fat, 0 g saturated fat, 14 g carbohydrate, 0 g protein, 1 g fiber, 0 mg cholesterol, 2 mg sodium, 6 mg calcium

Chocolate-Walnut Melt-in-Your-Mouth Cookies

Makes 30

PREP TIME: **25 minutes**
COOK TIME: **12–15 minutes**

A wonderful treat or reward awaits you at the end of a busy day: A delightful hit of sweetness, with just the right crisp texture and rich chocolately goodness.

175 g	6 ounces semi-sweet chocolate chips
2	2 large egg whites, at room temperature
0.5 mL	1/8 teaspoon cream of tartar
2 mL	1/2 teaspoon vanilla extract
125 mL	1/2 cup packed light brown sugar
75 mL	1/3 cup finely chopped walnuts
50 mL	1/4 cup all-purpose flour
30	30 walnut pieces

1. Preheat the oven to 350°F (180°C). Coat two baking sheets with nonstick cooking spray.
2. Melt the chocolate chips in a small glass bowl in the microwave, 1 to 1 1/2 minutes. Cool slightly.
3. In a medium bowl, with an electric mixer, beat the egg whites together with the cream of tartar and vanilla until soft peaks form. Gradually beat in the brown sugar, 1 tablespoon (15 mL) at a time, to make stiff peaks.
4. Drizzle the chocolate on top of the egg whites and gently fold until thoroughly incorporated.
5. In a small bowl, stir the chopped walnuts and flour until blended. Sprinkle over the egg whites and gently fold until blended (batter will deflate slightly). Immediately drop the batter by rounded teaspoons onto baking sheets. Place a walnut piece in the center of each.
6. Bake, turning pans halfway through baking time to ensure even baking, until firm around the edges, 12 to 15 minutes. Remove the cookies from the pans and cool on wire racks.

Per cookie: 70 calories, 4 g total fat, 1 g saturated fat, 9 g carbohydrate, 1 g protein, 1 g fiber, 0 mg cholesterol, 5 mg sodium, 9 mg calcium

Lemon-Lime Yogurt Cake with Mixed-Berry Topping

Serves 10

PREP TIME: **25 minutes**
COOK TIME: **25 minutes**

Fresh, clean, summery flavors make this delicate white cake a winner. Change the berries used in the topping with any kind available fresh in the market. Consider using sliced peaches or nectarines in place of the berries, or use just one type of berry instead of a combination of three.

135 mL	1/2 cup plus 2 teaspoons sugar, divided
50 mL	1/4 cup unflavored vegetable oil
5 mL	1 teaspoon grated lemon zest
2 mL	1/2 teaspoon grated lime zest
2 mL	1/2 teaspoon vanilla extract
125 mL	1/2 cup plain low-fat yogurt
250 mL	1 cup cake flour (not self-rising)
2 mL	1/2 teaspoon baking soda
2	2 large egg whites
0.5 mL	1/8 teaspoon cream of tartar

TOPPING

125 mL	1/2 cup unsweetened apple juice
25 mL	2 tablespoons sugar
1 mL	1/4 teaspoon grated lime zest
500 mL	2 cups hulled and chopped strawberries, blueberries, and/or raspberries or blackberries

1. Preheat the oven to 350°F (180°C). Coat an 8-inch (20-cm) cake pan with nonstick cooking spray and sprinkle with 2 teaspoons (10 mL) of the sugar. Shake to coat the bottom of the pan evenly.
2. Combine the remaining 1/2 cup (125 mL) of sugar, the oil, lemon zest, lime zest, and the vanilla in a large bowl. Beat until well-blended. Add the yogurt and stir to combine. Sift the flour and baking soda together in a small bowl and fold into the wet ingredients.
3. In a medium bowl, with an electric mixer, beat the egg whites and cream of tartar until soft peaks form. Add to the batter and gently fold with a rubber spatula until blended. Spoon into the pan and smooth the surface. Bake until the cake is golden and a toothpick inserted in the center comes out clean, about 25 minutes.
4. Meanwhile, prepare the topping. Combine the apple juice, sugar, and lime zest in a small saucepan and heat to simmering. Cook, over low heat, stirring occasionally, for 5 minutes. Remove from the heat and let cool to room temperature, about 30 minutes.
5. Place the berries in a medium bowl and pour the apple juice mixture on top. Refrigerate until ready to serve.
6. Cool the cake in the pan for 10 minutes. Loosen the sides with a knife and invert onto a wire rack. Cool completely. Serve in wedges topped with the fruit.

Per serving: 177 calories, 6 g total fat, 1 g saturated fat, 30 g carbohydrate, 3 g protein, 1 g fiber, 1 mg cholesterol, 84 mg sodium, 33 mg calcium

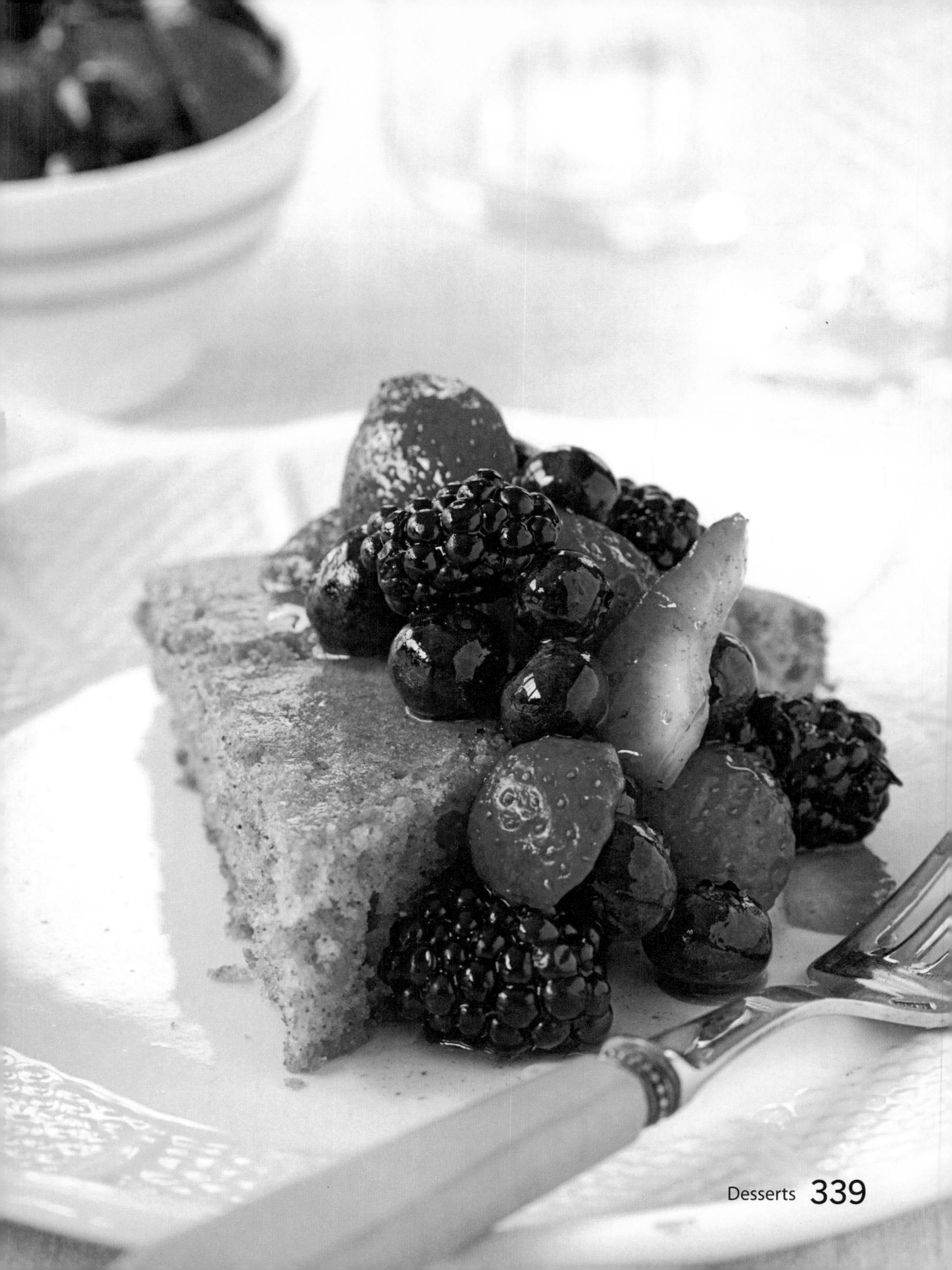

Chocolate-Peanut Butter Brownies

Makes 20

PREP TIME: **20 minutes**
COOK TIME: **25–30 minutes**

125 mL	1/2 cup sifted cake flour (not self-rising)
75 mL	1/3 cup unsweetened cocoa powder
50 mL	1/4 cup finely chopped unsalted dry-roasted peanuts, divided
2	2 large eggs
125 mL	1/2 cup packed light brown sugar
50 mL	1/4 cup smooth peanut butter
50 mL	1/4 cup unsweetened applesauce
50 mL	1/4 cup unflavored vegetable oil
5 mL	1 teaspoon vanilla extract

Who can resist the winning combination of chocolate and peanut butter in a moist yet cakey interpretation of the quintessential brownie? Not many. Here we have both in a heart-healthy version of the chocolate brownie made with a double whammy of smooth peanut butter and crunchy peanuts.

1. Preheat the oven to 350°F (180°C). Coat an 8-inch (20-cm) square baking pan with nonstick cooking spray.
2. Combine the flour and cocoa in a large bowl and stir to blend. Add in 2 tablespoons (25 mL) of the peanuts.
3. Combine the eggs, brown sugar, peanut butter, applesauce, oil, and vanilla in a food processor and process until smooth. Pour over the flour mixture and fold together with a rubber spatula until evenly moistened. Spread in the pan and sprinkle with the remaining 2 tablespoons (25 mL) of peanuts.
4. Bake until the edges pull away from the sides of the pan and a toothpick inserted in the center comes out clean, 25 to 30 minutes. Cool in the pan. Cut into 20 squares.

Per brownie: 101 calories, 6 g total fat, 1 g saturated fat, 10 g carbohydrate, 2 g protein, 1 g fiber, 18 mg cholesterol, 23 mg sodium, 10 mg calcium

Fig, Raisin, and Walnut Oatmeal Cookies

Makes 30

PREP TIME: **25 minutes**
COOK TIME: **15 minutes**

Chewy dried fruits and nuts add natural sweetness to these tender little cookies. Make short work of chopping figs by first brushing the blade and interior of the food processor bowl with oil or nonstick cooking spray. Figs are high-fiber and, along with raisins, are a good source of iron. These are good keepers.

125 mL	1/2 cup unsalted butter
125 mL	1/2 cup pure maple syrup
5 mL	1 teaspoon vanilla extract
500 mL	2 cups old-fashioned oatmeal
125 mL	1/2 cup whole-wheat pastry flour
5 mL	1 teaspoon baking powder
5 mL	1 teaspoon ground cinnamon
125 mL	1/2 cup packed chopped dried Black Mission or Calimyrna fig pieces (1/2 inch/1 cm
125 mL	1/2 cup raisins
125 mL	1/2 cup chopped walnuts

1. Preheat the oven to 350°F (180°C). Coat 2 baking sheets with nonstick cooking spray.
2. Melt the butter and syrup in a small saucepan over low heat. Pour into a large bowl and stir in the vanilla.
3. Pulse the oatmeal, flour, baking powder, and cinnamon in a food processor 3 or 4 times. Add to the maple syrup mixture along with the figs, raisins, and walnuts. Stir with a spatula until thoroughly blended.
4. Drop by half-tablespoons (making 30 equal portions) onto the baking sheets. Bake until the bottoms are lightly browned, about 15 minutes. Transfer to wire racks to cool.

Per cookie: 90 calories, 5 g total fat, 2 g saturated fat, 11 g carbohydrate, 2 g protein, 1 g fiber, 8 mg cholesterol, 37 mg sodium, 20 mg calcium

Recipe List

Breakfast

Walnut-Topped Blueberry-Bran Muffins 214

Blueberry-Orange Yogurt Smoothies 215

Strawberry, Pineapple, and Almond Smoothies 215

Whole-Grain French Toast with Sautéed Apples 216

Cooked Oatmeal-and-Bulgur Cereal with Apples and Dates 218

Strawberry, Oatmeal, and Whole-Wheat Pancakes with Strawberry Maple Syrup 219

Individual Breakfast Tortilla 220

One-Egg Omelets with Chopped Broccoli, Tomatoes, and Cheddar 222

Smoked Salmon and Asparagus Frittata 223

Appetizers and Snacks

Deviled Eggs with Black Olives 224

Avocado, Tomato, and Cucumber Dip with Steamed Shrimp 225

Crisped Potato Skins with Veggie Salsa 226

Cranberry-Peanut Cereal Bars 228

Endive with Curry-Walnut Cream Cheese 229

Olive and Dried Fig Tapenade 230

Smoked Trout Pâté with Dill 232

Curry-Spiced Nuts 233

Stuffed Dried Apricots with Chopped Pistachios 233

Roasted Red Pepper and Chickpea Dip with Pita Chips 234

Salads

Main Dish

Tuna, Red Cabbage, Green Bean, and Caper Salad 236

Chicken, Arugula, Avocado, and Tomato Salad with Lemon-Garlic Dressing and Black Olives 238

Sardine and New Potato Salad with Spinach and Dill-Mustard Dressing 239

Quinoa, Shrimp, and Fresh Corn Salad on Curly Leaf Lettuce with Toasted Cumin-Lime Dressing 240

Side Dish

Sweet Potato, Green Apple, and Peanut Salad with Apple-Cider-Vinegar Dressing 242

Asian Coleslaw with Ginger and Two Sesame Flavors 243

Chopped Mango, Broccoli, Tomato, and Romaine Salad with Herbed Buttermilk Dressing 244

White Bean, Fennel, and Onion Salad with Red-Wine Vinaigrette 245

Black Bean, Corn, Tomato, Avocado, and Cilantro with Lime and Jalapeño Dressing 246

Hot Smoked Salmon, Celery, and Egg with Creamy Mustard Dressing 248

Lentil, Roasted Red Pepper, and Spinach Salad with Walnuts, Olives, and Sherry Vinaigrette 249

Mixed Greens with Sliced Pears, Toasted Almonds, and Shaved Parmesan 250

Cantaloupe and Watercress Salad with Feta Cheese 251

Soups

Mushroom, Spinach, and Wild Rice Soup 252

Barley, Chicken, and Spring Vegetable Soup 253

Roasted Tomato Soup with Toasted Cumin and Brown Rice 254

Creamy Curried Carrot Soup 256

Butternut Squash and Apple Soup 257

Asian-Flavored Chicken, Shiitake, and Bok Choy Soup 258

Black Bean Soup with Chipotle Chiles 260

Two-Fish Soup with Fennel and Roasted Tomatoes 261

Entrées

Poultry

Curried Chicken Breasts with Butternut Squash, Green Beans, and Tomatoes 262

Pan-Seared Chicken Thighs with Chimichurri Sauce 263

Braised Chicken Breasts with Garlic, Lentils, and Asparagus 264

Hazelnut-Crusted Turkey Cutlets with Parmesan and Rosemary 266

Herb-Roasted Turkey Breast 267

Tandoori Chicken 268

Lamb

Lamb Stew with Artichoke Hearts and New Potatoes 269

Marinated Lamb Kebabs with Zucchini, Tomatoes, and Red Onions 270

Pork

Rosemary-Crusted Pork Tenderloin with Roasted Tomatoes and White Beans 272

Pork Tenderloin Medallions with Lemon and Honey Mustard Sauce 273

Beef

Grilled Flank Steak and Sweet Potatoes with Dried Tomato, Caper, and Parsley Sauce 274

Zinfandel Beef Stew with Roasted Vegetables 276

Orange-and-Soy-Glazed Beef Stir-Fry with Green Beans, Mini Bell Peppers, and Peanuts 277

Seafood

Pan-Seared Shrimp with Lemon Orzo Primavera 278

Orange-Glazed Roasted Salmon with Tricolor Bell Peppers 280

Broiled Fish Steaks with Tomato, Peach, and Orange Salsa 281

Oven-Fried Fish Fillets with Chunky Low-Fat Tartar Sauce 282

Salmon and Asparagus Farfalle with Walnut-Feta Sauce 284

Cornmeal-Crusted Trout Almondine on Smothered Greens with Lemon 285

Sautéed Salmon Fillets with Tomatoes, Zucchini, and Green Olives 286

Oven-Roasted Mackerel with Cherry Tomatoes, Potatoes, and Smoked Paprika 288

Pasta

Whole-Grain Pasta Primavera with Ricotta 289

Soup Bowl Lasagna with Spinach, Turkey Sausage, and Three Cheeses 290

Cheesy Curly Macaroni with Broccoli and Cherry Tomatoes 292

Fusilli with Pinto Beans, Kalamata Olives, Tomatoes, and Broccolini 294

Vegetarian

Barley Risotto with Mushrooms and Spinach 295

Roasted Eggplant, Zucchini, and Red-Pepper Parmigiano 296

White Bean and Roasted Vegetable Casserole with Millet and Crumb Crust 298

Three-Bean Vegetarian Chili with Tomato, Avocado, and Corn Topping 299

Vegetables and Grains

Roasted Asparagus with Orange Gremolata 300

Green Beans with Ground Toasted Almonds 301

Oven-Roasted Beets with Herbed Vinegar Dressing 302

Honey-and-Soy-Glazed Broccoli, Cauliflower, and Red Peppers 304

Oven-Roasted Brussels Sprouts with Smoked Ham and Peanuts 305

Broccoli Rabe with Sautéed Cremini Mushrooms 306

Stir-Fried Cabbage with Tamari and Ginger 308

Carrots and Sugar Snaps with Tarragon and Orange 309

Roasted Carrots, Red Onions, and Bell Peppers with Lemon 310

Oven-Roasted Cauliflower with Madras Curry Powder 312

Braised Mixed Greens with Slow-Cooked Garlic and Dried Currants 313

Velvet Spinach with Sesame 314

Oven-Roasted Sweet Potatoes and Butternut Squash with Pecans 316

Rough-Mashed Olive Oil and Garlic Potatoes 318

Summer Squash, Edamame, and Leek Sauté with Lemon and Thyme 319

Blistered Tomatoes with Corn, Green Beans, and Basil 320

Orzo Pilaf with Spinach and Walnuts 321

Lentils with Dill and Sun-Dried Tomatoes 322

Quinoa Pilaf with Dried Apples and Sliced Almonds 323

Wild Rice with Two-Mushroom Sauté and Toasted Hazelnuts 324

Bulgur Pilaf with Dried Cranberries and Pistachios 326

Double Corn Polenta Toast with Cilantro 327

Desserts

Toasted Almond and Chocolate Soufflé Cake 328

Whole-Grain Scones with Dried Currants and Walnuts 329

Fresh Fruit and Cheese Tartlets 330

Pistachio and Chocolate Chip Biscotti 332

Apple Streusel Pie 333

Three-Berry Oatmeal and Almond Crisp 334

Fresh Pineapple-Mango Sorbet 336

Chocolate-Walnut Melt-in-Your-Mouth Cookies 337

Lemon-Lime Yogurt Cake with Mixed-Berry Topping 338

Chocolate-Peanut Butter Brownies 340

Fig, Raisin, and Walnut Oatmeal Cookies 341

Index

A

aerobics, "steps" per minute from, 181

Alaskan pollock, omega-3s in, 125

albacore, omega-3s in, 125

almonds, 120

alpha-lipoic acid (ALA), 210

amino acids, best sources of, 94

anchovies:
- omega-3s in, 125
- as protein rich, 104

angina, supplements to treat, 206–7

antioxidants, fruits and vegetables high in, 73

Apo-B (apolipoprotein B):
- Healthy Heart Miracle Diet and, 32–33
- as heart disease indicator, 31–33

apples, as heart healthy, 31

arctic char, omega-3s in, 125

arginine, 210

arugula, simple prep for, 85

asparagus, simple prep for, 85

aspirin, risks and benefits of, 44–45

Atkins diet:
- low-fat diet vs., 16–17
- rise of, 16–17

Atlantic cod, omega-3s in, 125

Atlantic herring, omega-3s in, 125

Atlantic mackerel, omega-3s in, 125

avocados:
- healthy fats in, 121–22
- multiple benefits of, 122

B

baby beets, simple prep for, 85

bad fats, 127–33
- purging kitchen of, 131–33
- saturated fat, 127–28
- trans fats, 129–30, 133

barley, 74–75

basketball, "steps" per minute from, 181

B-complex vitamins, 202–4

beans, as protein source, 94–95

beef:
- choosing cuts of, 167
- leanness of, 99
- lean vs. extra lean, 100
- as protein source, 99–100
- recipes, 274–77

blood pressure, lowered with exercise, 180

blood pressure drugs, risks and benefits of, 43–44

blood sugar, carbs and, 18

body fat:
- as health factor, 36–39

measuring, 38
see also visceral fat; weight

bok choy, simple prep for, 85

Brazil nuts, 120

bread, advice for choosing, 64–65

breakfast:
carb correcting in, 78–81
carb plan for, 78
fats fix for, 134–35
fats plan for, 134
protein in, 106–7
protein plan for, 106
recipes, 215–33
suggestions for, 80, 107, 135

broken heart syndrome, 187

buffet, smart choices at, 161

bulgur, 75

butter, healthy use of, 128

C

calories:
from processed vs. natural foods, 74
used by NEAT activities, 175

canoeing, "steps" per minute from, 181

canola oil, healthy fats in, 118–19

carbohydrates:
adding good, 71–77
correcting your, 60–89
as dietary culprit, 18
emotional cravings for, 50–51
havoc wreaked by, 62–63
meal-by-meal plan for, 78–89
plan at a glance, 60
purging bad, 63, 64–71
quiz on, 61
shopping for good, 76–77
swaps for bad, 64
see also good carbs

carnitine, 210

cashews, 120

catfish, omega-3s in, 125

cereal, advice for choosing, 65

chicken nuggets, trans fats in, 130

Chinese restaurants, healthy eating at, 160–62

chocolate, dark, healthy fats in, 122–23

cholesterol:
Apo-B as measure of, 31–33
as dietary obsession, 15–16
good (HDL) vs. bad (LDL), 17–18
improved by exercise, 181–82
levels in low-fat diets, 15–16
levels on Atkins diet, 16–17
saturated fat and, 127–28
supplements to improve, 204–5, 208–9

chopping wood, "steps" per minute from, 181

clams, omega-3s in, 125

Coenzyme Q10 (CoQ-10), 205–6

coffee, and heart health, 80–81

collard greens, simple prep for, 85

cooking oil, 116–18
choosing the right, 118
storage of, 117

corn chips, as healthy choice, 138

cottage cheese, protein from, 103

crab, omega-3s in, 125

crackers, trans fats in, 130

cycling, "steps" per minute from, 181

D

dairy, as protein source, 102–3

dancing, "steps" per minute from, 181

danish, trans fats in, 130

deli meats, home-cooked meats vs., 102

depression, 196–97
getting help for, 197
health impact of, 196

dessert:
carb correcting in, 88–89
carb plan for, 88
fats fix for, 139
fats plan for, 139
recipes, 328–41
suggestions for, 89, 139

diabetes, risk lowered with exercise, 180

dietary fats, *see* fats

dinner:
carb correcting in, 83, 86
carb plan for, 83
fats fix for, 136–37
fats plan for, 137
protein in, 108–10
protein plan for, 109
suggestions for, 83, 110, 137

dinnerware, downsizing, 154

doughnuts, trans fats in, 130
drugs:
consulting doctors about, 199
for heart disease, 40–45
lifestyle vs., 40–42
managing dosage of, 45
risks and benefits of, 42–45
see also specific drugs

E

edamame, as protein rich, 105
eggs:
as protein rich, 98, 104
understanding labels on, 98
emotional eaters, 50–53
carbs craved by, 50–51
solutions for, 51–53
emotional health, in healthy lifestyle, 186–97
enchiladas, trans fats in, 130
endothelial dysfunction:
foods to reduce risk of, 31
Healthy Heart Miracle Diet and, 31
as symptom of heart disease, 30–31
entrée recipes, 262–99
everyday eating, 48–59
choosing simpler foods for, 66
focusing on meal, 154
healthy leftovers for, 86
quiz to assess, 49
resisting temptations and, 56
scheduling meals for, 157–58
see also healthy heart lifestyle; Healthy Heart Miracle Diet
exercise:
barriers to, 176–77
health impact of, 36–37
for lower stress, 194
NEAT activities as, 174–75
overcoming obstacles to, 178–79
as part of healthy lifestyle, 172–85
preparation for, 182–83
6 week interval workout, 184–85
see also activity levels
extreme eaters, 53–57
solutions for, 54–57

F

fast food restaurants, healthy eating at, 166–67
fats:
in Atkins diet, 16–17
bad, *see* bad fats
at breakfast, 134–35
in desserts, 139
as diet fundamental, 114
at dinner, 136–37
fixing your, 112–39
grassfed livestock and healthy, 101
healthy, *see* healthy fats
in low-fat diets, *see* low-fat diets
at lunch, 135–36
meal-by-meal plan for, 134–39
plan at a glance, 112
in snacks, 138
see also MUFAs; PUFAs; saturated fat; trans fat
feasts, meals as, 57–58
fiber, best sources of soluble, 72
fish:
choosing fresh, 137
omega-3 fatty acids in, 124–26, 199
as protein source, 99
see also seafood
fish oil, fats managed with, 124
fish sandwiches, trans fats in, 130
fitness, as health factor, 36–39
flaxseed oil, as fish oil alternative, 200
food diary, 151–53
football, “steps” per minute from, 181
14-day eating plan, 140–49
about menus on, 141
French fries, trans fats in, 130
friendship, as heart healthy, 192
fruits and vegetables:
as good carbs, 71–73
natural sugar in, 73–74
top antioxidant, 73
tropical, 71

G

gardening, “steps” per minute from, 181
garlic, 207–8
glassware, downsizing, 154
golf, “steps” per minute from, 181

good carbs:
adding, 71–77
at breakfast, 78–81
for dessert, 88–89
at dinner, 83, 86
in fruits and vegetables, 71–73
in grains, 74–76
at lunch, 81–82
shopping for, 76–77
in snacks, 86–88
grains:
good carbs in, 74–76
recipes for vegetables and, 300–327
grapeseed oil, 118
green beans, simple prep for, 85
greens, good carb choice of, 84–85

H

haddock, omega-3s in, 125
halibut, omega-3s in, 125
hawthorn, 206–7
hazelnuts, 120
healthy fats, 114–26
in avocados, 121–22
in canola oil, 118–19
in dark chocolate, 122–23
in nuts and seeds, 119–20
in olive oil, 116–18
from olives, 119
in peanut butter, 119–20
healthy heart lifestyle, 171–211
activity levels in, 179–80
eating out and, 159–67
emotional health in, 158, 186–97
exercise as part of, 172–85, 194
at holiday time, 167–69
lowering stress for, 190–95
maintaining, 150–69
NEAT activities for, 174–75
6-week interval workout for, 184–85
supplements in, 198–211
tips for staying on, 151–56
weekend strategies for, 157–59
work/life balance in, 194–95
Healthy Heart Miracle Diet, 47–149
correcting carbs in, 60–89
dietary fats as part of, 112–39
drug dosages and, 45
everyday eating in, 48–59
flexible food choices in, 154–55
14-day eating plan, 140–49
monitoring progress in, 155–56
protein in, 90–111
heart attacks:
causes of, 22–35
quiz for risk of, 35
heart disease:
medications, 40–45
quiz for risk of, 35
heart-healthy diet:
elements of, 14–21
quiz, 19–21
heart rate monitors, 183
heart supplements, 198–211
high blood pressure:
as cause of heart attacks, 22–24
Healthy Heart Miracle Diet and, 24
salt levels and, 24
high protein diets, debate over risks of, 93
home cooking, cutting salt with, 25
homocysteine:
Healthy Heart Miracle Diet and, 30
heart disease signaled by high, 29–30
supplements to lower, 202–4
horseshoes, "steps" per minute from, 181
hummus, as protein rich, 105
hunger, as motivation for eating, 58–59

I

ice skating, "steps" per minute from, 181
Indian restaurants, healthy eating at, 164
inflammation:
Healthy Heart Miracle Diet and, 28
heart health impact of, 26–28
lowered with exercise, 180
supplements for, 205–6, 209–11
Italian restaurants, healthy eating at, 162

J

Japanese restaurants, healthy eating at, 164–65
juice, advice for choosing, 69–70

K

kale, simple prep for, 85

L

lamb:
- as protein source, 99–100
- recipes, 269–70

laughter, as heart healthy, 191

leftovers, as healthy eating tip, 86

leisure, planning for, 191

lemon juice, glycemic levels lowered by, 67

lifestyle:
- dieting vs., 38–39
- drugs vs., 40–42
- weight loss as part of, 36–37
- *see also* healthy heart lifestyle

livestock, healthy fats from grassfed, 101

lobster, omega-3s in, 125

low-fat diets, 15–18
- Atkins diet vs., 16–17
- cholesterol levels in, 15–16
- evidence against, 17–18
- extreme, 16
- as misguided, 15, 16

low-glycemic grains, 74–76

lunch:
- carb correcting in, 81–82
- carb plan for, 81
- fats fix for, 135–36
- fats plan for, 135
- making time for, 82
- protein at, 107–8
- protein plan for, 108
- social activities as substitute for, 158–59
- suggestions for, 82, 108, 136

M

macadamia nuts, 120

mahimahi, omega-3s in, 125

margarine, trans fats in, 130

martial arts, "steps" per minute from, 181

meals, making time for, 82, 154

medications, *see* drugs

mercury, in seafood, 126

metabolic syndrome:
- Healthy Heart Miracle Diet and, 29
- as heart disease symptom, 28–29

Mexican restaurants, healthy eating at, 163

mopping, "steps" per minute from, 181

MUFAs (monounsaturated fatty acids), 114–23
- in avocados, 121–22
- body fat burned by, 115
- in canola oil, 118–19
- in dark chocolate, 122–23
- health benefits from, 115–16, 123
- in nuts, 119–21
- in olive oil, 116–18
- in olives, 119

multi-tasking, as bad eating habit, 154

mussels, omega-3s in, 125

mustard greens, simple prep for, 85

N

NEAT (nonexercise activity thermogenesis), 174–75
- calories burned by, 175

niacin (vitamin B_3), 204–5

nuts and seeds:
- healthy fats in, 119–20
- MUFA levels in, 120
- as protein rich, 96–97, 105

O

olive oil:
- healthy fats in, 116–18
- safe storage of, 117

olives, healthy fats from, 119

omega-3 fatty acids:
- in fish, 124–26
- supplements, 199–201

oysters, omega-3s in, 125

P

packaged snacks, advice for choosing, 70–71

painting, "steps" per minute from, 181

parties, healthy lifestyle prep for, 15

pasta:
- advice for choosing, 65–66
- recipes, 289–94

peanut butter:
- healthy fats in, 119–20
- as protein source, 97

peanut oil, 118

peanuts, 120

peas, simple prep for, 85

pecans, 120

pets, and lowering blood pressure, 194

photographs, as motivators, 152

pie, trans fats in, 130

pistachios, 120

pork:
as protein source, 100–101
recipes, 272–73

portion sizes, 152

positive thinking, as anti-stress solution, 192

potatoes, healthy ways to eat, 68

poultry:
home cooked vs. deli, 102
as protein source, 101–2
recipes, 262–68

progress tracker, 156

protein, 90–111
amino acids from, 94
at breakfast, 106–7
at dinner, 108–10
health benefits from, 91–93
at lunch, 107–8
meal-by-meal plan for, 106–11
plan at a glance, 90
from plant sources, 96
recommended levels of, 93
snacks with, 110–11
sources of, 94–103
sources to avoid, 95
stocking up on, 104–5

PUFAs (polyunsaturated fatty acids), 123–26
in fish, 124–25

push-ups, health benefits of, 182

Q

quinoa, 75–76

quizes:
on danger carbs, 61
eating habits, 49
exercise barriers, 176–77
heart attack risk, 35
heart-healthy diet, 19–21
sitting disease, 173
stress protection, 195

R

racquetball, "steps" per minute from, 181

red meat, as protein source, 99–100

red yeast rice, 208–9

relaxation techniques, for lowering stress, 193–94

restaurants, healthy eating at, 160–67

rice, advice for choosing, 67

rollerblading, "steps" per minute from, 181

rowing, "steps" per minute from, 181

S

sablefish, omega-3s in, 125

salad dressing, myth of fat free, 116

salads:
recipes, 236–39
see also greens

salmon, canned, as protein rich, 104

salmon, omega-3s in, 125

salt:
high blood pressure and, 24
in home cooking vs. pre-packaged foods, 25

sardines:
omega-3s in, 125
as protein rich, 105

saturated fat, 127–28
good vs. bad meals for, 127

scallops, omega-3s in, 125

seafood:
choosing fresh, 137
omega-3 levels in common, 125
recipes, 278–88
see also fish

sesame oil, 118

shortening, bad fats in, 131

shrimp:
health myths and benefits of, 28
omega-3s in, 125

side-dish, recipes, 242–51

sitting disease quiz, 173

6-week interval workout, 184–85

skiing, "steps" per minute from, 181

snacks:
bad fats in, 132–33
carb correcting in, 86–88
carb plan for, 87
carbs in packaged, 70–71
fats fix for, 138
fats plan for, 138
with protein, 110–11
protein plan for, 110
suggestions for, 87, 111, 138

snapper, omega-3s in, 125

snowshoeing, "steps" per minute from, 181

soccer, "steps" per minute from, 181

socializing, as anti-stress solution, 158, 190–91

soft drinks, advice for choosing, 68–69

sole, omega-3s in, 125

soluble fiber, best sources for, 72

soup, recipes, 252–61
sourdough bread, as low-glycemic choice, 65
soy, benefits and risks of, 97
spices, antioxidants from, 86
spinach, simple prep for, 85
squid, omega-3s in, 125
statins:
  effectiveness rate for, 42
  risks and benefits of, 42–43
stress, 187–95
  damage from chronic, 187
  emotional eating from, 187–88
  judging levels of, 188–90
  quiz, 195
  solutions for, 190–95
  of working mothers, 193
stroke, quiz for risk of, 35
success checklist, 153
sugar, as empty calories, 74
supplements, for heart health, 198–211
swimming, "steps" per minute from, 181
Swiss chard, simple prep for, 85

T

temptations, resisting unhealthy, 56
tennis, "steps" per minute from, 181
Thai restaurants, healthy eating at, 165–66
tilapia, omega-3s in, 125
tortilla chips, as healthy choice, 138
trans fats, 129–30
  common sources of, 130, 133
  myth of zero, 131
  in restaurant food, 130
triglycerides:
  Healthy Heart Miracle Diet and, 34
  as heart disease indicator, 33–34
tropical fruits, health benefits of, 71
tropical oils, bad fats in, 131–33
trout, omega-3s in, 125
tuna, canned, as protein rich, 104
tuna, omega-3s in, 125
turmeric, 209–11
turnip greens, simple prep for, 85

V

vegetarian, recipes, 295–99, 300–327
vinegar, glycemic levels lowered by, 67
visceral fat:
  health impact of, 25–26
  Healthy Heart Miracle Diet and, 26
  how to check for, 38
vitamin B_1 (thiamine), 202
vitamin B_3 (niacin), 204–5
vitamin B_6 (pyridoxine), 202–3
vitamin B_9 (folate), 203
vitamin B_{12}, 203–4
vitamin D, 201–2
volleyball, "steps" per minute from, 181

W

walking, "steps" per minute from, 181
walnut oil, 118
walnuts, 120
waterskiing, "steps" per minute from, 181
weight:
  benefits of extra, 39
  exercising to lose, 181–82
  as health factor, 36–39
  impact of fad diets on, 38–39
  losing vs. working to lose, 36–37
weightlifting, "steps" per minute from, 181
women, heart disease in, 193
working mom syndrome, 193

Y

yard work, "steps" per minute from, 181
yoga, "steps" per minute from, 181
  yogurt, as protein rich, 105